Asbestos, Its Properties, Occurrence & Uses

You are holding a reproduction of an original work that is in the public domain in the United States of America, and possibly other countries. You may freely copy and distribute this work as no entity (individual or corporate) has a copyright on the body of the work. This book may contain prior copyright references, and library stamps (as most of these works were scanned from library copies). These have been scanned and retained as part of the historical artifact.

This book may have occasional imperfections such as missing or blurred pages, poor pictures, errant marks, etc. that were either part of the original artifact, or were introduced by the scanning process. We believe this work is culturally important, and despite the imperfections, have elected to bring it back into print as part of our continuing commitment to the preservation of printed works worldwide. We appreciate your understanding of the imperfections in the preservation process, and hope you enjoy this valuable book.

ASBESTOS
ITS PROPERTIES, OCCURRENCE, AND USES

"Of steely colour and of wondrous might
 Arcadia's hills produce th' asbeston bright;
 For kindled once it no extinction knows,
 But with eternal flame unceasing glows;
 Hence, with good cause, the Greeks asbeston name
 Because, once kindled, naught can quench the flame."
                                       "LAPIDARIUM."

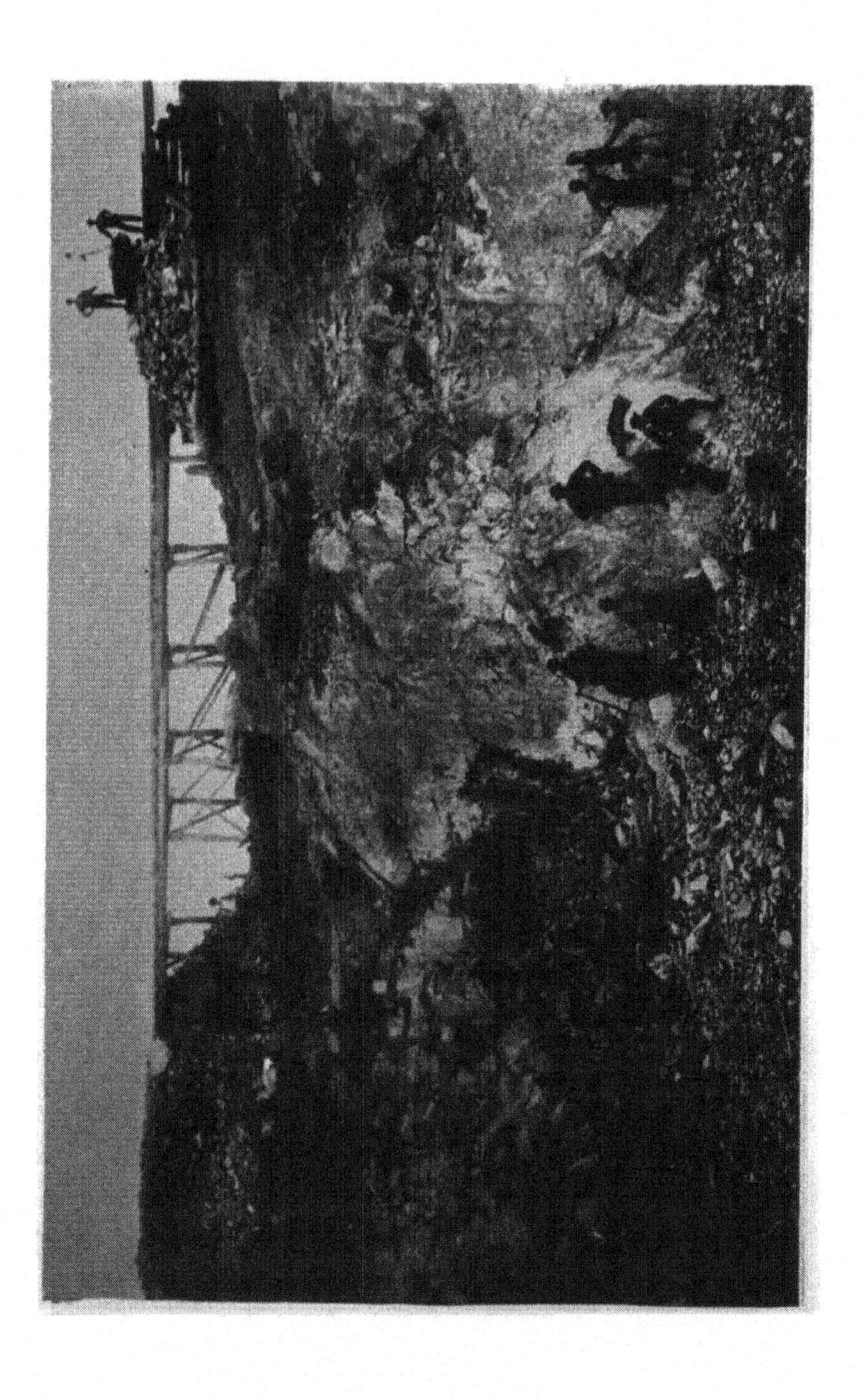

ASBESTOS

ITS PROPERTIES, OCCURRENCE, & USES

WITH SOME ACCOUNT
OF THE MINES OF ITALY AND CANADA

By ROBERT H. JONES

With Eight Collotype Plates and other Illustrations

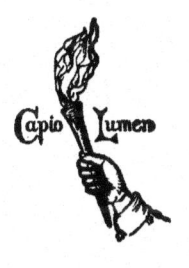

LONDON
CROSBY LOCKWOOD AND SON
7, STATIONERS' HALL COURT, LUDGATE HILL
1890

TN
930
.J66
1890

PREFACE.

SOME three years ago the writer of the following pages issued, in pamphlet form, a short account of the Canadian Asbestos Mines, appending thereto a few pages descriptive of the more important uses to which asbestos was found applicable.

Taking a keen interest in the subject, and believing that, in the near future, there would be few branches of practical mechanics, of art or of industry, in which asbestos would not find a place, he has carefully noted the new uses which are continually suggested, and the processes of manufacture which are from time to time devised for its further utilisation.

He trusts that in endeavouring to weave the contents of a somewhat voluminous note-book into a connected and readable form he has been in some degree successful; his object being to give a synopsis of all that is known on the subject generally, so that those who, like himself, are interested in this singular mineral, may find all the details ready to hand without the labour and time he has had to expend in looking them up. Much of the most important of these are buried in blue books, pamphlets, and articles in magazines and scientific journals, published in England, America, and on the Continent of Europe, a considerable part of which are not at all times readily accessible to the general reader. He hopes by this means to stimulate a spirit of enquiry which will lead to a search for the mineral in other lands, and tend to develop the uses of some of those varieties which now are assumed to possess but little commercial value.

A very large amount of information is derived from the Geological Reports from time to time issued by the Dominion Government, and from the writings of the members of the Geological Survey of Canada, especially those of Dr. Ells, a very high authority on all that relates to Canadian asbestos.

In every case the writer has sought the highest and best authorities for the statements made, which, wherever possible, he has given in the writer's own words, indicating at the same time the sources from which his information has been derived, so that the reader may better appreciate its authenticity and value than if it were given as his own.

In preparing the following pages for the press he is glad to have an opportunity of expressing his grateful acknowledgments to Mr. E. W. H. Eady, of Southampton, whose scientific acquirements and practical skill in photography and photo-micrography have been freely placed at his disposal, and have thus enabled him by pictorial delineation more clearly to indicate many points which would have been somewhat difficult of elucidation without such generous assistance.

R. H. J.

LONDON,
  1st *September*, 1890.

CONTENTS.

INTRODUCTORY.

NATURE AND PROPERTIES OF ASBESTOS—Essential Characteristics—Charlemagne's Tablecloth—Cremation Wrappings—Difficulty of Weaving — Napkins — The Sudarium — Marco Polo — Indian Dresses—Cere-cloth—Sacred Fires—Rock Crystal—Lamps—Gibbon—Amianthus—Potstone—Madame Perpenti—Dr. Bruckmann—Aldini—Canadian Asbestos 1

CHAPTER I.

VARIETIES AND QUALITIES OF ASBESTOS.

DERIVATION—Name—Varieties—Description—Granular and Fibrous Structure — Variations — Occurrence — Chrysotile Spinning — General Use 13

CHAPTER II.

PRESENT SOURCES OF SUPPLY.

GENERAL RANGE OF DEPOSITS — Intermediate Varieties — United States—California—Russia—Siberia—The Ural—China—Africa —Blue Asbestos—Crocidolite — Natal — Barberton—Italy and Canada—Future Supply 32

CHAPTER III.

ITALIAN ASBESTOS AND THE ITALIAN MINES.

ITALIAN ORE A DISTINCT VARIETY—Essential Characteristics—Mr. J. Boyd's Paper—Italian Exhibition—Quantitative Analysis—The Mines—Varieties of Ore—The United Asbestos Company and its Operations—The Industry as carried on in France—The New Asbestos Company 45

CHAPTER IV.

CANADIAN ASBESTOS (Chrysotile, Schillernder Asbest).

FIRST APPEARANCE UNPREPOSSESSING—Hydrous Character—Colour—Description—Amianthus—Foliated and Fibrous Serpentines—Sources of Supply—Eastern Townships—Minerals found there—Position and Climate—Great Geological Fault—Serpentine Belt—Decomposed Serpentine—Dykes—Shickshock Mountains—Veins Irregular—Surface Influences—Trial Borings—Classes of Ore—Local Conditions—Prospecting—Chromic Iron—Impurities—Discolouration—Marketable Value—Ornamental Serpentines . 58

CHAPTER V.

THE CANADIAN MINES OR QUARRIES.

THE THETFORD GROUP—Discovery—The Johnson Mine—The Boston Packing Company—Bell's Asbestos Company—Ward's Mine—King's—Quality of Thetford Ore—Western Limit Theory exploded—THE COLERAINE AND BLACK LAKE GROUP—Anglo-Canadian Company—The Scottish Canadian Asbestos Company—Frechette's Mine—The United Asbestos Company—Bell's—Wertheim's—Megantic Mine—White's Asbestos Company—Broughton—Danville—South Ham—Antimony—Wolfestown—Profitable Nature of Asbestos Mining 84

CHAPTER VI.

OUTPUT, COST OF PRODUCTION, WAGES, ETC.

RAPID ADVANCE OF THE INDUSTRY—Upward Tendency of Prices—Progressive Output—America the Largest Consumer—Commissioner's Report for 1889—Percentage of Output—Old Methods of Work discontinued—Cost of Cobbing—French Canadian Labour—Drink—Points for Consideration—Causes of Failure . 114

CHAPTER VII.

NEWFOUNDLAND AND NORWAY.

GENERAL RESEMBLANCE OF STRATA TO GASPÉ—Granite, Serpentine, Asbestos, and Picrolite—Pseudo-Chrysotile—Crocidolite—Coarse Asbestos—Minerals found in Norway 127

CHAPTER VIII.

THE USES OF ASBESTOS: APPLICATION TO ENGINEERING PURPOSES.

EARLY EXPERIMENTS—Causes of Failure—Engineering Purposes—Packings—Boiler Coverings—Fire-felt—Fire-felt with Superator Covering—Cement—Asbesto-Sponge—Joints of Hot-air Pipes . 132

CHAPTER IX.

APPLICATIONS OF ASBESTOS TO MILITARY AND FIRE PREVENTIVE PURPOSES.

BIG GUNS—Miners' Safety Lamps—Torpedoes—Time Fuses—Dynamite Shells—Ironclads—Military Aeronautics—Safes and Deed Boxes—Carriage of Explosives—Lint—Building Operations—Bâches—Theatrical Curtains—Protection Shields—Fires in Theatres—Captain Shaw's Book—A Yankee Yarn—Fire Kings—Firemen's Clothing—Appareil Aldini—Barnum's Show . . 144

CHAPTER X.

MISCELLANEOUS APPLICATIONS OF ASBESTOS.

COLD STORAGE—Retention and Exclusion of Heat—Deck Cabins—Filtration—Filter Papers—Water Filters—Filtration of Sewage—Pipe Joints—Furnace and Kiln Linings—Crucibles—Gas Stoves—Open Fires—Fletcher's Stoves—The Leeds Stove—Plastic Stove Lining—Asbestos Paint—Insulation—Paper for Battery Plates—Gloves—Aprons—Stove Piping—Rope—Ladders—Rods in Dye-Houses—Lamp Wicks—Gas Shades—Wall Papers—Writing Paper—Cigarette Papers—Tobacco Paper—Pulp-Boards—Cork Soles—Moulds for Type—Silversmiths' and Jewellers' Moulds—Covering for Woodwork—Fireside Rugs . 163

CHAPTER XI.

SUBSTITUTES AND SIMILARITIES.

SLAG WOOL—Origin of Pele's Hair—Properties of Slag Wool—Defects—Rock Wool—Patent Fire and Sound Proof Plastering—Infusorial-earth or Fossil-meal—Woodite—Whaleite—Wood Wool 184

CHAPTER XII.

FIBRE SPINNING.

ORGANIC AND INORGANIC FIBRES—Powers Employed—Wool—Cotton—Silk—Spider's Web—Spun Glass—Quartz—Chrysotile—Italian Asbestos—Delicacy and Strength of some Mineral Fibres 211

LIST OF ILLUSTRATIONS.

PLATES.

Asbestos Mine		*Frontispiece*
Italian Grey		*To face page* 13
Italian Flossy		,, 45
Italian Silky		,, 53
Chrysotile		,, 59
Picrolite		,, 83
Surface Veins		,, 93
Mountain Wood		,, 129

ENGRAVINGS.

	PAGE
Sketch Map showing Position of Eastern Townships of Quebec	*Facing* 63
Sketch Map of the Lake Nicolet Estate	108
Asbestos Wick and Braided Packings (Chalmers-Spence Company, New York)	133
Round Rope	135
Round Core	135
The "Duriflex"	135
The "Manhattan"	136
Fire-Felt (Chalmers-Spence Company)	137
Patent Roll Fire-Felt (Do.)	138
Patent Removable Covering (Do.)	139
Fire-Felt with Canvas Flap	139

LIST OF ILLUSTRATIONS.

	PAGE
Fire-Felt with Superator Jacket	140
Sheet Fire-Felt with Superator Jacket	141
Cement, with Air Space left	142
Filter	165
Asbestos Cloth Filter Suspended	166
Asbestos Rope Ladder	175
Asbestos Watch-Case Soldering Block (Chalmers-Spence Company)	181
Patent Ring-Block for Soldering Stone-set Rings (Do.)	182
Spectacle Block (Do.)	183
Slag Wool under the Microscope.—English Make	194
,, ,, ,, American Make	195
Silicate Cotton under the Microscope (Frederick Jones & Co., Kentish Town)	196
Mineral Wool under the Microscope (Western Mineral Wool Company, Cleveland, Ohio)	197
Cottage Residence, having Walls, etc., protected by Silicate Cotton (Frederick Jones & Co.)	200
Portable Anti-thermal and Anti-septic Hut (Do.)	202
Fibre of Sheep's Wool, magnified 600 diameters	212
Filaments of Raw Cotton	213
Fibres of Raw Silk	214
Radial Thread of Garden Spider	216
Spun Glass	217
Quartz Fibre	217
Asbestos Fibre under the Microscope.—Thetford Ore	219
,, ,, ,, ,, ,,	220
,, ,, ,, ,, ,,	221
,, ,, ,, Italian "Silky" Fibre	222
,, ,, ,, Italian "Flossy"	223
,, ,, ,, Italian "Grey"	224
,, ,, ,, Corsican Fibre	225

ASBESTOS.

INTRODUCTORY.

NATURE AND PROPERTIES OF ASBESTOS—Essential Characteristics—Charlemagne's Tablecloth—Cremation Wrappings—Difficulty of Weaving—Napkins—The Sudarium—Marco Polo – Indian Dresses—Cere-cloth—Sacred Fires—Rock Crystal – Lamps—Gibbon—Amianthus – Potstone — Madame Perpenti — Dr. Bruckmann — Aldini — Canadian Asbestos.

ASBESTOS is one of the many marvellous productions of inorganic nature. It is found in a singular variety of forms, and in some shape or other in almost every part of the world. Some few, only, of the many varieties known, are at present found useful, but those few are applicable to a surprising number of very dissimilar uses. In itself asbestos is a physical paradox, a mineralogical vegetable,* both fibrous and crystalline, elastic yet brittle, a floating stone, but as capable of being carded, spun, and woven as flax, cotton, or silk.

Occupying the position of a connecting link between the animal, vegetable, and mineral kingdoms, it possesses some of the characteristics of all three. Whilst in appearance as light, buoyant, and feathery as thistledown, it is, in its crude state, as dense and heavy as the solid rock in which it is found; ostensibly as perishable as grass, it is yet older than any order of

---

* "All stones, metals, and minerals are real vegetables, that is, grow organically from proper seeds, as well as plants."—Locke's "Elem. Nat. Hist.," c. viii.

"Whenever a unit, an individual, develops in nature, growth is the first condition. This is equally true of inorganic as of organic bodies. . . .

animal or vegetable life on earth. So little, indeed, is it affected by the dissolving influences of time that the action of unnumbered centuries, by which the hardest rocks known to geologists are worn away, has had no perceptible effect on the asbestos found embedded in them. Whilst the greater portion of its bulk is composed of the roughest and most gritty materials known, it is really as smooth to the touch as soap or oil. Apparently as combustible as tow, the fiercest heat cannot consume it, and no combination of acids will affect the appearance and strength of its fibre, even after days of exposure to its action.*

Its peculiar properties thus endow it with practical indestructibility, and enable it to resist decay and destruction under almost every condition of heat and moisture, even preserving it from undergoing any deleterious change when brought into contact with superheated steam or grease; nor is it even worn away or rendered useless by the severe treatment it undergoes in connection with marine, hydraulic, or other engines. So little influence of a chemical nature does it exert over any metal with which it is brought in contact that, if a joint be broken, the surfaces will be found entirely free from corrosion. Its incombustible nature and slow conduction of heat render it also a complete protection from flames. In its crude state, therefore, it is keenly sought for, whilst, as a manufactured article, it must necessarily command a high price until more extensive sources of supply than those at present available are discovered.

The most important characteristic of asbestos is its fireproof quality, which was well-known to and appreciated by the ancients. In our own time it is also known as a useful non-

Growth, the addition of homogeneous body substance, is absolutely universal. The inorganic crystal grows by absorbing homogeneous matter from the surrounding fluid medium, which then passes from a fluid into a solid condition. The only difference between the growth of a crystal and that of the simplest organic individual, the cell, is that the former adds the new substance externally, while the latter absorbs it internally."—Hæckel's "Evolution of Man," i., 156.

* Simmonds on "Waste Products and Undeveloped Substances."

conductor of heat and electricity, as well as for its important property of practical insolubility in acids. Some varieties are said to have resisted a temperature as high as 5,000° Fahr.: but, although it is absolutely infusible, except at very high temperatures, in the hydrous varieties its fibres lose their flexibility and become brittle at a temperature sufficiently high to effect, even partially, its dehydration.

In former days, cloth made of asbestos was cleansed by passing it through fire,* by which, of course, a charcoal fire is understood. It is related of Charlemagne (or, according to some writers, Charles V.) that having one of these cloths in his possession he, to the astonishment of his guests, occasionally amused himself by throwing it on the fire and afterwards withdrawing it, cleansed but unconsumed.†

Its fire-resisting properties were, however, known long before Charlemagne's day, although the difference between the manners and customs of ancient and modern times has caused it, like many other things, to be somewhat differently appreciated by us.

The Romans, who drew their supplies from the Italian Alps and from the Ural, believed it to be of vegetable origin, the

* "Amiantus alumini similis nihil igni deperdet."—Pliny, 36. "Quod ignis adeo non inquinet ipsius splendorem, ut etiamsi in eum conjicitur sordidus, nihil deperdens, nitidus et splendens extrahatur."—Agricola, 609.

† As a modern pendant to this well-known legend, the following is current in Quebec. A labouring man, who had left the old country to seek a better fortune in the Dominion, found employment at once on arrival in one of the many lumber yards on the St. Lawrence, where his energy and activity, supplemented by great bodily strength, soon secured for him a good position. It so happened, however, that one evening, on returning from their daily toil to their common apartment, some of his fellow-workmen saw him deliberately throw himself into a seat, kick off his boots, and then pull off his socks, and, having opened the door of the stove, coolly fling them in on to the mass of burning wood. Possibly no particular notice would have been taken of this, judged as a mere act of folly and waste on the part of the new-comer; but when, almost immediately afterwards, they saw him again open the stove door, take out the apparently blazing socks, and, after giving them a shake, proceed just as deliberately to draw them on to his feet again, that was a trifle too much! Human nature could not stand that. Consequently the horrified spec-

silky appearance and unctuous feel of the fibre contributing to the idea that it was an organic substance; silk itself, according to Herodotus (3, 106), being a kind of wool which grew on trees. According to him, they made a kind of cremation cloth of asbestos, in which to enwrap the bodies to be consumed on the funeral pyre, so that the ashes and unconsumed particles of bone might be kept separate from the remains of the fuel, for preservation in vases or in the family urn. In this wrapping, apertures were of necessity left to allow of a free passage for the flames. It would not appear, however, that such a cloth as this could very frequently have been so used on account of its expensiveness. Pliny specially mentions it as a rare and costly cloth, the funeral dress of kings.* Assuming its vegetable origin, he calls it linum vivum,† the difficulty

tators, having for a moment looked on aghast, fled precipitately from the room. To them the facts were clear enough. This, they said, was no human being like themselves; such hellish practices could have but one origin. If not the devil himself, this man certainly could be no other than one of his emissaries. So off they went in a body to the manager and demanded his instant dismissal, loudly asseverating that they would no longer eat, drink, or work in company with such a monster. Enquiry being at once set on foot, it turned out that some time before leaving England the man had worked at an asbestos factory, where he had learned to appreciate the valuable properties of the mineral; and being of an ingenious turn of mind, he had managed to procure some of the fiberised material and therewith knit himself a pair of socks, which he was accustomed to cleanse in the manner described. He was, as has been said, an unusually good workman, consequently his employers had no wish to part with him. Explanation and expostulation, however, were all in vain; nothing could remove the horrible impression that his conduct had made upon the minds of his superstitious fellow-workmen; go he must and did, nor could the tumult be in any way allayed until he had been dismissed from his work and had left the yard.

* "Des suaires dans lesquelles on enveloppait le corps des grandes personnages."—Jagnaux, "Traité de Min." "Die Gewänder, deren man mehrere wieder abgefunden hat, waren aber so kostbar als Perlen."—Quenstedt.

† "Plinius handelte ihn als linum vivum bei den Pflanzen ab;—'nascitur in desertis adustisque sole Indiæ, ubi non cadunt imbres, inter diras serpentes, assuecitque vivere ardendo.'"—Quenstedt, "Handb. der Min." "Lana montana."—Agricola.

of weaving which, he says, was very great on account of the shortness of the fibre, which is a somewhat singular reason to give, seeing that he was not speaking of chrysotile, to which that remark might have applied, but to the Italian mineral, amianthus. Judging, however, from modern experience it would seem that shortness of fibre could not have been the only, or indeed the main cause of the difficulty, and it would be singularly interesting to know how the difficulty, whatever it was, was in those days surmounted. It is supposed that the weaving process was achieved by mingling organic fibres of some kind, probably flax, with the asbestos, and then, aided by a liberal supply of oil, weaving both fibres together, the oil and flax being afterwards got rid of by exposing the cloth to a red heat; which, in point of fact, was the mode actually adopted in modern times, until, after long-continued experiment, means were found of overcoming the refractory nature of the fibre.* In one of the asbestos cloths shown at the Vatican Museum, Mr. Boyd could plainly distinguish the vegetable matter woven in with the mineral fibre. Varro and others also make mention of these cloths, but give us no information on the point of manufacture. "Most kinds of asbestos," Mr. Simmonds says, "cannot be spun or woven without the intermixture of cotton or linen fibre, as the asbestos fibres are not quite long enough. The intermixture of longer fibre makes the operation

---

* "There is nothing more wonderful in the intellectual history of mankind than the skilful management (by the ancients) of many processes in the arts, the true nature of which was not understood till ages and ages afterwards. Thus, although zinc was scarcely known as a distinct metal until almost a century since, and almost within the same period, one of its commonest ores, calamine, was held in so little estimation in Great Britain, that it was frequently used as ballast for shipping, yet that same ore was used before the time of Aristotle for the purpose of making brass, and to that purpose it is principally applied at the present day."—Second Bridgewater Treatise. In regard to which it may be remarked that Pliny noticed that if copper was placed in close proximity to calamine, it, on being exposed to heat, increased in weight by absorption of the calamine, thus anticipating the conversion of copper into brass by cementation.

quite easy, and when the fabric is entirely ready it is simply placed in the fire, when the combustible linen or cotton is burned out and the incombustible texture remains." Such cloths as these, after all, must have been very wretched-looking skeletons of what was intended, and perhaps were objects rather of curiosity than of any practical utility.

In regard to the so-called napkins, which are often mentioned, there can be no doubt that these, as well as some articles of dress, were, in ancient days, when wood was the principal fuel used, occasionally made of asbestos, and cleansed in the manner described. Pliny, referring to this practice (19, 1), avers that thereby "such things were returned far fairer and whiter than they could possibly be rendered by the air or water." Some of these napkins, supposed to have been used by the Emperors, are still to be seen in the Vatican library, and in the Museums at Naples; in the latter case having been found at Pompeii, and in the former there is a shroud of considerable length which was found perfectly intact in a sarcophagus in the Via Prænestina, in 1702. Some of the cloth of which these are made is so identical in appearance with that manufactured at the present day that only an experienced eye could detect the difference. The Pope is said to have a cloth of the kind in his possession, in which he keeps the Sudarium of Our Lord, the cloth having been sent to one of his predecessors as a costly gift by the Great Khan.

That asbestos cloth was really manufactured in the country of that potentate is corroborated by Marco Polo, who tells us that when (about A.D. 1250) he was traversing the region then known as the Great Empire of Tartary, but which now forms part of Russian Siberia, where, as we know, the mineral exists in abundance, he was shown some cloth which withstood the action of fire, and which the people told him was made from the skin of the salamander. But Marco was far too old a traveller to be caught by any fable about a woolly lizard, so he very carefully examined the material, which he then found to be made of "a fibrous mineral called amianto." Following up his enquiries, he elicited the information that when the ore, from the fibres of which the cloth was made, was first dug out from the mountain and broken up, it strung together, and formed a thread similar to wool; this was then dried and pounded in a mortar, when, after washing out the impurities, the clear thread remained behind. This thread was afterwards woven into cloth, which, at first, had a somewhat dingy appearance, but, after being subjected to the action of fire, became "white as snow, and without a stain."

When the mode adopted, at the present time, of extracting the mineral from the rock, and preparing it for use, comes to be considered, we shall see with what singular accuracy the process has been thus described. It is matter of regret, therefore, that the painstaking traveller did not push his enquiry still further, or find an opportunity of witnessing the manufacture, so that he might have told us, in the same lucid manner, how the weaving of the fibre was accomplished. The dinginess of colour he refers to is easily accounted for by the handling.

Under the Pharaohs a coarse kind of cloth was specially made as a cere-cloth, to cover the relics of humanity, and so help to preserve them from the ravages of time, the body having been first embalmed, by the undertaker, with aloes and subtle essences, in order to prevent the survivors from suffering from the pestilential exhalations, which would otherwise have emanated from them.

The religious care with which the ancients guarded from extinction the Sacred Fires, in the Temples of the Gods, caused them to use asbestos as an auxiliary, the flame having been first started by means of a crystal sphere. * The lamps, also,

* Rock crystal, a pellucid quartz, pure silica. From κρύος, ice, κρύσταλλος, pure ice. This latter term was first applied to crystals of quartz only, which, by reason of its transparency, freedom from colour, and frequent enclosures, was thought to be water congealed by intense cold.—Pliny, 27, 9; Sen., "Nat. Quæst.," 3, 25. That it has once been liquid is proved by its enclosures. Boyle, however, showed it to be heavier than an equal bulk of water, by more than two to one, ice being bulk for bulk lighter than water. Pliny says that "the best cautery for the human body is a ball of crystal acted on by the sun" (37, 10); but

which were used by the Vestal Virgins are stated to have been furnished with asbestos wicks, the fine fibres of which would well serve to draw up and feed the flame with oil, * whilst themselves remaining unconsumed. Strabo † and Plutarch ‡ both speak of these lamps, calling them ἄσβεστα (perpetual). Pausanias § also mentions them, specially alluding to one made of gold, for Minerva, by Callimachus, an Athenian artist, respecting which he says that, although it was kept ever burning, both by day and night, it was only supplied with oil once a year. The wick, he says also, was made of Carpasian linen, "the only linen which is not consumed by fire," the name being derived from Carpasius, in Cyprus, where it was first manufactured; no doubt being the same as that mentioned by Strabo, as made of Carystian stone, an asbestos found at Carystus, in Euboea. ||

With one more instance of its use by the ancients, we may leave this part of the subject. We are told by Gibbon ¶ that, at the Siege of Auximum, the Roman General, in order to poison the waters, and thereby tame the stubborn spirit of the defenders of the place, cast into the stream (among other

the following extract from the "Lapidarium" indicates a still more singular virtue supposed to be inherent in rock crystal:—

> "Crystal is ice, through countless ages grown
> (So teach the wise) to hard, transparent stone;
> * * * * *
> Dissolved in honey, let the luscious draught
> By mothers suckling their lov'd charge be quaffed,
> Then from their breasts, as sage physicians show,
> Shall milk abundant, in rich torrents flow."

* "Le mot asbeste vient de ce que dans l'antiquité on employait cette substance pour faire des mèches qui, alimentée *par une source de bitume,* fournissait des lampes perpetuelles."—Jagnaux, "Traité de Min.," 551.
† P. 396.   ‡ "De Def. Orac.," v. 2, 410 B.   § Lib. 1, 26.
|| When Caron was experimenting on magnesia, in 1868, with a view to its application as a refractory material for crucibles, he used the native carbonate of magnesia from Euboea, where it occurs compact and tolerably hard, with traces of lime, silica, and iron, and occasionally, he says, "matières serpentineuses," which would greatly lessen its fusibility.
¶ "Decline and Fall," c. 42.

noxious things) "quicklime, which is named, says Procopius, *
titanos by the ancients, by the moderns *asbestos*, meaning by
the moderns the men of his own time, *i.e.*, the sixth century."
But what Procopius here calls asbestos was evidently not
amianthus; possibly it was a variety of gypsum, which
occasionally has an asbestiform appearance, although it may
be easily distinguished from asbestos by its softness and by its
becoming an opaque white powder immediately, and without
fusion, before the blow-pipe; whereas, although a single fibre
of asbestos will fuse to a white enamel, the material itself is
unaffected by fire. When, however, dealing with such statements as these, we must bear in mind that mineralogy, as
we understand it, was only very imperfectly known to the
ancients; consequently, things quite distinct from one another
were, in former days, often comprehended under one generic
term, and this not only because their appearance was very
similar, or because they might possibly agree in some striking
quality, but sometimes even on account of their place of origin,
and, in a few special cases, because the uses to which they were
applied were somewhat similar. It has always, therefore, been
a matter of extreme difficulty to identify the names of minerals,
as formerly employed, with those they were intended to indicate. † To give one instance, white clay or chalk, quicklime
and the sulphate of lime, were one and all occasionally called
gypsum, although, as a matter of fact, that word was used
generally to signify sulphate of lime only. "Calci res gypsum
est," Pliny says; but Theophrastus, ‡ who was a far better
mineralogist than Pliny, uses the term with a more general
signification, as of an earth prepared by fire, in doing which
he evidently confounds it with quicklime, as in the paragraph
where he says:—"Its heat, on being moistened, is surprising;
and, when used for building purposes, the builders break it
up, pour water on it, and stir it about with sticks, its heat
being such that they cannot touch it with their hands." In
another place he compares amianthus to rotten wood,§ and

* Lib. 2, c. 29.   † Moore, "An. Min."
‡ περι λιθων, c. 29.   § αμιανθος λιθος, v. 155.

even such dissimilar minerals as iron ore, quartz, emery, and the diamond were occasionally comprehended under the single term *adamas*.

Professor Ansted, in his "Rambles in Search of Minerals," tells us that certain tribes of Indians make dresses of asbestos, which they cleanse by throwing them into fire.

The variety of asbestos spoken of by Marco Polo as amianto (amianthus) has always been regarded as the most valuable kind, on account of its beautifully long, white, flexible, and delicately arranged fibres. In whatever part of the world it occurs, it is found embedded in the older crystalline rocks. It is seldom found in the United States; never, so far as I know, in Canada. Very beautiful specimens are brought from Savoy and Corsica; indeed, so plentiful is it in the latter island that formerly (its mercantile value being unknown) it was often used, instead of tow, for packing. Dana says that Dolomieu, when there, made use of it for packing up the other minerals of his collection. There is also a fibrous kind of potstone * found there (which, like asbestos, is a silicate of magnesia †), with which the inhabitants manufacture certain kinds of pottery by mixing it with the ordinary potter's clay, obtaining thereby a lighter and more durable vessel than they could get by the use of clay alone.

Referring to the use by the ancients of asbestos in lamps and fires, the mineral, being abundant in Greenland, is used there now by the inhabitants for lampwicks, and certain kinds of lamps are made in England having asbestos wicks, whilst the very common use of it in gas stoves, where the appearance of fire is desired, will be at once called to mind. These modern adaptations of the fibre, therefore, can only be looked on as so many exemplifications of the truth of Solomon's saying that "there is nothing new under the sun."

* Ollite (*lapis ollaris*) from *olla*, a dish. This is an impure soapstone of a greyish green or dark green colour, and usually of a slaty structure. It is found abundantly at Potton in the Eastern Townships of Quebec. See *post*, p. 200.

† So called from a city in Thessaly. There was another city, also of the same name, where, Pliny says, the mineral called magnet was found,

In the general application of asbestos, in modern times, to the several branches of practical mechanics and industrial manufactures, it is to Italy that we are indebted for leading the way. Previous isolated experiments are recorded, but these do not seem to have been followed up, until long afterwards. In the last century, for instance, Professor Bruckmann, of Brunswick, was successful in the manufacture of asbestos paper, on which he caused to be printed a natural history of the mineral, some copies of which book are said to be still preserved in the museum at Wolfenbuttel. And early in the present century Madame Perpenti, of Cône, successfully employed asbestos, not only in the manufacture of paper, but of cloth also, as well as of a kind of coarse lace, with many other articles of a useful character. And it is worthy of note, that in her make of cloth, she made no use of any other fibrous ingredient as an admixture; her process simply consisting of softening the asbestos in water, beating and rubbing it, and finally separating the fibres by means of a comb furnished with fine steel points.

Apart, however, from these and other isolated cases, which no doubt pointed out the way for later experimenters, the important industrial capabilities of asbestos were neglected until quite recently, and not seriously taken in hand until 1850, when the Chevalier Aldini and others conducted a series of experiments, in which they were to a great degree successful, with the object of turning its fire-resisting properties to account for the protection of firemen. And soon after this a Florentine priest, one Giuseppe della Corona, brought to a successful issue his experiments for the manufacture of asbestos millboard.

When, however, we turn to Canada we find that, although the valuable variety of asbestos which occurs in the Dominion was well known to geologists for many years prior to 1877, yet, for all practical purposes, its true economic importance

which he describes as being of a whitish colour, somewhat resembling pumice and not attracting iron. A purer form of magnesia was no doubt meant by Hippocrates ($\tau\eta\varsigma\ \mu\alpha\gamma\nu\eta\sigma\iota\eta\varsigma\ \lambda\iota\theta o\nu$) which he mentions as being prescribed as a cathartic, possibly native carbonate of magnesia.

remained unrecognised until that date; and even so recently as 1882 its value may be said to have been generally unknown. In Rand and Macnally's Great Atlas of the World, we do not find asbestos even mentioned, in the copious dissertation to be found there on the trade and manufactures of the Province of Quebec: iron and copper alone being named as the chief mineral productions of that part of the Dominion. And when, in 1886, a little book was prepared, with great care and at considerable expense, for gratuitous distribution in the Canadian section of the Colonial and Indian exhibition of that year, in order to enlighten the world on the capabilities, productions, and mineral resources of Canada, no mention was made of asbestos among the mineral productions of the country, although some good specimens were to be seen there, notably an exhibit by the Johnson Company of Thetford.

From the foregoing it would seem that, even at so recent a date as 1886, no very great importance was attached to this mineral in the country of its production. Now, however, all this is changed: land on the serpentine belt (where the mineral is alone found) is daily increasing in value, and new mines are being sought for and opened; whilst, as the demand for the raw material increases, fresh capital is being furnished, and improved machinery invented and brought into use, for increasing the production, greater care being at the same time used in the cobbing and preparation for market of the raw material.

The uses of asbestos, in the arts and manufactures, are now of so important and varied a character that the main features of these must be treated of in a separate chapter, as even a mere enumeration of the principal among them would run to a considerable length. Indeed, now that it has been demonstrated that a fairly abundant supply of the raw material can, with tolerable certainty, be relied on, at a fairly reasonable cost, there would seem to be no limit to the growing demand, especially as new uses for the mineral are being daily found. This demand will, of course, still more rapidly increase, as the value and almost universal utility of the fibre becomes, by its more extended use, more clearly and widely known.

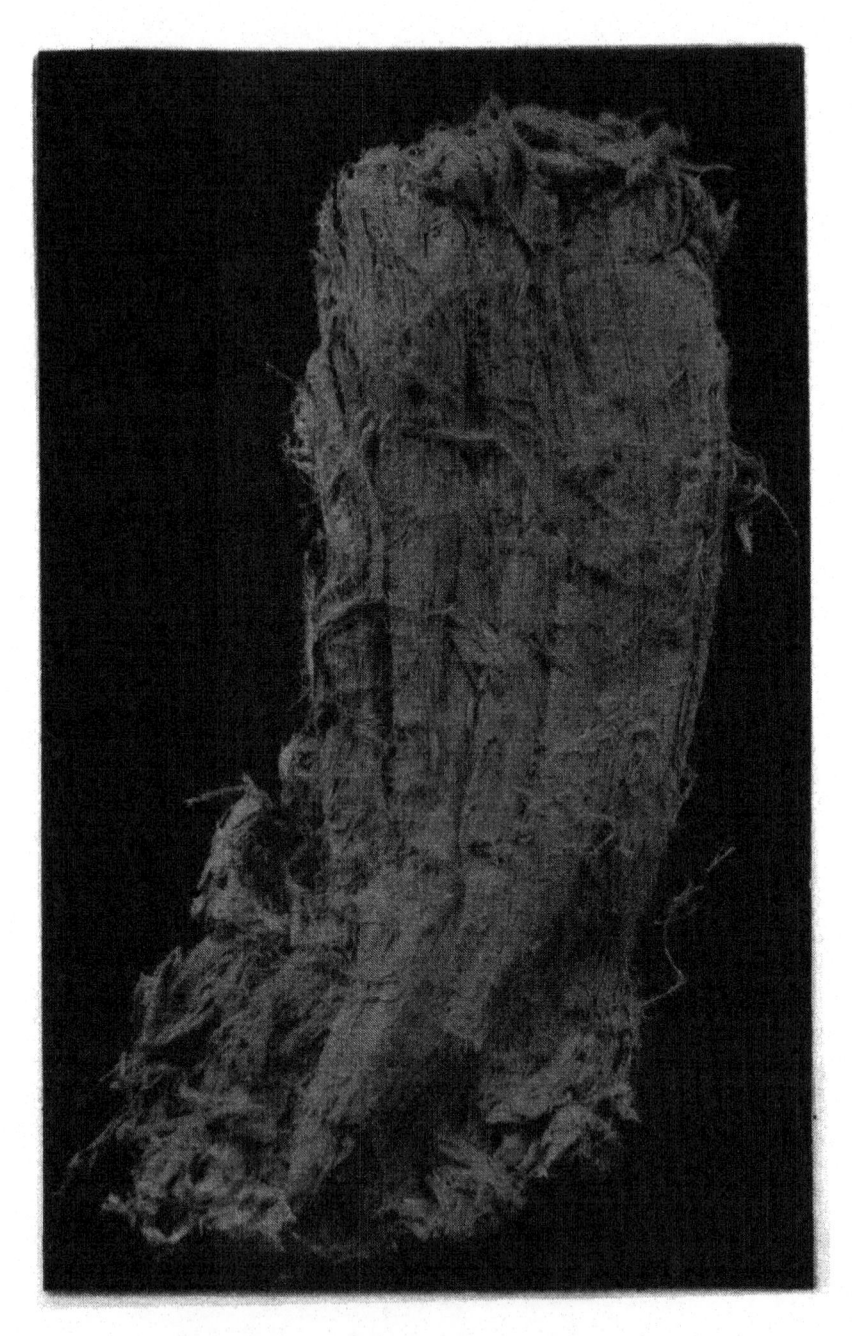

ITALIAN ASBESTOS. "The Grey."

CHAPTER I.

VARIETIES AND QUALITIES OF ASBESTOS.

DERIVATION — Name — Varieties — Description — Granular and Fibrous Structure — Variations — Occurrence — Chrysotile Spinning -- General Use.

DERIV.: ἀ, Priv., and σβεσω, I quench.

CALLED by mineralogists asbes*tus*, the name in its Greek form, as commonly used, ἄσβεστος, signifies unquenchable, unconsumable, endless, "qui peut dure un temps infini." * In Spain and Portugal it is called asbesto, whence asbestino (asbestine), a name applied to asbestos cloth. The French, using the same derivation, call it asbeste (minéral filamenteux et incombustible). In Germany it is termed Steinflachs (stone-flax); and in Italy, amianto (amianthus, from ἀμιαντος, pure, incorruptible), so named because of the simplicity of the means of restoring it, when soiled, to its original purity, by the agency of fire; and in the local vernacular of the French Canadian miners it is pierre-à-coton (cotton-stone), perhaps as expressive a non-scientific designation as can be found, the fibre itself being commonly spoken of as cotton.

Asbestos is a term of a generic character applied to the peculiar fibrous form assumed by several minerals, and not a name given to any one particular species, the asbestiform condition being simply a peculiar form under which many minerals, especially serpentine, occasionally present themselves.

The varieties of asbestos are very numerous. They are all silicates of lime and magnesia or alumina; compounds of silica

* "Αγάπη 'Ασβεστος" (a memorial of) Eternal affection.—Archbishop Benson, *Daily Graphic*, 4th April, 1890. *Vide ante*, p. 8.

(silicic acid) with an earthy base, and the greater part of them hydrated. The bases, lime and magnesia, with the protoxides of lime and magnesia, being mutually replaceable in many of the magnesian silicates, these latter are subject to great variations in colour, density, and other characteristics.* Nearly all the forms are distinguished by having a crystalline fibrous structure, and most of them possess both flexibility and elasticity; in some of them the whole mass is flexible and elastic, in others the fibres only are so.

What may be termed *asbestos proper*, or *true asbestos*, is a fibrous variety of hornblende, or pyroxene, and differs materially from the so-called asbestos of Canada, this last being a fibrous form of serpentine containing 12 to 14 per cent. of water, true asbestos being essentially anhydrous. The anhydrous silicates of magnesia have nothing of the soapy feel, so common among the hydrous species, excepting talc, which is often hydrous.†

The sub-varieties known as mountain wood, mountain leather and paper, and mountain cork, differ in many ways from the more valuable kinds, one of their principal peculiarities being that their fibres, instead of lying parallel across the vein, are so matted and interlaced, that the fibrous structure is not at all times readily apparent. The three first-named are so called from similarity of appearance to the substances after which they are named, and the latter from its extreme lightness, which enables it to float on water, as if it were really cork; its lightness being caused by the loose interlacement of its fibres, forming multitudinous air cells.

Mountain Wood (*Ligniform asbestos, Bergholz, Holzasbest, Xylotil*) is hard and close grained, and will take a high polish. It is generally of a brownish colour and often bears an exact resemblance to petrified wood, for which, at first sight, it might easily be mistaken, especially when sufficient iron is present to give it the ruddy tinge of decayed wood or bark. Under the microscope, however, the crystal fibre is easily detected, as is also the absence of the vegetable cells which are always to be

---

* Dana, "System of Min.," 1850, 265.   † Dana, *ibid.*

found in petrified wood. The fibres of this variety, though it varies very much in texture, are generally long, curved, and compact, and these will melt to a black slag. Rammelsberg thinks it may be an altered chrysotile.

Mountain Leather (*Bergleder, Bergfleisch*), which contains little or no alumina, originates in cases where the fibres "felt" by interlacement, instead of lying parallel. This usually looks and feels very much like kid leather. The varieties which feel greasy and cold contain a mixture of talc, and are called Bergfleisch; when they are poor and warm they become light enough to float on water, and these may sometimes be mistaken for meerschaum.*

Mountain Paper is merely a finer and thinner variety of the last named. It is a papery-looking sub-variety of asbestos, sometimes called fossil paper.

Mountain Cork (*Rock-cork, Bergkork*) is a spongy elastic form of asbestos, which has a texture like felt. It is similar to mountain leather, but more elastic and thicker. It possesses the lightness and elasticity of cork, and is usually of a dingy white colour. The composition of mountain cork is as follows:—

Silica	57·20
Peroxide of iron	4·37
Magnesia	22·85
Lime	13·39
Water	2·43
	100·24

Sp. gr., 0·68 to 0·99. Professor Heddle includes these two last under the name of pilolite (πιλος λιθος, feltstone). He procured seven specimens from as many different localities in Scotland, and, having analysed them, found they were essentially hydrated silicates of alumina, magnesia, protoxides of iron and manganese, with some lime, for which the calculated formula is given as $Mg_4 (Al_2) Si_{10} O_{27} 15 H_2 O$. These seven specimens were found in granular limestone, and in veins in granite, sandstones, and slates.

* Quendstedt, 332.

Mountain Flax (*Bergflachs, fossil flux*) is merely a popular name for amianthus.

Chrysotile (*Schillernder asbest*), the form mostly found in Canada, differs materially from some of the other varieties, and is of so important a character that it will be separately described, as will also the principal Italian species.

Blue Asbestos (*crocidolite, krokidolit, Blaueisenstein*) is a totally distinct variety, being a silicate of iron, iron in this replacing magnesia, in the same way as is the case with alumina in the Natal species. It occurs in micaceous porphyry in the Vosges; and very abundantly, in association with beds of iron ore, in the asbestos mountains, Great Orange River, South Africa, about 700 miles from the Cape of Good Hope. It is found in two forms, fibrous and earthy; the former is of a peculiar lavender-blue or leek-green colour, in appearance much like chrysotile, and possessing long, delicate-looking fibres, which are somewhat elastic and easily separable by the fingers. The colour is caused by the large proportion of oxide of iron it contains. The enclosing rock is a dark brown and purplish shale. A good deal of diopside also occurs in the same formation. The technical description of crocidolite is as follows: "Silicate of iron, sodium (magnesium and aluminium), 3 R″ O$_1$ R″$_2$ O$_3$. H=4. Sp. gr., 3·2 to 3·6, lustre, silky." But, although described as silky, the fibres generally have the appearance of stocking-wool rather than silk, as would seem to be indicated by its name, which is derived from κροκις (pro κροκύς, Ger. Flocke), woof, in evident allusion to its wool-like fibres. Its composition is given as—

Silica	51·1
Protoxide of iron	35·8
Soda	6·9
Magnesia	2·3
Water	3·9
	100·0

De Lapperent, in alluding to this form, says: "Masses souvent asbestiformes composées de fibres parallèles très fines, faciles à separer, paraissent être à l'Arfvedsonite ce que l'asbeste est à l'actinote. Les fibres sont tendres, elastiques et flexibles. Bleu indigo ou bleu-gris ; poussière bleu lavande. Les fibres très déliées fondent à la flamme d'une bougie en devenant rouges ; au chalumeau elles fondent facilement en globule noir magnétique : dans le matras degage de l'eau. Se dissout facilement dans le borax en donnant un verre verte olive. Dans le sel de phosphore laisse un squelette de silice. N'est pas sensiblement attaquée par les acides. On peut la considerer comme un Arfvedsonite dont la chaux aurait disparu."* His analysis does not differ in essential particulars from that given above :—

Silice	51·22
Oxide ferreux	34·08
Oxide manganeux	0·10
Magnesia	2·48
Chaux	0·03
Soude	7·07
Eau	4·50
	99·48

Crocidolite occurs in both its forms in Greenland in association with sodalite,† and at Stavern, in Norway. The fibrous seams or masses of this variety, make an angle of 106° with the opposite surfaces of the seam, according to Haussmann,‡ who states that a cylinder of it $\frac{7}{100}$ of an inch in diameter supported ninety-one Hanoverian pounds without breaking, whereas one of asbestos $\frac{7}{100}$ of an inch in diameter broke with a weight of 6 oz. This marvellous tensile strength, which is attributable to the large amount of iron in its composition, is neutralised (for present purposes) by a corresponding deficiency of fireproofness, occasioned by the want of lime or magnesia. It is difficult, therefore, to see how this variety is to be usefully employed, in competition with the light-coloured, elastic, but less tenacious, varieties, which usually contain, with a small proportion of iron, a correspondingly larger amount of lime and magnesia.

* "Cours de Min.," 84. † Dana. ‡ "Handb.," 1847, 743.

Breislakite is a woolly-looking variety of fibrous pyroxene, named after Breislak, an Italian mineralogist. This is sometimes called cyclopeite, and is found at Vesuvius and Capo di Bove. The fibres are flexible and the colour reddish brown: it contains silica and alumina, but does not appear to possess any economic value.

Byssolite (from Byssus) is an old name for asbestos, now seldom used. Des Cloizeau says: "On avait donné autrefois le nom de Byssolite à une asbeste gris-jaunâtre qui accompagne souvent les crystaux d'albite du Dauphiné."* And Bauer, speaking of it, says: "Byssolit gleicht graue und blondfarbigen Menschen haaren, aber trotz deiser Feinheit bleibt er glasig spröde, weil er auf Feldspathgesteine mit Adular und Bergcrystals in den Hochalpen einbricht."† It is of an olive-green colour, coarse and stiffly fibrous. It occurs associated with a black oxide of manganese.

A dark green coloured asbestiform mineral, found near the Cow Flat Copper Mines in New South Wales,‡ was shown to have the following composition, and is consequently unworkable:—

Hygroscopic water	1·084
Combined water by difference	1·941
Silica	49·447
Alumina	9·688
Iron sesquioxide	16·330
,, protoxide	5·151
Manganese protoxide	4·389
Magnesia	traces
Lime	11·970
	100·000

Another mineral of a more valuable character is picrolite.§ This occurs in many places, amongst others at Bolton, in the Eastern Townships of Quebec.‖ Its ore is separable into long,

* "Manuel de Min.," 80. † "Lehrbuch," 425.
‡ Liversedge's "Min. of New South Wales," 1888, 181.
§ From πικρος, bitter; "ou qui a une saveur désagréable," in allusion to the magnesia or Bittererde present.
‖ Dr. Sterry Hunt, "Physiology and Physiography of Minerals," 334.

rigid, somewhat elastic fibres; it has a specific gravity of 2·607, and the following composition :—

Silica	43·70
Magnesia	40·68
Ferrous oxide	3·51
Oxide of nickel	traces
,, chromium	,,
Water	12·45
	100·34

Dana describes this as "columnar, the fibres or columns not easily separable, or affording only a splintery fracture." He gives several analyses, from different localities, differing slightly according to the place where found, but all in practical accord with that given above, and all showing important characteristics.

Mr. Donald thinks it probable that movements of the rocks, and resulting heat, may have been intimately connected with the formation of picrolite.

This mineral, called by the miners bastard asbestos, is generally found along the lines of faults in all the asbestos mines, sometimes in very considerable quantities; notably at Broughton, where large heaps of it, some showing singularly fantastic forms, have been thrown out on the dumps.

Another mineral of some value, which is sometimes called non-fibrous asbestos, may, perhaps, be mentioned here. This is really actinolite,* which is found in the State of Maine and many other places in America, at Arendal in Norway, and elsewhere; also in a radiated form (radiated actinolite, the coarse circular fibres in this case being radiated or divergent) in Central Ontario, notably at North Hastings, where it is being worked. It is found in magnesian rocks, such as talc,

* From ακτιν, ακτινος, a ray of light, "trait de lumière," the crystals being arranged in the form of rays (actinote, Strahlstein). "To nourish the vegetation of this earth the *actinic* and luminous rays of the sun must penetrate our atmosphere."—Tyndall. The actinic rays are violet and blue.

steatite, or serpentine, and is used for one or two purposes, for weighting paper and various forms of adulteration, also by Mr. James, of Bridgewater, Ontario, on whose land there is a considerable deposit, for the manufacture of a "patent actinolite cement roof," which seems to have met with considerable success. The roofing material prepared from this actinolite having, for some time, withstood the test of the Canadian climate, with its extremes of heat and cold, may consequently be deemed fit for use in any part of the world.

In order to prepare it for use, the mineral is pulverized in attrition mills, in such a way as to preserve the fibres as nearly intact as possible. It is then put up in bags, which each contain sufficient material, when mixed with a proper proportion of coal tar, to produce the quantity of cement required for a square of roofing, the fibre preventing any cracking or running in the composition. It is entirely fireproof, the coal tar being so effectually absorbed that there is nothing left to burn. It is obvious, therefore, that the material can be used for a variety of other purposes equally valuable, and there can be little doubt that, as the price of chrysotile rises to prohibitive proportions, these forms of actinolite, as well as the tremolite of the New York State, will be more sought after, and will increase in value in proportion as attempts are made to find a substitute for the higher-priced mineral. The specific gravity of actinolite is 3 to 3·2. Asbestiform actinolite resembles the radiated, but the fibres are more delicate. Tremolite graduates into actinolite by an increase in the proportion of iron, but is easily distinguishable by its colour.

There are many varieties besides the above, but these will no doubt be sufficient to show the diversity of form assumed by asbestos in various localities and in different regions; ranging from the silky flexibility of amianthus to the density of mountain-wood and the extreme tenacity of crocidolite. But, in whatever part of the world it may be found, it will be seen that too much attention cannot be paid to its composition, or to its immediate surroundings, so much depending on this for its usefulness in the arts and manufactures.

VARIETIES AND QUALITIES OF ASBESTOS.

Both pyroxene * and hornblende † are sometimes called asbestos, the latter most frequently, the former more rarely assuming an asbestiform character. The name, moreover, is frequently used with especial reference to certain amphibolic minerals, such as actinolite, tremolite,‡ and marmolite,§ in

---

* "Pyroxene is one of the most common minerals. It is a constituent in almost all basic eruptive rocks, and is principally confined to crystalline and volcanic rocks. In different localities it is associated with granite, granular limestone, serpentine, greenstone, basalt, or lavas. The name is derived from πυρ, fire, and ζένος, stranger, Haüy's idea being that this mineral 'was a stranger in the domain of fire,' whereas in fact it is, next to the feldspars, the most universal constituent of igneous rocks."—Dana, "Min. et Lith.," ed. 1879.

† "Hornblende is generally dark green, brown, or black in colour, and often occurs in stout or more slender prisms, or in irregular-shaped granules or patches. It is an essential constituent of syenite or diorite, and is met with likewise as an accessory mineral in many other igneous rocks. Its cleavage is more perfect than that of augite, and often gives it a platy-like structure, the angles between the cleavage planes being 124° 30″ and 56° 30″."—Geikie, "Geol.," 146.

"Pyroxene and hornblende have the same formula, and under this there is but one difference of any importance, viz., that lime is a prominent ingredient in all the varieties of pyroxene, while it is wanting, or nearly so, in some of those of hornblende. It is difficult to distinguish hornblendic asbestos from the pyroxenic, except by noting its association with known varieties of one or the other minerals."—Dana.

"La hornblende ne diffère de l'actinote que par une proportion plus forte de l'oxyde de fer ; à mesure que le fer augmente, la couleur verte de l'actinote devient de plus en plus foncée, passe au noir par degrès insensibles de telle sorte qu'il est impossible d'établir une ligne de démarcation bien nette entre ces deux substances."—Jagnaux, 554.

‡ "So called from the name of the place, Tremola, Mont St. Gothard, where it was found. It commonly occurs in dolomite or granular limestone. Actinolite is found in the greatest perfection in talcose rocks. Tremolite and the pale varieties of hornblende, containing no iron, fuse readily to a glass, nearly transparent to a milk-white; the lighter coloured varieties, containing iron, fuse to a dark yellowish glass."—Dana.

"La tremolite lorsqu'elle s'altère et devient hydratée manifeste une tendance marquée à se deviser en fibres flexibles, à éclat soyeux, capable de former par leur enchevêtrement de veritables tissus minéraux."—De Lapparent, 376.

§ A thin foliated variety, so called before it was known to be serpentine ; it contains a good deal of water.

which long capillary crystals occur, forming a compact fibrous mass, the individual crystals generally lying side by side, in parallel lines, at right angles to the walls of the vein, i.e., to the cooling surfaces. But it must be understood that these conditions will be found in very varying degrees in different varieties of the mineral. In amianthus,* for instance, the fibres of which are of a singularly delicate character and beautifully arranged, the crystals are very flexible and are easily separated by the fingers; whereas, in the commoner varieties, the crystals are of a much coarser character, are more difficult to separate, are frequently interlaced or irregularly disposed, and possess but little flexibility. Many of these last are of such a brittle siliceous texture as to be of little or no economic value: they usually exhibit a dull green colour, are somewhat unctuous, and occasionally, but only rarely, display a pearly lustre. Sp. gr. usually about 2·7.

One of the most valuable properties of asbestos is its infusibility. Under the blowpipe a single fibre will fuse into a white enamelled glass or opaque globule, but in the mass some varieties have been known to resist the most intense heat without any visible effect. Chrysotile, however, if exposed for some time to long-continued heat will lose somewhat of its tenacity and silkiness, and become rough and brittle.†

When of a light colour, or some light shade, it is usually found to be tremolite or actinolite. The ore found in the celebrated seam at East Broughton was, like the serpentine in which it was enclosed, of a singularly light (yellowish green) shade, but this was fully equal, if not superior, to any that has since been found in the darker rock, which usually carries the finest quality.

Tremolite, the magnesia-lime variety, is especially common in limestones, particularly magnesian or dolomitic; the compact tremolite, called nephrite, is found in talcose rocks or schists; actinolite, the magnesia-lime-iron variety, in steatitic rocks;

* ἀμίαντος λίθος, Dioscor., v. 155.
† See *post*, p. 94.

and brown, dark green, and black hornblende, in chloritic schists, mica schist, gneiss, and in various other rocks.

Asbestos commonly occurs in crystalline rocks of metamorphic origin,* its infusibility being due to the large proportion of magnesia in its composition; which, like lime, has proved absolutely infusible at the highest temperatures attainable in furnaces or otherwise. The more delicate varieties, presenting the lustre of satin, as we have seen, are usually termed amianthus, though much so called is chrysotile † or fibrous serpentine, both of which are hydrous. As a mineral it has been often described, but apart from its igneous origin,‡ no satisfactory theory has yet been advanced to explain its occurrence, or the conditions which have led to its assuming this peculiar form. Dr. Ells,§ whose intimate knowledge of all that relates to Canadian asbestos is well known, says, "it is still an open question."||

* "Metamorphism consists in the re-arrangement of the component material of rocks, and notably in their re-crystallisation along particular lines or laminæ. It is usually associated with evidences of great pressure, the rocks in which it occurs having been corrugated and crumpled, not only in vast folds, but even in such minute puckerings as can only be observed with a microscope."—Geikie's "Geol. Sketches," 326.

† "L'amiante, que l'on emploie dans l'industrie, provient généralement du Canada; il est fibreux, blanc et tres réfractaire."—Jagnaux, 1885, 551.

‡ "Prestwich divides igneous rocks into *volcanic*, or such as have been ejected or have welled out on the surface and have, therefore, cooled and consolidated rapidly, and *plutonic*, or such as have been formed under conditions of depth and pressure and have cooled slowly, thereby receiving a more or less distinct crystallisation of the component minerals."—"Chem. and Phys. Geol.," 34.

"Plutonic rocks are of igneous or aqueo-igneous origin, formed at a great depth and under great pressure of superincumbent rocks; they have melted and cooled very slowly so as to permit them to crystallise. They contain no tuffs or breccia, like the volcanic rocks, nor have they pores or cellular cavities. They comprehend granites, syenites, and some porphyries, diorite, tonalite, and gabbro."—Lyell.

"The plutonic (granitoïde) rocks and the volcanic and porphyritic (trachytoïde) present evidence of two distinct periods of crystallisation, the products of which may be easily discriminated."—Levy.

§ Dr. R. W. Ells, of the Geol. and Nat. His. Survey of Canada.

|| Geol. Report, 1886.

One of the highest living authorities on geology and mineralogy remarks that there is very little to be said in regard to chrysotile that is special to this particular mineral; it is an example of fibrous crystallisation due to crystallising across a fissure, but why it is so finely fibrous cannot at present be explained, except by stating that this is the way with serpentine. When first formed the serpentine is probably in a soft or pasty state* and contracts as it hardens (as if from drying) and in thus contracting breaks into thin, irregular, usually nearly parallel, plates, flat, incurving; and in the intervals between these plates the serpentine crystallises in the fibrous form we call chrysotile. Sometimes there are many such layers to an inch, and in other cases the fibres are several inches long.

Professor Dana refers, but only in a general way, to this important point. In his chapter on Theoretical Crystallogeny,† he says:—"In aggregated crystallisations there is a mass of material entering into the solid state together, and no opportunity exists for single crystals to perfect themselves. While a liquid mass is cooling, whenever the temperature of solidification is reached, at numberless points throughout the mass, crystallisation will begin, and together an aggregation of crowded crystals or grains is produced, with no external regularity of form; in other words the *granular structure*. The same will happen in a crystallising solution if the process goes on rapidly.

"When a solution is spread thinly over a large surface minute crystalline points encrust the whole, and if the solution be gradually supplied as crystallisation goes on, it is obvious that the minute points may elongate into crowded prisms of fibres, producing a *fibrous structure*. Such a structure is common in narrow seams in rocks, and the fibres are usually elongated across the seam."

---

* Serpentine is frequently found in a pasty state in Italy. Also at the Megantic mine in Coleraine, Quebec. It is here so soft when first taken out as to be compressible between the thumb and finger, but hardens on exposure to the atmosphere.

† "System of Min.," 1850, 124.

This latter paragraph would seem to refer to chrysotile rather than to asbestos; the crystals of the former being elongated across the seam in the precise mode described, whereas the capillary or filiform fibres of the latter are frequently tufted or bundled up in irregular masses, and are often so compactly cemented together by some foreign substance as to require treatment in the boiling tanks and thorough beating and rubbing to rid it of the cementing material before submission to the carding machine.

It is much to be regretted that this interesting subject has not yet received more attention from scientists; we can only hope that ere long (in the words of Professor Dana) "the entrance to one of the innermost recesses of the works of nature will be thrown open, and that the qualities of atoms and molecules, their forms and peculiarities, will soon be understood."*

The phenomena of crystallisation are an intensely interesting study, not only on account of the great beauty of some of the forms, but also of the mathematical regularity and precision with which the process is accomplished.† Although ignorant of the manner in which the majority of crystals are formed in the vast laboratory of nature we can crystallise an immense number of substances, watch their numerous intricate modes of formation, and that even in the smallest appreciable quantities, when aided by the microscope. The formation of artificial crystal may be readily effected, and the process seen, by simply placing a drop of the saturated solution of any salt upon a previously warmed slip of glass.

Mr. Simmonds, when referring to fibrous minerals possessing the chemical composition of augite or amphibolite, says:—"In all these minerals a portion of the magnesia is displaced by

* "System of Min.," 1850, p. 125.
† "Here is a solution of common sulphate of soda or Glauber salt. Looking into it mentally we see the molecules of that liquid, like disciplined squadrons under a governing eye, arranging themselves into battalions, gathering round distinct centres, and forming themselves into solid masses, which, after a time, assume the visible shape of the crystal now held in my hand."—Tyndall's "Fragments of Science."

basic water, and it is exactly the presence of this water which appears to give to these minerals the fibrous structure, and in general causes the crystalline structure to be found with one long axis, obliterating all sideward aggregations of molecules." *

When the prismatic concretions become very narrow the fibrous structure originates. Minerals may have either a parallel-fibrous structure, as is seen in gypsum, calc-spar, &c.; an irregularly-fibrous structure, as in augite or hornblende; matted, as in rock-cork, or radiated, as in actinolite, &c., where the fibres radiate from central points.

Minerals presenting a fibrous structure are sometimes said to be the result of a disturbed crystallisation, although the systematic perfection of some of them would seem to be at variance with this idea. Possibly the fibres of asbestos, like those of some other fibrous minerals, have been produced by the same process of crystallisation which has given rise to the long acicular crystals occasionally found in quartz; and asbestos may perhaps be considered an extreme example of crystallisation in the fibrous form; the crystallisation having evidently taken place under conditions of high temperature and extreme pressure. This pressure may have been caused either by the weight of the superincumbent mass, or by the action of gas, in the same way as liquid steel is compressed in hermetically-sealed ingot moulds by carbonic acid introduced into the top of the mould, the heat of the molten metal, in that case, evaporating the acid when the confined gas exerts a very high pressure upon the metal. M. Gosselet, referring to crystalline minerals generally, says they owe their origin to the action of superheated water in the rock,† in this agreeing with Professor Dana, who says that the great promoter of metamorphic changes is subterranean heat, acting in conjunction with moisture and, usually if not always, under pressure.‡ It is admitted that rapidity of cooling tends to produce the glassy condition of minerals, whilst slow cooling

* "Undeveloped Substances," p. 467.
† Report of Geol. Congress, 1888. ‡ 1850, p. 124.

is the condition most favourable to crystallisation; it may, therefore, be that the more intense the previous heat, the more extreme the pressure, and the slower the process of cooling, the finer would be the resulting crystallisation. And this view seems to be supported by the fact that the heat, by which the production of the fibrous mass was generated, necessarily proceeded from below upwards, whilst it is a matter of daily observation at the mines that the deeper the fibrous veins are followed down into the rock, and the harder and more compact the rock becomes, the finer and purer the fibre is found to be. This is a matter of no slight importance to the miner, because the proportion of the inferior grades, which are of much less value, diminishes in a corresponding ratio; the inferiority of these mainly resulting from surface influences acting upon the shattered rock.

When Mr. Moseley was watching the molten lake at Kilauea,* he saw the smooth surface become cracked in all directions by contraction on cooling, whilst all below was glowing hot. It may be that cracks such as these, formed by contraction of the cooling crust of the earth, originated the fissures in which the asbestos lies, and that when the molten mass below had, by gaseous agency or the explosive power of steam, been forced upwards, so as to fill the fissures, the cooling process commenced. The walls of the vein, that is, the cooling surfaces, or rather the wall, for the fibres grow from one side only, would first become drusy, the point of the minute crystals thus formed on the inner cooling surface forming the poles of attraction; and these, becoming gradually elongated, would eventually reach and then become stopped by the opposite wall of the vein, the result being layers of the filiform or capillary crystals constituting the asbestos mineral, compacted into a solid mass, as we find them, by the intense pressure. The difference in the quality of the asbestos would result from the component parts of the molten mass which had thus become crystallised; hence, the lower veins would of necessity be of finer quality and freer from impurities than those nearer

* "Notes by a Naturalist on board the *Challenger*," 501.

the surface, where extraneous matters would be more likely to intrude, and where solutions of metallic oxides, resulting from surface exposure, could by infiltration through the shattered rock, or by the planes of cleavage, exercise a deleterious effect on the cooling mass.

In regard to metallic veins, M. Simonin remarks that metallic emanations reach the fissures in one of two ways. Either they are deposited in the fissures, which constitute the veins, in the state of vapour, which he calls *the dry method*, as in the craters of volcanoes or the chimneys of smelting furnaces; or in a state of chemical precipitation by *the wet method*, as in the solutions of our laboratories. The rich family of precious stones, he adds, seem to owe their perfection to the same cause. Volatilised in the clefts of the igneous rocks, these stones are there turned into brilliant crystallisations—"the tears of nature." *

Turning from theories of formation to the mineral itself, it may be remarked that, as a general rule, asbestos of good quality is only found in serpentine; sometimes, but rarely, it is met with in limestone, and in that case is often found to give an asbestiform appearance to large masses of the rock, or the gangue that contains it. It occurs thus occasionally, as already mentioned, in a pasty state, and then hardens on exposure to the air. It is also found, in masses, in feldspathic and chloritic rocks.† One instance has been noted of its occurrence in quartz;‡ but here, when six feet of the rock had been blasted away, the inevitable serpentine was found cropping through. In the Coleraine and Black Lake district of the Eastern Townships of Canada, it is occasionally found in contact with granite, which is not held to be a good sign. For some as yet unexplained reason (although granite, like porphyry, is one of the richest metalliferous rocks), the granite seems to detrimentally affect the quality of the fibre. Granulite, on the other hand, as will be seen later on, has quite the contrary effect. At East Broughton, the asbestos

* "La Vie Souterraine," 406. † Davies on "Earthy and Other Minerals."
‡ James Boyd on "Italian Asbestos."

occurs along the contact between the serpentine and black Cambrian slates; and here, although the asbestos is remarkably good, there is a striking difference in its appearance. Another divergence is that of a case cited by the State mineralogist for California, where the asbestos vein occurs in a belt of slate enclosed in granite; but the asbestos here, like most of that found in California, is brittle and wanting in elasticity. Many specimens have been sent me for trial from this part of the world, but none of them have as yet been found to possess much commercial value. The enclosing rocks must, consequently, always claim the highest consideration of the explorer, because it is certain that, although some rocks are highly favourable to the formation of good fibre, others are just as much opposed to it. The serpentine, in which it generally occurs, is, in most cases, a product of the hydration of rocks containing olivine, augite, hornblende, and other intrusive or erupted igneous masses. It is essentially a hydrated silicate of magnesia, resulting from the alteration of magnesian rocks. Containing some protoxide of iron and other impurities, these frequently cause a change in colour from a dull green to brownish or reddish brown, often marked with red or purple. In olivine, under the action of carbonated waters, the iron is frequently carried off instead of being peroxidized, some of the magnesia being removed at the same time; hence comes serpentine, which frequently retains the crystalline form of chrysotile.

Most minerals, even when their general nature and component parts are very nearly identical, are found to vary very considerably in appearance and character, according to the different conditions of climate and locality; sometimes, even in adjacent localities, they will vary with the nature and surroundings of the rock in which they occur. Asbestos forms no exception to this rule. It is widely disseminated over the globe, but the deposits are not found to repeat themselves in different regions, even in strata of the same age, but both in appearance and composition will be found to vary very greatly. This difference may occasionally be caused by variation of constituents, as in some of the South African varieties, but in others it may be the result of formation under different temperatures, or according to different rates of cooling.

To be of any economic value, the essentialities of asbestos are length and fineness of fibre, tensile strength and flexibility, combined with great power of fire resistance. Some of these qualities are often lacking, and the value of the mineral consequently diminished, even when it has the most promising outward appearance, as in that from Griqualand.

The main point in which asbestos differs from other minerals lies in its being both fibrous and textile. Subject to what is stated above, its quality is determined by the greater or less proportion of siliceous matter with which the fibre is associated. When crushed out from the rock, and freed from all harsh or gritty particles, its fibres vie in delicacy with silk, and, after carding, are spun and woven in precisely the same way. For a long time they obstinately resisted all attempts in this direction, the difficulty arising, as will be explained subsequently, from the peculiar formation of the fibre, which, possessing a perfectly smooth surface, and being much less elastic than fibres of organic origin, would seem of necessity to require the admixture of some foreign material to enable it to be spun into a yarn. That difficulty, however, has now been so entirely overcome, that yarns capable of withstanding great tensile stress can be readily produced by machines constructed for the purpose. The difficulty of twisting it into a thread becomes at once apparent when its behaviour in the breakers and carding engines is seen, and this difficulty will be more fully explained presently. Instead of leaving these in a sheet or "lap," it drops out in separate fragments just as it entered, except that the fibres are combed out straight and laid side by side parallel with each other. The carding is, however, ultimately accomplished in several successive machines, each set to a finer gauge than the preceding. The entire process consists of one long brushing and combing, in which cylinders, covered with teeth of gradually increasing fineness, pass the fibres from one to another, continually drawing them out, until all the knots and irregularities are eliminated, and they lie straight and parallel.*

Regarding the general use of asbestos, Germany is a large consumer. In France the consumption is not so great, though some very good qualities of paper were some time ago made there. The industry is, however, apparently reviving in France, an energetic attempt having recently been made by a company, calling itself La Société Française des Amiantes, at Tarascon-sur-Rhône, for the production of the usual qualities of asbestos goods, accompanied by some others of a novel character. Paris was the first to set an example, by following out Aldini's idea of protecting firemen by a dress of asbestos cloth, which has since been followed up in London, after conclusive proof of its practical utility, in Paris.

But America is as far way ahead of any other country as a consumer of asbestos, as she is also in her manifold applications of it. A good deal is used in England in the manufacture of some valuable kinds of packing for engineering work, millboards, felts, lubricants, paint, and the like; but in England we lack in some degree the readiness which is found on the other side of the Atlantic, in the adaptation of new materials, and the adoption of new methods of working up those in use.

Whether it be that Englishmen are influenced by climatic or other causes, certain it is, that they are slow to adopt new systems, to cultivate novel ideas, or to move out of old grooves. Consequently, when new materials, or even novel applications of those long used, are suggested, they ponder over them, hesitate, and weigh the chances, and, in so doing, not infrequently let slip valuable opportunities; whilst the keener and more enterprising American, once he sees the drift of the new matter, will, to use his own expression, "catch hold" at once. It by no means follows, however, that in England this is the fault of the manufacturers alone; they have naturally to gauge the requirements of their customers, and prefer to limit their make to what they know they can sell.

* *Engineering*, 6th March, 1885.

CHAPTER II.

PRESENT SOURCES OF SUPPLY.

General Range of Deposits—Intermediate Varieties—United States—California—Russia—Siberia—The Ural—China—Africa—Blue Asbestos—Crocidolite—Natal—Barberton—Italy and Canada—Future supply.

As already mentioned, asbestos, in one form or another, and in more or less abundance, is pretty well diffused over the whole surface of the globe. It occurs in England, in Aberdeenshire in Scotland, and at Lough Foyle in the north of Ireland. It is not found in any great abundance in France; but is plentiful in Portugal, Spain, Italy, and Savoy. It occurs in profusion and singular purity in the Island of Corsica, where, however, the condition of land tenure forms an obstacle to working the deposits. It is found in Switzerland and in Germany; in the Pyrenees, and also in Greece, Turkey, Asia Minor, and Russia. It occurs also in Greenland and Iceland; in some parts of South America, notably in Brazil; in Australia, Tasmania, and New South Wales. In North America it is frequent, occasionally abundant, but often of a coarse character. In south Norway it is found in association with the apatite-bearing rocks; in other parts of Scandinavia it mostly takes the form of mountain wood or cork.

Specimens from all these places are to be found in England, in the museums, or preserved as curiosities in private collections; but, in by far the larger number of cases, their brittleness, coarseness, or want of flexibility deprive them, for present purposes, of any commercial value. In many localities where the quality is good, the quantity available is not sufficiently abundant to pay for working. The seams vary very greatly in different regions, not only in length of fibre, colour, and general appearance; but whilst they have, almost universally, the same dip and inclination, they differ very greatly in composition.

The intermediate varieties, the produce of different lands, are many of them not only singular, but, in some cases, singularly beautiful. The asbestos of different countries is as varied as the characteristic foliage. What, for instance, can be more strange than the bluish aspect of the Australian trees, compared with the soft, delicious greens of the English foliage, when luxuriating in the moist, but clear, atmosphere of early summer? And how different this from the gorgeous hues of the Canadian maple, which can be likened to nothing but a succession of gigantic bouquets of tropical flowers, often thrown prominently into relief, by a deep background of pine—a never-ending source of delight to the traveller! Then contrast the smooth and white, rock-like, form of asbestos from the Pyrenees with the harsh and brittle tremolite of Servia, unpleasant to handle, its fine needle points insidiously penetrating the skin, just like the particles of slag wool; and compare this with the long, soft silkiness of the Corsican variety, the hanks of which look like skeins newly wound from a cocoon, the resemblance being all the more perfect from some of these being a silvery white, whilst others are of a pale gold colour; then turn, again, to the singular Scandinavian forms, which are rough and rugged as the country from which they come.

That asbestos of good quality is not found in the United States, in workable quantities, is shown by the fact that, whilst America is by far the largest consumer of the mineral, her supplies of crude ore are almost entirely derived from Canada. Out of a total export from the Dominion of 3,936 tons in 1888, no less than 3,612 tons were taken by America. It may certainly be that some portion of this large quantity was bought by dealers in New York, who afterwards exported it at enhanced prices; but of this we have no data. In 1889, under the stimulus of the high prices then ruling, the exportation from Canada was much larger; but for that year the proportion of the amount exported will work out very differently, as four of the mines have been purchased, and are now worked, by English and German manufacturers, who require the whole produce for their own special use; the output of these mines, therefore, is practically withdrawn from the market.

But even if it could be said that the quality of the ore found in America was good, the deficiency in quantity is shown by the official returns. According to these, the total production of asbestos in the United States for 1888 [*] is stated to have been 150 tons only, the value of which is put at about £6 per ton, which sufficiently indicates the quality. Moreover, the figures for recent years show a continual falling off in production in precise accord with the rise in price of Canadian, which can only be attributed to the growing appreciation of the merits of Canadian ore for manufacturing purposes.

In 1882 the produce was returned at		1,200 tons,	valued at	$36,000	=£7,422
,, 1883	,,	,,	1,000 ,,	,,	30,000	6,185
,, 1884	,,	,,	1,000 ,,	,,	30,000	6,185
,, 1885	it fell to		300 ,,	,,	9,000	1,855
,, 1886	,,		200 ,,	,,	6,000	1,237
,, 1887	,,		100 ,,	,.	4,000	824

whilst, as we have already seen, in 1888 it was 150 tons, valued, like the foregoing, at little over £6 per ton. This shows clearly enough that American manufacturers do not rely on home production, and as they make no use of Italian ore, their dependence at present is necessarily on that of Canada to meet their rapidly increasing requirements. Probably the official returns refer to amianthus alone, under the head of asbestos, because it is well known that large quantities of a coarsely fibrous mineral (talc or tremolite) are used in New York, for instance, and also exported thence to England, and of course

[*] "Mineral Resources of the United States for 1888."

under the pressure of the high prices now ruling the production and sale of this form, under whatever heading it may be classed, will be largely increased.

In 1887, there was a good display, of the economic minerals of the United States, on exhibition at Earl's Court, Kensington; but my journey thither was fruitless, so far as asbestos was concerned, there being, in the whole collection, but one small tray of amphibole,* and even that was of no commercial value.

In California, that rich storehouse of the economic minerals, asbestos occurs in many places, and sometimes in deposits of considerable extent, but out of numerous samples forwarded from that state, none have yet been found that, with our present limited knowledge of the capabilities of the mineral, would pay for working. In San Diego County, asbestos of a coarsely fibrous kind occurs in a belt of slate enclosed in granite, an unusual formation. Here the strike is north 70° west magnetic, and the dip nearly vertical; the ore is exposed in an open cut 15 to 20 feet long by 6 or 8 deep. There are deposits also in Placerville, El Dorado, and Lake Counties. Some of them possess sufficiently good fire-resisting qualities, but they are mostly deficient in tenacity. It is not to be said that these forms are worthless—their value will no doubt presently be discovered—but at this moment, when the practical uses of the mineral are so far undeveloped, it is only the more silky fibres that are in special demand. For grinding, the manufacture of cement, boiler and pipe coverings, roofing materials, and similar purposes these Californian varieties may be useful; but generally the supply of refractory minerals for use in this way is sufficient to meet the demand.

In Wyoming considerable deposits have been discovered but these are all of a coarse character, and although it is reported that a good deal has found a market it does not appear to be of much value, though somewhat different in character from the foregoing.

* "On attribue généralement à l'amphibole les mineraux fibreux, et plus ou moins flexibles, que l'on a désigné sous le nom d'asbeste ou d'amiante."
—Jagnaux, 550.

Writing on undeveloped substances in 1876, before the introduction of Canadian asbestos, Mr. Simmonds, editor of the " Journal of Applied Science," remarked, that an examination of the several varieties of asbestos (from America) appeared to indicate a gradual increase in the tenacity of the fibre found in a direction proceeding from Georgia to Vermont, where the quality appeared to culminate in the asbestos found in the northern part of that state. Now, we know that, passing over the border, from Vermont into the Eastern Townships of the province of Quebec, the fibre is found in the highest state of purity and perfection in the great belt of serpentine traversing those townships, especially in Wolfe, Megantic, and Beauce.

Asbestos occurs abundantly in various parts of Russia, especially in Siberia and the Ural, but up to the present time little use has been made of it there, on account of the prevailing ignorance respecting its peculiar properties. An amusing instance of this occurred some time ago at some iron works in the interior with which I was at the time connected.

The iron ore, in the district referred to, is found in bunches and nodules, near the surface of the ground; and in order to get it, the peasants dig out pits about seven or eight feet in depth, and then burrow, rabbit-like, into the surrounding earth in all directions below. When all the ore is got out from one spot, they dig another pit further afield, and so they go on until the particular patch of ground they are working on is exhausted. On the occasion referred to, some of our men, in their burrowing, threw out a considerable quantity of asbestos. They had not the slightest idea what it was. In fact, they knew nothing at all about it, except that it was not what they were in search of; and, consequently, as it obstructed their work, they threw it all out in a heap, near the piles of ore. Presently, one of the foremen or overlookers saw it, and wanted to know what that rubbish had been put there for. "Here," said he, to some of the men, "just clear up all that mess at once, and fling it into the furnace, and get rid of it." And this was immediately done, with what result may be easily imagined.

At the present time, St. Petersburg possesses the only manufactory for the use of asbestos in Russia, but probably the time is now ripe for a change. Recent information has been received, of the discovery of enormous deposits of the mineral, in one or two places, which, it is said, as usual in these cases, are of the finest quality. Its value commercially will be dependent, first, on the quality, and then on the nearness of the mines to an available market, transport being necessarily an important factor in the element of cost. But as a matter of fact, the specimens of the mineral sent from Russia hitherto, have not been up to the mark. There is some reason, however, for believing that the new discoveries are of a different character from those previously made.

Siberia, being so well known for its rich mineral treasures, and the formation of some parts of the country giving indications of the whereabouts of asbestos, the recent discoveries there are by no means surprising. It seems, moreover, that the inhabitants are now realising the value of the discovery, for the protectionist papers are clamouring for the imposition of a prohibitive duty on imported asbestos, so as to encourage local industry. For many reasons, not the least of which is difficulty of communication, the rich mineral treasures of Siberia have not yet attracted much attention from European capitalists. This important question of communication is, however, now being gradually overcome, and means of establishing a trade will soon be found by the German merchants who overrun the country in every direction.

Some little while ago the Technical Society of Moscow announced the fact of its having received some unusually fine specimens of asbestos from Ekaterinburg, accompanied by scientific reports which seem clearly to establish the existence of large deposits of the mineral. From Orenberg to Ekaterinburg the whole country is reported to be traversed by rocks containing deposits, culminating near the Verkin Tagil Ironworks, in the vicinity of which is a hill called by the peasants Sholkovaya Gora (hill of silk), which is said to be entirely composed of asbestos. The principal of these deposits lie close to the railway, the facilities afforded by which, aided by those of the Volga River system, will materially assist in opening up an export trade, as soon as these deposits are properly worked. Further deposits have also been disclosed in the Gorobtagsdat and the Neujansk districts of Perm. Similar announcements were, some short time back, made of discoveries in South Russia, but the local excitement died away when it was found that the quality was not as represented.

Asbestos has been found in Alaska, but, there also, difficulty of communication blocks the way.

Chrysotile has been found at Ilfracombe in Tasmania, in Australia, and New South Wales. Asbestos in long, white, silky fibres, occurs at Jones Creek, Gundagai, where fine specimens of pyrophyllite are found; with meerschaum at Bingera, Murchison County, and picrolite is found at Kelly's Creek, Gwydir River. Jagnaux gives the following analysis:—

Silice	55·19
Magnesie	31·58
Chaux	—
Oxide ferreux	1·70
,, manganeux	—
Alumine	1·40
Eau	10·62
	100·49

The value of the asbestos raised in 1885 and preceding years, however, amounted only to £3,216. The serpentines in Australia, as elsewhere, in which the asbestos is found, are in close association with deposits of chrome iron and other minerals.[*] Those with which the asbestos deposits are most commonly associated are soapstone, magnetic or chromic iron, and occasionally mica and enstatite; chromite is less frequently met with, but generally all iron found in the workings is called by the miners chromic. The colour of Australian asbestos is usually white or a light dingy blue, the form densely

[*] "Minerals of New South Wales," by A. Liversedge, F.R.S., 1888, p. 180.

compact, but the fibres easily separable. The Native Asbestos Company is located in Flinders Street, Melbourne, Victoria.

In China also asbestos occurs; but, apart from the manufacture of a coarse kind of cloth, we know little of any purpose to which it is there applied. One singular use of it may, however, be mentioned, which Dr. Hobson, of the London Medical Mission, brings to our notice. He says that it is used by the Chinese as a medicine and figures, in their pharmacopœia, in company with such uncanny things as "dried spotted lizard, silkworm moth, human milk, the parasite of the mulberry tree, asses' glue," &c.; and, this being so, we are quite prepared to take Cobbold* at his word when he tells us that the native practice of medicine in China is not easy for a foreigner to understand. Before, however, we smile, or turn with disgust from the medical practice of the "heathen Chinee," it will be well to call to mind, that it is less than 200 years ago since such horrible things as "toads, vipers, centipedes and worms, found a place in the official pharmacopœia of the London College of Physicians."† Hippocrates prescribed asbestos as a cathartic, but it is probable that under this name he referred to native carbonate of magnesia.

Now if we turn to Africa, "the land of sparkling gems," which, in all ages, has been celebrated for its mineral wealth, and which now, as in the days of Aristotle, "has always something new to show," we shall find her true to her reputation and showing several new, or rather unfamiliar, varieties of asbestos. Africa has (perhaps in some moment of despondency) been stigmatised as "a country of samples," but when we remember that she has furnished the world with *six tons* weight of diamonds, a thousand tons of ostrich feathers,‡ with gold, and other produce, in equally fabulous quantity, it must be admitted that her samples are of rather a portentous character. And even now, whilst her wealth of gold and gems is being distributed in such lavish abundance, news is flashed

* "Pictures of the Chinese Painted by Themselves."
† "English Folk Lore," by the Rev. F. T. Thiselton Dyer.
‡ "The Land of Gold, Diamonds, and Ivory," by J F. Ingram, F.R.G.S.

home that she again "has something new to show," asbestos having been discovered, according to report, of a quality and in such abundance, as has never before been seen.

Crocidolite (blue asbestos) has long been known to exist in the neighbourhood of the Great Orange River; both crocidolite and soapstone were among the mineralogical specimens brought home, from the Kalahari Desert, by Mr. Farini; and a special variety of asbestos, of a highly aluminous character, occurs in Natal.* This last is imported into England for use in the potteries as a refractory material for lining furnaces and kilns, and for the making of crucibles, for which it seems to be well adapted, alumina being both insoluble and infusible.† Asbestos is also found in abundance in the Somali fields, about a hundred miles beyond Kimberley; and yet another discovery was announced in September, 1889, of a "gigantic asbestos farm," (whatever such an expression may be taken to mean), on the property of the Griqualand West Copper and Mineral Syndicate. The find here was, with the usual exultation, announced to be amianthus of the finest quality, beautifully white in colour, and many feet in length. The first samples sent over, however, by no means bore out this description, being comparatively short and brittle. The produce of deeper workings soon followed; some of these in my possession are very beautiful in appearance, in fineness of colour and length of fibre not to be surpassed by the best Italian, but, at the same time, they are so deficient in tensile strength as to be practically useless for any present purpose. But although for

* Alum is often found efflorescent or in feathery masses; and in many parts of Africa, notably at Lagoa Bay, it occurs in fine crystallisations like asbestos with a silky lustre; in a cave near the Bosjesmans River it is said to cover the floor to a depth of six inches. Sapphire is pure alumina crystallised; but the sapphire of the ancients was lapis lazuli, as appears from Isidorus: "Sapphirus cœruleus est cum purpura, habens pulveres aureos sparsos," particles of iron pyrites disseminated through it and looking like gold.

† "The magnesian silicates are only fusible at very high temperatures, but the silicates of alumina are probably quite infusible."—Pickett's "Useful Metals and their Alloys," 624. *Vide post*, 169.

this particular kind there is no demand now, it must not be forgotten, that every year brings to light new mineral combinations, or new varieties of those with which we are already acquainted, and usually the practical application of them soon follows.

When these African discoveries were first announced, simultaneously with those in Russia, and those anticipated, with less probability of realisation, from Servia, fears were expressed lest the markets would be glutted and prices so reduced, as to make it scarcely worth while to work the mines, but it must not be forgotten that

> "Le globe est un vaisseau frété pour l'avenir
> Et richement chargé . . . . ,"

and that as new scientific discoveries are made, so the great mineral reserves which, year after year, are brought to light, readily find their place, without much disturbance, in the great economical relations of the world.

The important question of transport, from these distant regions, will be one of the first difficulties to present itself; but granted a practical acquaintance with the mineral, no great difficulty need be apprehended on this head.

Bearing in mind the great number of places, in the neighbourhood of the gold mines, where both asbestos and crocidolite abound, it would not appear at all unlikely that, in the near future, a good quality of asbestos will be discovered, and that Africa may become one of the main sources of supply. The elevation of Griqualand West is about 4,000 feet above the sea level, a not unimportant factor in the case.

In addition to the African localities already indicated as the whereabouts of the mineral, travellers seem to have been frequently on the verge of discovery. Anderson [*] found in the Kuruman range, at Blaaw Klip, a soft stone, which the natives dug out from the hillside and formed into pipes, plates, &c., no doubt a kind of ollite, or potstone, which would seem to indicate a promising locality for asbestos. And

[*] "Twenty-five Years in a Wagon," vol. 1.

Dr. J. W. Matthews,* who spent a considerable time in that region, reports that the calcite, which runs through the blue ground in all directions in the diamond district, was covered with a coating of a "greyish-white substance, very soapy to the touch, and resembling steatite."

The importance of the subject, in view of the probability of the South African asbestos mines coming prominently to the front at an early date, will perhaps justify the insertion here of an extract from Dr. Schenk's report on the formation at Barberton. The Doctor, an eminent geologist, who has paid several visits to the goldfields, says that the formation there consists of very old, and, in most instances, highly metamorphosed rocks, composed of slate and sandstone, with interposed eruptive rocks of greenstone (diorite, serpentine, &c.). These rocks are highly erected, dipping invariably at great angles, often perpendicular, and run from east to west. It is in this formation that the gold-bearing reefs are situated, and these, with few exceptions, run in the same direction, nearly always accompanying the eruptive rocks. The gold, in his opinion, came with the eruptive rocks from the interior of the earth to the surface, and there became concentrated in reefs, which consist of quartz, and often contain iron with the gold. There is no young formation overlying these rocks at Barberton but, in the Drakensburg and Witwatersrand, a younger formation lies unconformably over the older rocks, which he concludes to be of Devonian age. The younger formation has subsequently been folded in the same way as the Barberton rocks, though it is not so highly erected. †

In a country where the hitherto usually recognised features of the mineral seem to be so diversified in colour, texture, and component parts, we should not, perhaps, be surprised at any further distinctive feature; yet it seems somewhat strange to be told of an "asbestos farm"; and, again, to find it stated, on the authority of "an eminent engineer, late Surveyor of Lands to the German Government," that on part of the ground

* "Ingwadi Yami," 148. † "Ingwadi Yami," Appendix.

where some of the new discoveries have been made he traced four distinct "*asbestos reefs*, three feet wide, and running parallel to each other at regular distances for many miles,"* a description calculated to make an asbestos expert open his eyes in wonderment.

Crocidolite in its earthy form occurs abundantly in the same region, varying in colour according to the mineral oxide which may happen to be present. Much of it is of the kind called " Tiger-eye," from its tawny-coloured, streaky brilliancy. It is of a densely compact nature, from its exceeding hardness difficult to work, but susceptible of high polish. The grain is very fine, and, even in the rough state, the fibres are singularly distinct. Some other minerals possess this peculiar shining lustre, though none in so fine a degree. Cat's-eye (Katzenauge), for instance, a chalcedonic quartz, when cut *en cabochon*, exhibits a like opalescence, or glaring internal reflection, like the pupil of a cat's eye, which is caused by the fibres of asbestos running through it. The same peculiarity, but in a lesser degree, is sometimes found in satin spar, when cut in the same way.

Chrysotile has been found on the Stewart River, British Columbia, where the occurrence of large masses of serpentine tends to justify the expectation that workable deposits will presently be found. †

In the district of Lake Temagami, to the north of Lake Nipissing, asbestos has been found from half an inch to nine inches long. One of the veins here shows about a foot wide, running in trap in the same direction as the quartz.‡

Although the statement with which this chapter opened that asbestos, in one form or another, is found in most parts of the world, has now been substantiated, Italy and Canada, which at present constitute the chief sources of supply, remain to be

---

* *The Diamond Fields Advertiser*, quoted in the *Weekly Bulletin*, September 7th, 1889.

† Report on the Yukon District, N.W.T., by G. M. Dawson, 1888.

‡ Report of the Royal Commission on the Mineral Resources of Ontario, 1890, p. 57.

considered; but so distinct and so important are the productions of these two countries that they need to be separately dealt with.

As to the more immediate outlook, it must be remembered that although, for their own special productions, these two countries are, for the present, the undoubted masters of the field, it is scarcely probable, in view of what is now taking place in many other parts of the world, that they will permanently remain so. So far as Italian produce is concerned, the company, which practically monopolises this, requires all the asbestos it can get for its own use, and in order to supplement the produce of its Italian mines, has recently bought a mine in Canada, and there also it will, in future, be a producer as well as a consumer. Indeed, the large consumers of the Canadian mineral, feeling the pinch of continually increasing prices (in consequence of supply not keeping pace with demand), are gradually buying up all the present best-known mines and turning miners themselves, the natural effect of which is that the produce of the mines so bought is withdrawn from the general market. It therefore becomes increasingly difficult for those consumers who are not also mine owners to obtain the supplies they want. A natural consequence of this state of things is further increased price and greater exertions to find fresh sources of supply. It is only, therefore, to be expected that new discoveries will continue to be made, and it may turn out that Italy and Canada will presently find both Russia and Africa formidable competitors. Dealings with the former country may, from many causes, remain somewhat difficult for the present, but with Africa the case is different. Given the requisite quality, the question of transport will soon be overcome, and it is only fair to assume, from what we have seen, that the right quality will presently be found there, and when that is the case, if the mines are only intelligently handled, methods, which almost indicate themselves, will speedily be adopted to settle the transport question.

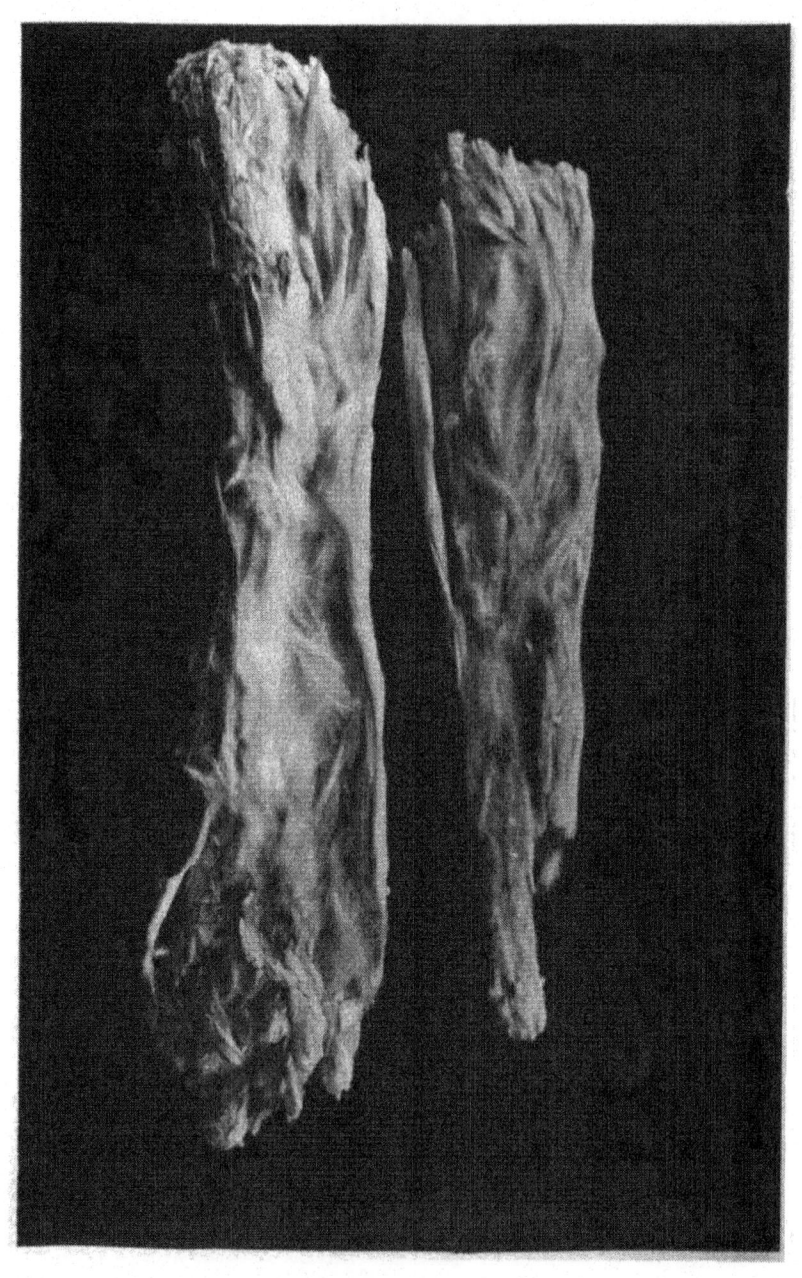

ITALIAN ASBESTOS. "The Flossy."

CHAPTER III.

ITALIAN ASBESTOS AND THE ITALIAN MINES.

ITALIAN ORE a Distinct Variety—Essential Characteristics—Mr. J. Boyd's Paper—Italian Exhibition—Quantitative Analysis—The Mines—Varieties of Ore—The United Asbestos Company and its Operations—The Industry as carried on in France—The New Asbestos Company.

IN the modern use of asbestos in practical mechanics and the industrial arts, Italy ranks first in order of time; it is only fitting, therefore, that the produce of the Italian mines should be first considered.

Asbestos, as found in the Italian hills, differs materially in appearance, form, and character from the mineral, so called, which is found in Canada: but the intrinsic features of the two kinds are practically the same, and the uses to which they are put are nearly identical.

It would serve no useful purpose now to revive the vexed question of their relative merits; practical experience in their use has shown that both possess undeniably good qualities, and that there is ample demand for both; those very qualities, in fact, which may render one of them less suitable for some particular purpose being precisely those which best adapt it for another.

Some fine specimens of Italian asbestos are occasionally to be seen in London, at the various exhibitions. One of the exhibits at the recent Italian Exhibition at South Kensington, of an unusual character, was described in the catalogue as a "Collezione d'amianti italiani in 70 vasetti"; these were sent from Rome by the "Impresa mineraria italiana" of that city, which company has an office in Leadenhall Street, London. Many of this large number of specimens were curious both in structure and colour; but it must not be supposed that they were so many distinct varieties; indeed, except as curiosities, their exhibition could scarcely be said to answer any specially useful purpose, as there were no analyses given, nor any facilities for their examination by experts.

In examining such a mineral as asbestos with a view to determining its economic value, too much importance cannot be given to its quantitative analysis. It is evident, however, that, when dealing with asbestos, accurate agreement between any two operations must not be looked for, unless the samples analysed are not only from the same mine, but from the same part of the same mine; because, though the constituents may be the same, the proportions may be different. In comparing, therefore, any two or more analyses made by different individuals, these can only be expected to agree approximately, unless we knew that they were the results obtained from analysing parts of the same piece of ore. To be of any commercial value, asbestos needs length and fineness of fibre combined with infusibility, toughness, and flexibility; some of these qualities are often wanting in a mineral of a very promising appearance. The qualities of length and silkiness can, of course, be determined by the eye, but why a beautiful silky specimen, such as some of those from South Africa, should be wanting in such essentialities as infusibility, tenacity, or elasticity, can only be determined by an accurate knowledge of the proportions of its constituent parts.

A consideration of this point will no doubt be sufficient to excuse the insertion here of one or two analyses, made by different gentlemen, all of them of sufficient eminence to justify the insertion of their work for comparative examination.

The first is taken from a very interesting paper * on Italian Asbestos, read before the Society of Arts in April, 1886, by Mr. James Boyd, from which paper the description of the Italian mines here given is mainly derived. In this paper the following comparative analyses of the Italian and Canadian

* *Jour. Soc. Arts*, No. 1743.

minerals are given, that of the Italian having been made by Prof. Barff.

	Italian.	Canadian.
Lime and magnesia	37·84	33·20
Silica	41·69	40·90
Oxide of iron	3·01	5·75
Potash	·85	traces
Soda	1·41	·68
Alumina	2·57	6·60
Moisture evaporated at 100 C.	3·04	—
Loss on heating to white heat, water of hydration, and organic matter	9·56	12·50
Chlorine	—	·25
Loss	·03	·12
	100·00	100·00

The professor, in a note appended to his analysis, remarks: "This asbestos contains nothing injurious to metal with which it comes in contact when used in connection with machinery, and the special character of Italian asbestos renders it vastly superior to that found in Canada." The first part of this sentence is just as applicable to Canadian as to Italian asbestos, but the concluding part is somewhat puzzling, as the professor does not tell us what the special characteristics he alludes to are, and they do not appear to indicate themselves by a comparison of the figures. Soon after the publication of this I had an opportunity of getting a sample of each sort analysed in Italy, through a friend there, the results of which were as follows:—

	Italian.	Canadian.
Magnesia	40·15	33·21
Protoxido de ferro	·75	5·77
Alumina	2·82	6·69
Silica	40·25	40·90
Acqua de hydrato	14·20	12·20
Soda	1·37	·69
Potassia	indicios	indicios
Cal.	,,	,,
Chlorina	·51	·22
Acido sulphurico	·31	indicios
	100·36	99·68

In regard to these the analyst remarks: "Although the Canadian sample shows a less percentage of magnesia, the difference is fully compensated for by the larger quantity of protoxide of iron and alumina."

The comparative analyses of the two ores which follow recently appeared in one of the American scientific journals, and were stated to have been made by Professor Durst, who has made a special study of the subject; and the concluding analysis of Canadian ore is one made by Mr. Donald, Professor of Chemistry at the McGill College, Montreal:

	Italian.	Canadian.	Canadian.
Silica	40·25	40·92	39·05
Magnesia	40·18	33·21	40·07
Water of hydration	14·02	12·22	14·48
Alumina	2·82	6·69	3·69
Protoxide of iron	0·75	5·77	(oxide) 2·41
Soda	1·37	·68	—
Potash, &c.	·15	·22	· —
Sulphuric acid	·31	traces	—
		Undetermined	·30
	99·85	99·71	100·00

Professor Durst expresses his opinion of the result of his work in this way: "Thus, while the Italian possesses a larger percentage of magnesia, it is poorer in alumina, and holds more water than Canadian. The Italian, obtained in long fibres, sometimes reaching 3 feet, cannot be worked with the same ease and evenness as the Canadian. The product likewise is not so uniform, while its greater density and weight renders it less desirable and more expensive for general use."

It seems clear, however, that, making all due allowance for difference of locality and surroundings in the samples analysed, the analyses are for all practical trade purposes in sufficient accord, whilst the balance of evidence is against Dr. Barff, both in precision of statement and in agreement with general commercial opinion.

The statement of Professor Durst, as to the superior ease with which Canadian fibre can be worked, seems to be corroborated by the following extract from a Canadian technical journal. Few people have had more practical experience, or can speak with greater authority than Mr. Boyd.

"Mr. James Boyd, managing director of the British Asbestos Company, writes to the London papers respecting the New Asbestos Company which has been formed to develop certain French and Italian properties as follows : ' I have recently heard that a Canadian asbestos property has been acquired by the Company holding the greater part of the Italian properties, or by parties interested in it. They could raise hundreds of tons from their Italian properties; and if they do not do so there must be a reason for it, and I believe the reason may be sought for in the fact that, whilst Canadian asbestos fibre can easily be spun into thread fit for manufacturing into rope or cloth, Italian can only be so spun on a commercial scale by the admixture of cotton, or some other material, owing to the want of cohesion amongst its fibres. Owing to the increasing steam pressures used in connection with triple expansion engines, a great increase has taken place in the consumption of packings made of asbestos cloth, and I believe it is practically impossible to make this of pure Italian asbestos. The English Admiralty have, I believe, persistently refused to put Italian asbestos packing on their list, for the reasons above stated. . . . The protective tariffs, so called, in France are not so high as to prevent both Italian and also English manufacturers of Canadian asbestos goods from selling their manufactures there; and as a matter of fact, the prices in France are lower than in England.'"*

The statements in the foregoing extract are singularly corroborated by the fact that the company first named, the "Impresa Mineraria Italiana," are now almost exclusively devoting their attention to the manufacture of various grades of asbestos cloth, which they make from the Canadian mineral alone.

There are three principal varieties of asbestos found in Italy, the grey, the flossy, and the silky. There is also an-

* *The Canadian Mining Review*, March, 1890.

other of a powdery character, of which a good deal is used, but to which not so much importance is attached.

The Grey variety, of which an illustration is given, is a rough-looking saponaceous fibre, of great tenacity and of considerable length. This is often found high up in the rocky face of the mountain, but occasionally on a lower level in the Alpine valleys. Sometimes it occurs in such difficult positions that, in the first stages of the work, the men have to be let down by ropes from above to bore the holes for making a working platform. The high table-land of Acqua Nera, 6,000 feet above the level of the sea, has its whole western face composed of rocks rich in asbestos, the seams of which run in a nearly vertical direction.

The Flossy form is dry, with a smooth silky fibre. This occurs generally in thick horizontal seams, which have a rapid dip when once the rock is opened. A large quantity of powdery material is found with it, in the centre of which lumps of quartz, and substances apparently of vegetable origin, are occasionally found.

The Silky variety is much like the flossy, but has a smoother texture, is longer in the fibre, and of greater tenacity. This is the kind mostly in use for gas-stove work.

The Powdery is found in the same range of mountains as the flossy, but generally at a much lower level. Like much of the mineral found in various parts of the world, it exhibits a pasty appearance when first opened up, but it rapidly dries and pulverises on exposure to the atmosphere. The Société Française des Amiantes claims that this powdery material is of great value to agriculturists as a manure, and to viticulturists for application to the vine stocks as a preventive of mildew and a destroyer of the phylloxera. It has been tried in England, with a similar object in view, in the hop gardens of Kent, but with no marked success; indeed, it is somewhat difficult to understand what there is in its composition to give it any efficacy for either of the purposes named.

Italian asbestos is rarely found at a lower level than 5,000 feet, ranging from this upwards to 12,000; in fact, up to the line of perpetual snow. It is usually got by running driftways into the face of the rock, when the seams, on being followed up, often abruptly end in pockets, which sometimes contain as much as a ton or a ton and a half of asbestos. When first taken out from the rock the ore is in lumps, forming hard, closely compacted, bundles of fibres, varying in colour from light grey to a dingy brown. With a little care threads of many feet in length may be drawn out from these bundles, the fibre closely resembling flax, but in appearance only, the difference being quickly perceptible to the touch.

In searching for asbestos on the Italian hills, the prospector is not guided by the same rules as those which guide the explorer in Canada; he looks in the perpendicular face of the rock for cracks, which may be filled with a white powdery substance which, when the surface is broken away, soon assumes a leathery appearance, and then, when further entry is made, the true asbestos is found. Mining for asbestos in Italy is, as a rule, carried on with greater difficulty than in Canada, and the supply of the mineral, if more abundant, is much more uncertain.

Mine owners in Italy, desirous of effecting a speedy sale of their property are, it is to be presumed, no better or worse than others in the same position elsewhere, in being apparently not averse to the practice of "salting." In Italy this salting process seems to consist in driving fine asbestos fibre into the crevices of the rock, and then, so far as possible, giving it the appearance of the real formation. Mr. Boyd tells us that in one instance of the kind which came under his notice, a sum of about £200 was actually paid for the right of extracting asbestos from the barren rock which had been so treated. Here, at any rate, the asbestos did not follow the usual course by running into a pocket, whatever might have been the case with the money.

Mr. Boyd, in the paper previously referred to, makes a statement of a very suggestive character as the result of long observation in Italy, which is worth recording. He says that " if asbestos be found on the surface of a rock exposed either to the south or south-west, the product is generally fairly abundant and of good quality. If exposed to the east there is fine quality, but very small quantity; whilst if exposed to the north the quantity is plentiful, but dry and hard, and on entering the rock all traces of it are lost."

Whether this be at all consistent with Canadian experience I cannot say. The lie of the ground and the course of the veins being so different, it is quite possible the theory may have no applicability at all to Canadian mining, but it is certainly worth the consideration of asbestos miners in other parts of the world, as well as in Canada.

Asbestos, as already explained, wherever it occurs, whether in Italy or any other part of the world, is found associated with other minerals, but occasionally, in the Italian deposits, minute crystals of a green-coloured garnet are found with the asbestos, which the miners call asbestos seeds (semenze dell' amianto).

It is now nearly twenty years ago since asbestos first began to be talked about in England, and attempts were very soon afterwards made to turn its peculiar properties to useful account. The time was getting ripe for such a business. Steam pressures had, for some time, been gradually rising. Although 30 lbs. to the square inch at sea, and 50 lbs. on land had hitherto been the average, these pressures were then beginning to be doubled, and consequently the old forms of packing for joints and glands were, under these new conditions, found to be incapable of withstanding the strain put upon them. Gasket rings and hemp gland packings had both to be superseded by more durable appliances, yet these were so far from being perfect that it was felt to be certain trouble would occur with them when exposed to the higher temperatures which were evidently coming.* Just about the same time asbestos millboard was being successfully made in Florence, and a good piston packing was made in America. Directly afterwards, a " Patent Asbestos Manufacturing Company" was established in Glasgow, for making piston packings after this American

* *Engineering*, March, 1885.

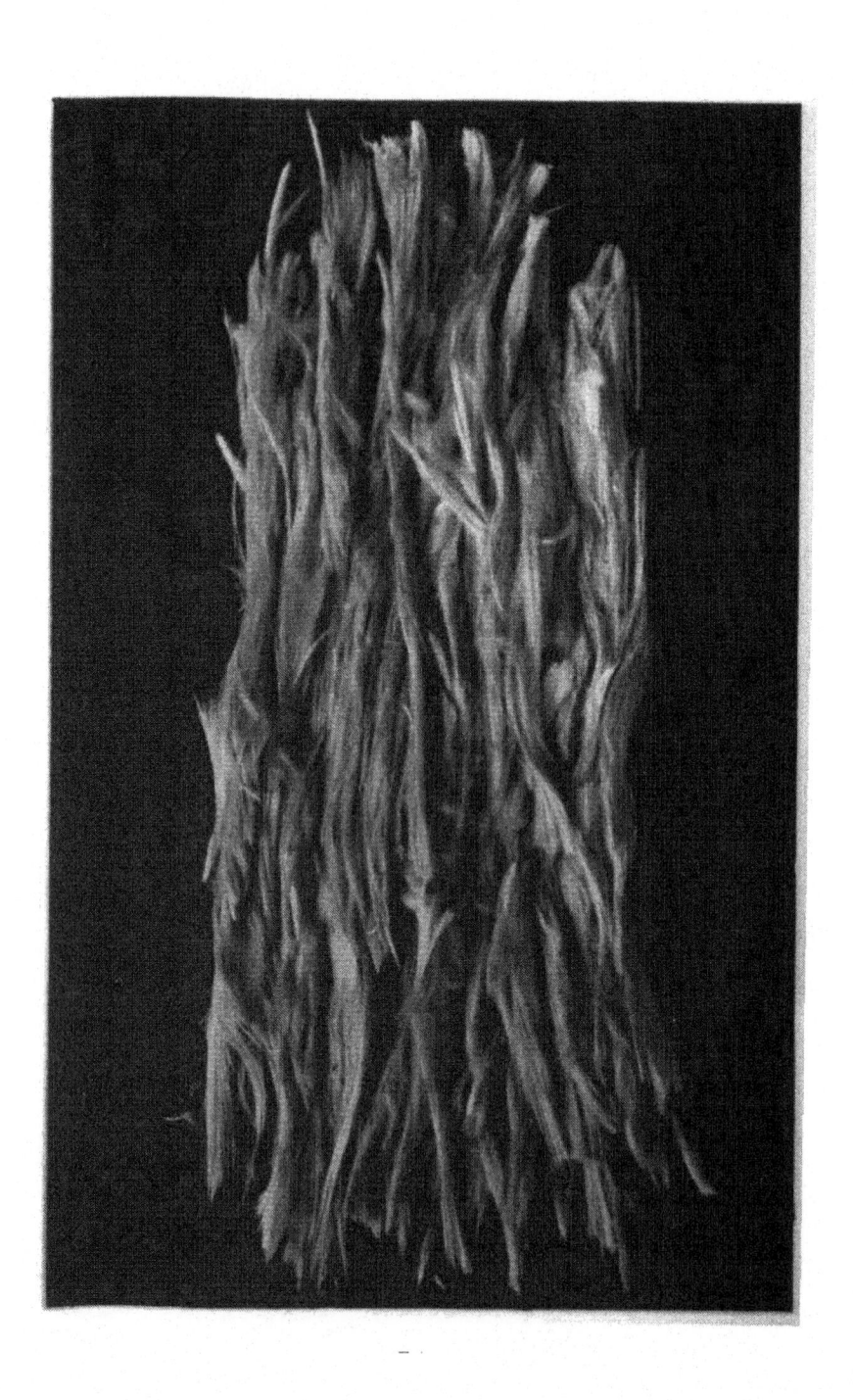

invention, and millboard after the Italian method. The peculiarity of the packing introduced by this Scotch company consisted in its being formed of a core of asbestos fibre, consolidated by machinery, and braided over with cotton to keep it together; and although this first attempt was somewhat crude, some wonderfully good results were obtained from it.

In 1879, one year after the opening of the first chrysotile mine in Canada, three firms which had made asbestos mining in Italy and the manufacture of asbestos goods a speciality, became amalgamated, as "The United Asbestos Company, Limited," of London; and this new company, having secured about 180 mining properties, covering 80 square miles, in the region of the Italian Alps, being nearly all the Italian mines then known, thereby at once, for the time being, obtained a practical monopoly of the trade.

The operations carried on by this company may be concisely stated as follows :—The crude asbestos, when extracted at the mines, is packed up in bags containing from one to two hundredweight each, and these bags are brought over to England, and discharged into lighters in the Thames, whence they are conveyed, by way of the Grand Junction Canal, to the company's works, at Harefield, in Hertfordshire. Here the bags, on being opened, are found to contain the asbestos in rough lumps, from the size of a man's hand to about as much as one man can lift. A sample of this crude ore can be seen at the company's offices, a remarkably fine specimen of the grey variety, brought from one of the company's mines in the Valtellina Valley.* This is a natural curiosity, and probably the finest piece of Italian asbestos yet seen.

When turned out of the bags the crude asbestos is, first of all, opened out by special machinery, constructed for the purpose, with the double object of loosening the fibres, and freeing these from the material by which they are compactly bound together. This is an operation which has no counterpart in the method of dealing with Canadian ore; nor for the

* A fine quality of alabaster (gypsum) is also found in this valley, so delicate as almost to resemble white wax.

Italian ore would any such opening machine as is in use in the shoddy or cotton waste trades do, as no tearing or cutting action can be permitted. Three machines, of gradually reduced sizes, are employed to open the asbestos, and then those portions which contain the longest fibres are taken to the boiling tanks, where they are rendered soft by heat and moisture. These tanks are each provided with a rotating beater, which maintains a thorough circulation, by first taking up the fibre, then opening and drawing it out, and afterwards sending it on to be soaked, until it comes round again to the beater. The short fibre, reduced to fluff, is taken to edge-runners and ground and prepared for the beating engines, where the binding material is added, and the whole thoroughly incorporated, after which it is drawn off into a receiving-tank, placed in the millboard machine-room. From this tank it is conveyed to the millboard machine, to which agitators are attached, to keep the fibre from settling. The water is drawn off through a fine wire gauze on a revolving cylinder, leaving a thin coating of the asbestos pulp on the cylinder. This is then taken off by an endless band, and transferred to a second solid rotating cylinder, where it steadily accumulates until the desired thickness has been reached. It is finally cut across, and removed in the form of a square sheet of millboard or paper.

This is much the same method as that adopted in France. Describing the mode of preparing millboard and paper there, Jagnaux says :—" Quant aux fils les plus courts, et ceux qui rest en pelotes on en fait de la bourre. C'est cette bourre qui, agglomérée au moyen d'un colle végétale, sert à la fabrication du papier et du carton d'amiante."

When the sheets leave the machine they contain a good deal of water, which is got rid of partly by pressure and in part by drying. They are then put between zinc plates and subjected to a powerful hydraulic press, which expels most of the remaining water, after which they are hung up, by spring clips in a steam-heated room, to complete the drying process, when, once more, the sheets are subjected to pressure, to flatten them out and improve the surface, after which the edges are trimmed and the manufacture is complete. When trimmed, the sheets usually measure 40in. × 40, their thickness varying by thirty-seconds from $\frac{1}{32}$in. to $\frac{1}{4}$. The board is then cut up into shapes and sizes suitable for the special purpose for which it is intended. It is mostly used for making joints not exposed to the action of moisture, such as dry steam, air, or gas.

The step from millboard $\frac{1}{74}$in. thick to paper is so small, that many attempts have been made to produce an asbestos writing paper, which, from its indestructibility, would be invaluable in case of fire, for preserving charters, policies, agreements, and other important documents. Such a paper is made, but generally it is too uneven in texture, and too much akin to blotting paper to permit of its use as a writing paper.

The other great division of the manufacture, consists of such articles as require the production of yarns. To the initial difficulty of this manufacture we have already alluded. When yarn is wanted, the raw material is discharged from the boiling tanks into hydro-extractors, where most of the water is thrown out, the drying process being afterwards completed by steam heat. The fibre is then passed through a shaking machine, which separates the long fibre from the short, the latter being sent to the millboard department, whilst the former is reserved for the carding-room, where it has to pass through several processes before the manufacture is complete.

Asbestos cloth is woven in a loom exactly like calico, except that the reeds and healds are much coarser. The narrow cloth or tape is woven in a smallware loom. Both the sheeting and the tape are used for making joints, and the former is sometimes rubber-proofed to render it water-tight. The asbestos and india-rubber woven tape is so constructed that it can be bent round a corner without puckering, and thus is particularly useful in making joints in manhole and mudhole doors. If the cloth or tape be rubbed with plumbago or powdered asbestos before it is used, the joint may be broken and re-made many times with the same packing. The cloth is also worked up into square gland packing, by being cut into strips and built into a square rope, with a backing of pure rubber to give additional elasticity. The edges of the strips lie in contact with the rod, and as the gland is screwed home, the compression of the rubber feeds the asbestos forward, so that a large proportion of the whole bulk can be actually worn away by the continual friction, before new packing is required.

It would carry this part of the subject to far too great a length, if even a summary account were given of the whole of the United Company's special machinery and manufactures; but it is evident that no one who has had an opportunity of considering the rapid advances made in the numerous and varied applications of this valuable material, will hesitate to admit that the persevering energy and practical skill exhibited by this Company have paved the way for other manufacturers, and that it can, consequently, claim to be the pioneer of most of the improvements which have been made in the machinery now in use for the manufacture of asbestos goods.

Before passing on to the consideration of Canadian asbestos possibly a few words may not be out of place here on the subject of the industry, as it is carried on in France, seeing that it is mostly Italian ore that is there used.

Attempts have more than once been made to establish the industry in France, at Mantes, Paris, and elsewhere, but, until recently, with no considerable amount of success. In the autumn of 1889, however, a more ambitious enterprise was set on foot by the establishment of the Société Française des Amiantes at Tarascon sur Rhone as a Société Anonyme. The business having been commenced on a scientific basis, was so far successful, that in order to obtain further capital, the undertaking was launched as an English Limited Liability Company in January, 1890, under the title of the "New Asbestos Company, Limited," capital £120,000. The asbestos deposits in the hands of this Company are 62 in Italy, covering an area of 700 acres, and 8 in France, extending over about eight acres. It has an establishment at Tarascon, for the manufacture of the general run of asbestos goods, and another at Gadagne on the Saône for the making of millboard and paper.

The Italian mines are situate in the Valleys of the Saone and d'Aosta. The deposits in this district are essentially pockety, some of the pockets occurring on the level; most of the works, however, are on the slopes of the mountain, extending up to 700 or 800 feet of altitude. A rather primitive method of work is carried on here at present; this is a species of isolated task work, each workman, at the close of his day's work, conveying to the store the quantity of mineral he has himself extracted from the mine. When brought in by the men, it is bagged up, and at once transported to the works at Tarascon, where the bags are emptied and the ore dealt with in much the same fashion as that already described, with the object of loosening the fibres and separating them from the very large quantity of powdery admixture which is found in this Company's mines. After this initial process the crude asbestos is separated into three divisions, each destined for its special purpose:—

1. The long fibred quality is set aside for spinning and weaving.

2. The shorter fibred material is sent to Gadagne for millboard and paper.

3. The powdery material, part of which is converted into cement, paint, &c., and a considerable quantity sold to agriculturists for manure, and to viticulturists for use in the manner described in another chapter, as a protection against noxious insects infecting the vines. In regard to which M. Ville, a Parisian professor of chemistry, states that he has discovered a new chemical manure, intense and almost miraculous in its effects. This is a mixture of phosphate of lime, carbonate of potash, and sulphate of lime, which if placed round vine growths will enable them to defy the onslaughts of phylloxera.

CHAPTER IV.

CANADIAN ASBESTOS (Chrysotile, Schillernder asbest).

FIRST APPEARANCES UNPREPOSSESSING. — Hydrous Character — Colour — Description — Amianthus — Foliated and Fibrous Serpentines — Sources of Supply — Eastern Townships — Minerals found there — Position and Climate — Great Geological Fault — Serpentine Belt — Decomposed Serpentine — Dykes — Shickshock Mountains — Veins Irregular — Surface Influences — Trial Borings — Classes of Ore — Local Conditions — Prospecting — Chromic Iron — Impurities — Discolouration — Marketable value — Ornamental Serpentines.

DERIV.: χρυσος, gold, and τιλος, fine hair.

JUST about the time of the establishment of the London Company referred to in the preceding chapter, Canadian asbestos was beginning to attract attention, and it is not difficult to understand, how it came about that a Company which had not only practically originated the trade, but, by securing a large proportion of all the then known Italian mines, had, as they supposed, become possessed of a practical monopoly of the business, should, at the outset, have viewed the claims of a younger rival with jealousy, not unmingled with some degree of contempt. Nor was this last entirely unjustified, as first appearances were decidedly against the new comer. The Canadian ore was not only of an entirely different character from their own, and such as required altogether different treatment, but the staple was ludicrously short in comparison, much of it was coarse, and the rough and careless manner in which some of the crude ore was prepared for market, might

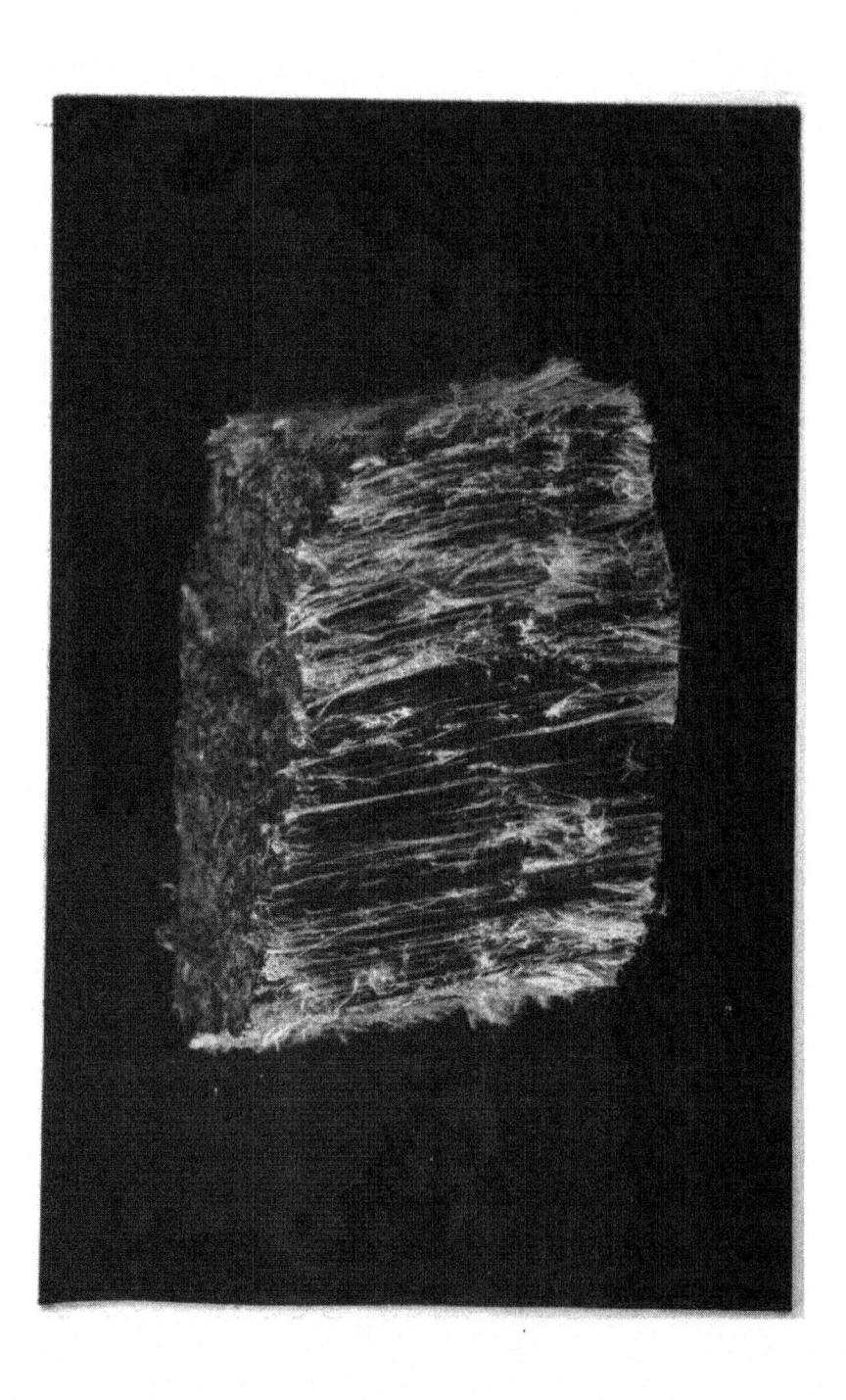

readily induce anyone to believe it to be a decidedly inferior article. All that, however, is now matter of history, and Canadian asbestos, since then, has taken high rank among the economic minerals of the world; its most strenuous opponents have not only adopted its use, but urged by the necessities of their trade, have secured a mine in Canada, and have thus become producers as well as consumers of Canadian ore.

Chrysotile, to give the Canadian mineral its technical designation, is usually said to be a fibrous form of serpentine,* one of several minerals which, under certain conditions, have a tendency to assume that peculiar structural form.

According to local surroundings, chrysotile varies in colour from a greenish white or olive green to a yellow or brownish shade. For reasons already explained its analyses will not always agree, but the differences are not great, and for all practical purposes its composition may be taken to be :—

Silica	43·50
Magnesia	40·00
Oxide of Iron	2·08
Alumina	·40
Water	13·80
	99·78

Sp. gr., 2·219. Optically it is bi-axial under polarized light.

Professor Dana says, it was first brought from Reichenstein, but, although it is found there, and in several other places, it is none the less the fact, that at the present time, it is not found of good quality, or in any considerable quantity, elsewhere than in Canada, and there only at present in one particular district.

A good popular description of the mineral was thus given in *Le Génie Civil* for September, 1883 : "La chrysotile du Canada n'est pas comme l'amiante ordinaire formée d'un paquet de fils d'un blanc verdâtre et remplissant des

* "Fibrous serpentine with a silky lustre is called chrysotile."—Dana, "Min. et Lith.," 1878. "On appelle chrysotil une serpentine en fibres soyeuses, d'un vert tirant sur la jaune d'or, qui se distingue de l'asbeste par sa solubilité dans les acides et sa teneur en eau."—De Lapparent, 408.

ciated are black, green, grey, and purple slates, with, occasionally, conglomerates and sometimes beds of hard quartzose sandstone. The diorites, with which it is also associated, frequently form great mountain masses, as at Orford, Ham, Thetford, &c., and in texture are both massive and concretionary, while in colour they range from different shades of green to brown.*

The main sources, from which the present supply of chrysotile is derived, lie within the province of Quebec, mainly within the counties of Wolfe, Megantic, and Beauce; the most productive of the mines, yet discovered, being situate in that part of the province which is known collectively as "The Eastern Townships of Quebec." Here the areas of serpentine are very extensive and prominent, but those portions on which the mineral abounds are comparatively rare, and are practically limited to two small sections lying about four miles apart. Other promising sections are being carefully explored, but these are as yet mostly covered with soil and forest, which obstruct investigation.

The district comprising the Eastern Townships, like the more southern part of the province of Ontario, which lies on the opposite side of the river, (notwithstanding that the rock formations of the two districts differ materially), is singularly rich in deposits of minerals, not only of vast extent, but of a very diversified character. In the Laurentian Strata of Ontario, as well as in the Ottawa district of the Quebec province, the rocks are mostly pyroxenic, and abound, the latter especially, in apatite,† whilst those of the crystalline and subcrystalline formations which traverse the Eastern Townships and run through the Gaspé peninsula, are mostly of a hydrous character, magnesian and chromiferous; and it is chiefly among these last that the serpentine, which forms the asbestos matrix, occurs. Asbestos is found in the serpentine limestones of the Laurentian series also, but little has yet been done there in

---

* Dr. Ells, "The Ottawa Naturalist," vol. iii., no. 2.

† "Apatite occurs, without exception, in association with pyroxenic or hornblendic rocks."—Penrose on "Apatites," 25.

e 63.]

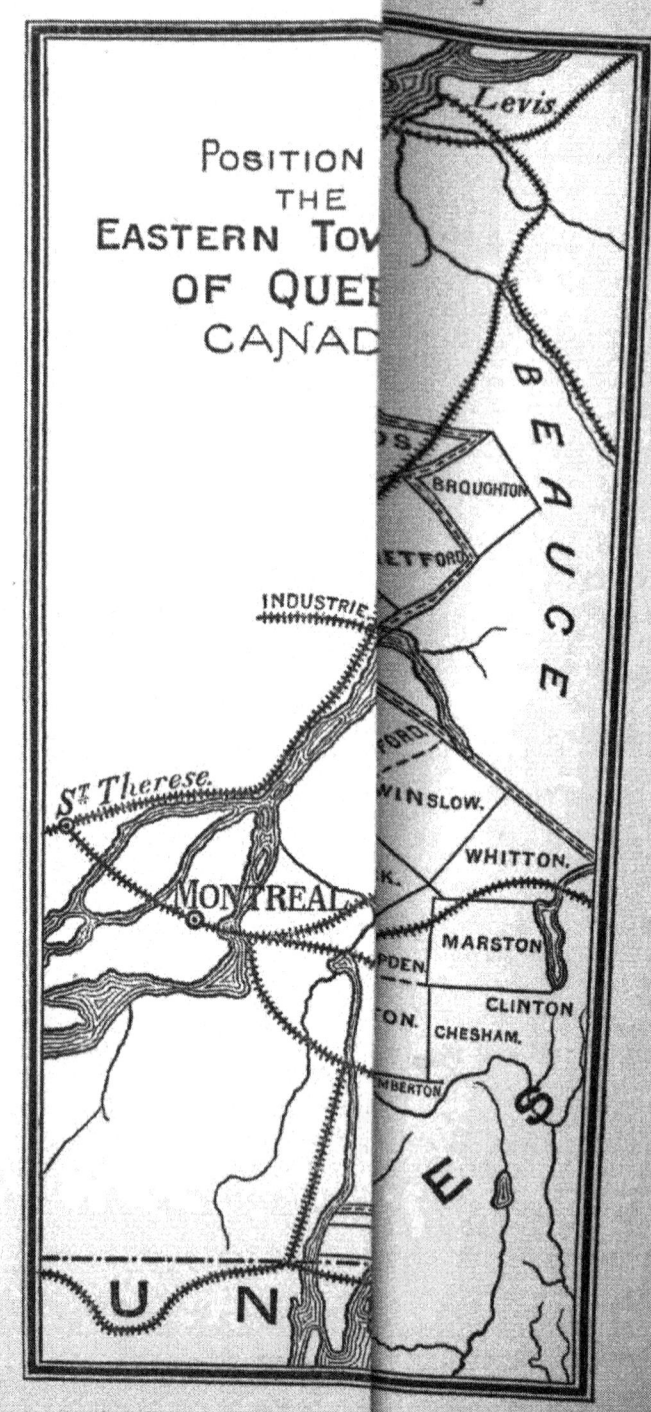

POSITION
THE
EASTERN TOV
OF QUEE
CANAD
Levis.
BEAUCE
BROUGHTON
ETFORD
INDUSTRIE
FORD
WINSLOW.
WHITTON.
St. Therese.
MONTREAL
MARSTON
PDEN.
CLINTON
TON.
CHESHAM.
MBERTON
E S
U N

the way of productive mining, although discoveries are likely to follow scientific prospecting.

Dr. Ells remarks that the areas of serpentine are very extensive in the two great geological formations of Canada; in the Laurentian, which stretches from the coast of Labrador to westward of the Great Lakes, covering an area of about 200,000 square miles, and the Quebec Group, which occupies a large portion of that province lying southward of the St. Lawrence, and between that river and the United States boundary. What may be termed the asbestos district in the Eastern Townships is a vast area of about 200 miles in length, by 6 or 8 miles wide,* the asbestos found here differing in many respects from that found in the Laurentian district.

That part of the country, which goes by the name of the Eastern Townships, includes the greater part of the province of Quebec, which lies on the southern side of the St. Lawrence. Its relative position as regards the cities of Montreal and Quebec and the river, will be seen from the sketch-map of part of the province annexed. It forms a narrow zone of metalliferous rocks, within which is comprised the greater part of the mineral wealth of the province. The deposits which occur in this part of the continuation of the Appalachian region, some of which are of great extent, comprise gold, silver, copper, galena, asbestos, antimony, nickel sulphide, pyrites, magnetic, chromic, and titanic iron ores, bog ore, steatite, and roofing slate; whilst many of the crystalline dolomites are intermixed with serpentine in such a way as to form black and gold, green and chocolate-coloured serpentine marbles, some of them of great beauty.

A general view of the mineral industry of the province is shown by the following table, which gives the production and value of the minerals for the year ending 30th June, 1889.†

* Dr. Selwyn, *Canadian Mining Review*, no. 6.
† "Rapport du Commissaire des Terres de la Couronne de la Province de Quebec pour les douze mois expirés le 30 Juin 1889."

	Tonnes.	Valur.
Phosphate	28,350	$460,950
Amiante (asbestos)	5,919	352,260
Cuivre	70,955	720,000
Fonte manufacturé avec bog-ore	4,000	120,000
Fer (minéral exporté)	3,000	15,000
Or	,,	,,
Graphite	450	23,500
Mica	,,	,,
Feldspath	250	1,750
Soapstone	150	1,200
Ardoises	20,300 square	90,000
Granit	30,000 pds. cub.	12,000
Calcaire à bâtir	200,000 vrg. cub.	200,000
Chaux	400,000 minots	70,000
Briques	30,000 milles	200,000
		$2,266,660

M. Mercier sums up the matter by stating that this mineral region contains about 1,000,000 acres of iron-bearing lands, 500,000 of apatite ground, 100,000 asbestos, 50,000 copper, 100,000 auriferous, and 10,000 oil bearing; forming a total of mineral wealth covering 2,000,000 acres of land, mostly in workable deposits.* The metalliferous zone covers the whole district, extending thence to the extreme east of the Gaspé peninsula. This latter region, on account of the dense forests which cover the greater part of it, the want of roads and other obstacles, has not yet been sufficiently explored to bring its mineral treasures to light. The Minister of the Interior, in 1882, reported to the Dominion Parliament, "We can affirm that this vast country constitutes the principal zone *minière* of the Eastern Townships. The zone extends from the frontier of the United States to the north-east of Quebec. Until now (owing to the difficulty of exploration) we have not found anything more than serpentine rocks and chromic iron in the region of Shickshock; but as these minerals are generally found with cotton-stone, brass, lead, antimony, and iron, also

* "General Sketch of the Province of Quebec," by the Hon. W. Mercier, Premier of the Province.

with gold and silver, it is not unlikely that we may find those minerals in the unexplored region of Gaspé."

The foregoing statement is corroborated by Professor Hunt, who, in 1865, wrote :—" The Eastern Townships are included in the rising zone, situated to the south of the St. Lawrence, as well as the more south-eastern region extending along the frontier, and forming a succession of valleys, which continues from the sources of the river Connecticut to the north-east of the Baie des Chaleurs. The Eastern Townships do not include this prolongation towards the north-east, but, as it geologically and geographically belongs to them, we may include it under the same name."

Since the above was written further progress has been made in the exploration of Gaspé, and it may be said that all the minerals found in the Eastern Townships abound there also, with rock oil in addition.

The volcanic range, which at the extremity of Gaspé is lost in the sea, practically passes under it, and rises again on the shores of Newfoundland, where the formation is the same, and where asbestos, gold, and many of the other minerals named, are also found.

Until the comparatively recent discovery of the chrysotile mines at Thetford, the district comprised within the Eastern Townships was but sparsely occupied, being, in fact, in much the same condition as Gaspé is to-day; but the discovery of asbestos, with the pecuniary success resulting from the working of the mines, has had the natural effect of attracting thither large numbers of the mining and trading classes, and continued success has so rapidly increased the population, during the last few years, that this district now promises to speedily become a populous, thriving, and most important part of the Dominion. And this result is likely to be a good deal facilitated, as well by the comparative mildness of the climate, as by the fertility of the soil, in this part of the province. It is unquestionably true, that the cold here is more rigorous than any experienced in England, the snow is deep and lasting, and the broad St. Lawrence is regularly frozen over. It is true, also, that no climate in the world can exceed that of England, in its pure balmy, delicious atmosphere during, perhaps, a few days in early summer and autumn; but when it is considered how lamentably few those days are, it may be that the balance of enjoyment might be awarded to this part of Canada; for, notwithstanding the rigour of winter, the air there is so dry and exhilarating, as to render the cold far less disagreeable and hard to bear than what we have to endure in England, where a warmer temperature prevails, accompanied by humid and foggy atmospheric conditions. As a rule, people suffer much less from cold in Canada, than they do in England,* and pulmonary and bronchial affections are not so prevalent. An unfortunate association of ideas, rather than actual fact, by which Canada is not the only sufferer, has caused the words Canadian, Siberian, and hyperborêan to be deemed interchangeable terms in popular estimation denoting the utmost severity of cold. †

In regard to fertility, we have the authority of Dr. Ells for stating, that much of the Eastern Townships district is underlaid by a broad band of slaty rock, with which a considerable development of limestone is associated, the decay of which produces a soil of great value to the husbandman.‡ The hard rocks of the Laurentides also are intersected in all directions by bands of crystalline limestone, of a soft and decomposing nature, which render the ground, especially in the valleys, very fertile.

Considered in relation to the mineralogy of this district, a matter of great importance is that nearly the whole of it is crossed, near the central line, by the great mountain range which forms, on the south of the St. Lawrence, a continuation of the Appalachian chain of the United States (of which the Alleghanies are an offshoot), and which, where it traverses

---

* Much the same may be said of the cold in Russia. Barry remarks: "I never suffered from the climate in Russia, even in the severest weather, so much as I do in England."—"Ivan at Home," p. 119.

† "Canada," 1886, p. 1.

‡ "Notes on the Economic Minerals of Eastern Quebec."

Canada, is locally known as the Notre Dame and Shickshock Mountain range. From Gaspé to Quebec this chain forms the watershed between the basin of the St. Lawrence and the Bay des Chaleurs and Bay of Fundy to the south ; and throughout the whole of this region serpentines abound.

The range, as it passes through the Townships, gradually approaches the river, running along its southern shore, at a distance varying from 10 to 30 miles inland, and terminating in the high tableland of Gaspé, at the eastern extremity of the province. It consists of several roughly parallel lines of mountainous country, showing one or two points of nearly 4,000 feet of altitude (the elevation in the Gaspé peninsula averaging 1,500 feet), which is cut by deep gorges through which the rivers flow; it is largely made up of crystalline magnesian rocks, including talcose and chloritic schists and beds of serpentine, in places associated with micaceous and gneissoid rocks and other crystalline deposits. Cambrian slates and other strata have here been thrown up by a great fault, into a position apparently higher than the Hudson River beds. This fault touches the boundary of the province, not over a couple of miles from Lake Champlain. From this it proceeds in a gently curving line to Quebec, keeping just north of the Fortress. Thence it coasts the north side of the Island of Orleans, leaving a narrow margin, on the island, of the Hudson River and Utica formations. From near the east end of the island it keeps under the waters of the St. Lawrence to within 80 miles of the extremity of Gaspé. Here it again leaves a strip of the Hudson River or Utica formation on the coast.*

Resulting from some mighty convulsion, which has left indelible traces behind it, the country, near the great fault, traversed by the mountain range, has evidently been subjected to enormous pressure, either arising from a shrinkage of the earth's crust, or by a forcing upward of the lower strata ; the whole of which, or that part of it which lies south and east of

* Second Report on the Geology of a Portion of the Province of Quebec, 1888.

the fault, has been greatly disturbed and broken up, and more or less altered by metamorphic agencies. Crystalline, gneissoid and magnesian rocks appear in part to underlie them and partly to be mixed up with them in intricate foldings, by which their stratigraphic relations become greatly obscured. In many places, also, they are broken through by trachytic and granitic masses. Whilst to the west and north of the great fault the strata are particularly undisturbed, those which lie directly east and south of it have been greatly tilted and uplifted, and generally reversed in dip. Towards the more central parts of the district, many of the beds have been altered and rendered crystalline by metamorphic agencies, and these have been folded up with one another and with an older system of crystalline rocks, forming the axes of the higher elevations in such a way as to produce great complications of structure. In its physical features the district is more or less of a mountainous character throughout, and in parts, as already stated, of considerable fertility. In this latter respect it differs remarkably from the mountainous Laurentian region of the northern part of the province.[*] The general features of the country, therefore, are very singular, having a rolling appearance, and, when viewed from any altitude, looking like an upheaval of mighty waves suddenly stilled and changed into stone. In his description of the mineral region east of the Rockies, Professor Geikie describes its peculiar uplifted formation, which is much similar to the region described above; there the ancient granitic and crystalline rocks [†] have been driven up like a huge wedge through the younger strata of the prairies, and now form the axis of the Colorado Mountains, respecting which the Professor remarks that, had it not been for this wedge, the "Centennial State" would have been

---

[*] Chapman on the "Geology of Ontario and Quebec," part 5.

[†] The author of "Les Schistes Crystallines" maintains that the designation of "crystalline rocks" is defective, inasmuch as we find associated with masses having a right to this title, and geologically confounded with them, other rocks, such as serpentine, obsidian, perlite, &c., which are not crystalline in character, but colloidal or porodic.

a quiet pastoral or agricultural territory, like the region to the eastward. The rise of the granite axis, however, has brought up with it that incredible mineral wealth which, in a few years, has converted the loneliest mountain solitudes into busy hives of industry. *

It is through the crystalline formations of the district bounded by the great fault that the belt of serpentine runs, in which the chrysotile is found. The serpentine itself is one of the altered igneous rocks of metamorphic origin, arising from the transmutation of magnesian limestone or some closely related strata. By the earlier geologists serpentine was called "a mysterious rock." In alluding to pikrite,† a bitter fibrous variety of serpentine, Cole says that perhaps among all the rocks of igneous origin, there are none which so much puzzle the petrologist in his attempts at a rational classification as the small group which seem to pass into serpentine. Comparatively few such rocks have yet been discovered, but whenever the stratigraphical details have been worked out, in conjunction with their mineralogical characters, they seem to establish the igneous origin of serpentine.‡ De Lapparent calls it a colloid mineral, which, he says, holds in suspension the fine fibres of the minerals at the expense of which it has been formed,§ these fibres being distinctly seen in the compact rock under polarized light.‖ Gages formed it artificially in a transparent amorphous mass by placing a solution of gelatinous silicate of magnesia in a dilute solution of potash, the serpentine being deposited after some months' standing.¶

The rocks from which serpentine is mainly derived by an aqueous process are called peridotites, though there are several varieties which receive distinctive names. They are all

* Geikie's "Geological Sketches," 216.

† Or picrīte, from πικρος, bitter, from the quantity of magnesia or bittererde present.

‡ "Studies in Micro. Science," art. "Pikrite."

§ "Cours de Min.," 408.

‖ "Im polarizirten Licht bemerkt man aber, dass auch das dichte Mineral aus höchst fein faserigen Theilchen besteht."—Tschermak., 494.

¶ "Report British Assoc., 1863," 203.

characterised by the predominance of the mineral peridote or olivine. Peridotites are not commonly found on the earth's surface, one reason being that olivine is an unstable mineral which readily absorbs water and passes into serpentine.*

As implied by its name, serpentine† (lapis colubrinus) is so tinted by association with other minerals, with chrome iron especially, as to exhibit a diversity of shades and colours which give it a mottled or spotted appearance, bearing a somewhat fanciful resemblance to the markings on a serpent's skin. For this reason Agricola named it serpentaria. It is also sometimes called ophiolite, and the commoner sorts ophite, both names being derived from ὄφις, a snake. The Italians look upon it as more froglike, and therefore call it rannócchia. Mineralogically it is a hydrated silicate of magnesia, something like talc, but with more water and less silica; it is somewhat soft and sectile, has a dull, splintery fracture, and a soapy unctuous feel. It occurs generally in compact granular, slaty masses, and when found disseminated through granular limestone it imparts to the latter a clouded green colour, forming what is called verd antique.

It is sometimes found, especially in Northern Italy, to be decomposed to a considerable depth, and frequently parts, in decomposing, with a large proportion of its magnesia and most of its alkalies. In addition to the formation of unctuous clays, this change sets free carbonate of magnesia and silica, which are deposited in veins traversing the altered rock. Bischoff proved experimentally that carbonated water is capable of decomposing the silicate of magnesia, and of carrying some of it off in the form of carbonate; and Rogers has shown that digestion in simple water for three days is sufficient to remove an appreciable amount of magnesia from even such minerals as hornblende.

The rocks in which the asbestos-bearing serpentine is found

* Major-General McMahon, "Discourse before the Western Micro. Club, 1890."

† Etym.: Lat., Serpentinus; Fr., Serpentine; Sp., Serpentin; It., Serpentino; resembling a serpent.

are closely associated with masses of diorite or doleritic rocks, of certain varieties of which, rich in olivine or some allied mineral, the serpentine is in many cases an altered product ;* and the asbestos, which is found in this serpentine, a still later product of alteration. These rocks are frequently associated with masses and dykes of whitish-looking rocks, composed of quartz and feldspar, with which there is occasionally a mixture of black mica, forming a granitoid rock, and almost always with magnetic and chromic iron ores. In St. Francis, Beauce County, the serpentine occurs in connection with magnetic and titaniferous iron ; in Roxton, Brompton, and some other places it carries copper pyrites and other copper ores.

The serpentine rock forms part of the great volcanic belt traversing the Eastern Townships, which can be traced with tolerable clearness, though with frequent and considerable interruptions, throughout a course of over 120 miles in length, in which it sometimes attains a width of more than 2,500 feet, bearing mostly from north-west to south-east, following in this respect the general trend of all fissures charged with metallic ores, which usually have an east and west direction, varying about 45° on either side.

That portion of the belt which more immediately concerns our subject, runs from the boundary of Vermont, in the State of Maine, to some distance beyond the Chaudière river, a little past the latitude of Quebec, traversing in its course the Townships of Potton, Bolton, Orford, Brompton, Melbourne, Cleveland, Shipton, Ham, Garthby, Coleraine, Thetford, and Broughton. The course of the belt, in its entire length, will be found elaborately traced out and described, in a very interesting report, by Dr. Ells on "The Geology of a Portion of the Eastern Townships," published by Dawson Brothers, Montreal, in 1887, by authority of the Dominion Parliament. Here it will be seen that in Cleveland and Shipton the belt assumes a transverse twist, which also affects the Cambrian and other formations in the vicinity, and changes the strike for some miles, in the townships of Wootton and Ham to an almost

* Dr. Ells' Report, 1886, Part III., p. 23.

easterly course. The prolongation of the Melbourne and Shipton ridge, which terminates in the Little Ham Mountain, after an interval of about five miles, occupied by slates and sandstones, reappears in the Big Ham Mountain, which rises boldly from the somewhat flat country at its base, to a height of 1,150 feet, forming a magnificent hill feature of the landscape.

The most important area is that which, terminating southward in Big Ham Mountain, extends north-easterly to and beyond the Chaudière. In this area serpentines are first seen in several hills, on the south side of the outlet of East Nicolet Lake, and both here and on the west shore (where a vein of magnetic iron occurs, having a thickness of 6 feet at the surface, increasing to 11 feet in the shaft at a depth of 12 feet), the serpentine is dark green, and contains a small quantity of grey copper ore. According to Mr. Coulombe, who first opened this mine in 1881, the serpentine extends south-east from this point to near the foot of the Ham Mountain. It occupies also all the islands in the lake, and the south and east shores, extending in a ridge to the road leading to Garthby village. On the south end of the lake there is a considerable area of soapstone. The principal mass of serpentine stops at Lot 55, but is found associated with diorites on the Garthby road. It again prominently appears on a ridge near the road leading from Wolfestown to Coleraine Station; on the north-east flank of which ridge the Belmina mine is situated. Here the serpentine is associated with considerable masses of the whitish granulite already mentioned. These appear occasionally to cut the serpentine after the manner of dykes, and to its presence may possibly be ascribed some of the frequent faults which affect these rocks, and which are disclosed in the asbestos workings. There can be no doubt that the presence of these dykes favourably affects the quality, as well as the quantity, of asbestos; in corroboration of which opinion may be alleged the well-known fact that the nearness of a fault may be often predicated by some sudden change in quality, whether for better or worse, in respect to the veins of many other minerals besides asbestos. This granulite, interstratified in a peculiar manner, is to be distinctly seen in some of the mines at Thetford as well as at Coleraine. In the latter place, it is found in all the mines on the western side of the serpentine ridge, and there the asbestos is abundant and good; but, directly the ridge is crossed, the granulite disappears, and the serpentine is found to be barren of fibre. This remarkable fact cannot at present be accounted for, nor is it known why the granulite exercises this influence over the serpentine. It is clear, however, that these intrusive rocks are newer than the serpentine which they traverse, as their intrusion is marked by the alteration and shattering of the mass traversed along the contact with these dykes. The white masses of these granulitic rocks, which are such an important feature in the serpentine areas of Coleraine and Thetford, form hills between Black Lake and Thetford, and are very conspicuous as seen from the railway.*

Crossing into the adjoining townships of Ireland and Coleraine, the serpentine forms part of a harsh, rugged-looking country to the west of the Quebec Central Railway, the boldly outlined peaks and ridges to the south-west of Black Lake forming also very prominent features in the landscape. These

---

* This semi-granite is the name of an elvanic or fine-grained rock containing in itself alkali, in the form of potash and soda, sufficient to melt the silica of which it is principally composed. It has been used for some time in the manufacture of glass, which, being the product of silica, a most refractory mineral, requires alkali and other fluxes to secure its fusion, whereas granulite requires no such flux to melt it beyond lime. The fine feldspathic granulite at Meldon, Dartmoor, is even finer than that found in Saxony; assays of this show—

Silica	69·34
Mixed oxide of iron and aluminium	3·56
Lime	1·34
Magnesia	1·00
Alkalies	23·36
Calcination loss	1·40
	100·00

ridges take their rise a short distance north of the boundary between Ireland and Wolfestown, extending thence into the Township of Thetford. In the vicinity of Black Lake Station, and between this point and Thetford, the serpentine is largely intermixed with granulite, and in so far as is yet known this area constitutes the richest asbestos ground in the province. The country rock in the great serpentine areas of Thetford and Coleraine is a black, greenish slate, with hard schistose quartzite ; but at Coleraine Station beds of dark red slates, mixed with conglomerates, occur.

Large areas of the volcanic rocks also occur in the Shickshock mountain range, in the northern part of Gaspé, in rear of St. Anne des Monts, the most easterly point being Mount Serpentine, about ten miles up the Dartmouth river from its outlet in the Gaspé basin. This district was partially explored by Mr. Obalski in the summer of 1889, and he states that Mount Serpentine, which rises 1,600 feet above the sea level, is not, as its name would lead one to suppose, composed of serpentine, but of hornblende. He, however, established the existence of a band of serpentine on Block 19 there, in which he saw numerous small veins of chrysotile. A specimen from this district in my possession cannot be distinguished from the usual run of Thetford ore, which proves the desirability of a thorough investigation of this as yet unknown region. The serpentine here is associated with limestone, and is surrounded by strata of Devonian age ; to the west lies the great mass of Mount Albert, whence the ridge extends westwards for some miles. Indications of asbestos are found at most points throughout the whole formation ; but, so far as is at present discovered, the mineral is most abundant in the localities named above, although there is certainly no reason why it should not be found in paying quantity at other points, especially as it is now well established that the masses and dykes of granulite already referred to favourably affect the presence of asbestos.

Traversing the serpentine in irregular veins, the fibre, unless affected by the dislocations of the containing rock, or distorted by pressure, always lies in parallel lines at right angles to the sides of the fissure. In many cases, the veins are rendered impure by the admixture of grains, or small, irregular threads, of chromic iron or of magnetite, which break the continuity of the fibre, and then the mineral has to be carefully cobbed in order to get rid of these impurities. Near the surface, also, the veins are occasionally affected, to some extent, by the infiltration of water, often impregnated with metallic oxides, the asbestos being thereby discoloured and its value diminished. This is especially noticeable where the serpentine is disintegrated or shattered at the surface, by the action of the weather, or other causes; but the discolouration ceases as soon as the rock becomes solid. The size of the veins varies greatly, and, like other mineral veins, as already mentioned, they are affected by faults or slides, which occasionally cut off completely a valuable working face. In these cases, the slickensided character of the faces of the fault is very marked, and sheets of impure or imperfectly formed asbestos (picrolite) are found lying among them along the planes of fracture. The veins have frequently the aspect of true segregation veins, and the containing walls have, in many places, a different aspect for a distance of half an inch to three inches on either side.

Mr. Obalski, Government Mining Engineer of Montreal, states that, when tracing out the bands of serpentine, he established the existence, north of Little Lake St. Francis, of a wide band of the dark-green rock containing asbestos not yet worked, or even explored. This crosses the Indian reserve, and a block not named in the map, which he calls Block K. It then enters Ranges B and A of Coleraine, and probably Range A of Thetford. Dark serpentine then ceases to be found, and a light-coloured variety appears in the neighbourhood of Lake Bécancourt, and in Ranges 8 and 10, where a little asbestos is found, but of inferior quality.

Asbestos of good quality has also been found at Shefford, on the line of the Quebec Central Railway, the deposits being pronounced by Professor Selwyn as very promising.

Good specimens have likewise been obtained at the Chaudière River, and a small quantity from the river Desplantes, one of its tributaries.

Some years ago a few tons were taken out of the Laurentian rocks in the Papineau Seignory; but, for some reason or other, the discoveries there made were not followed up.

On Lots 10 and 11, Range 8 of Templeton, there are two contiguous workings, from which a sample ton was sent to Ottawa in 1879, realizing 100 dols., a good price at that time.

A sample sent me from Lot 8, Range 10 of Templeton, is of a striking character. Like all that found in the Laurentian strata, it is essentially different from the Thetford or Black Lake ores, being of a singularly light colour and of such special brilliancy as almost to appear semi-transparent.

The company formed to work the deposits at Brompton Lake are now turning out some good material. The fibre, though comparatively short, is of good quality, and remarkably free from iron.

Traces, also, are to be met with at Chelsea, and on Meech's Lake, as well as in the hills running northward of Ottawa city. The indications thereabouts are so good that geologists are disposed to think that mining for asbestos in the Ottawa Valley will presently assume some importance.

Fibrous hornblende is plentiful at Cape Breton; but no true asbestos has yet been found there. Gesner[*] states that samples of asbestos were found in Clare Township, N.S., with fibres radiating from a common centre. These were found in veins penetrating a rock compounded of slate, quartz, and feldspar, and were probably radiated actinolite.

In its pure state, chrysotile is as heavy as the rock in which it is enclosed, so compactly are its fine crystalline fibres compressed together; but when once it has been disintegrated, it is quite impossible to pack or knit the fibres together again, in such a way that they cannot be easily separated by the fingers.

The veins nowhere present themselves in uniform abundance, although rich veins are sometimes opened up which have a

[*] Gesner's "Geology and Mineralogy of Nova Scotia," 1836.

certain continuity. As a general rule the quality of the ore improves, and the quantity increases, as the workings are prosecuted to greater depth; nor is it difficult to comprehend why this should be so. Moreover, as has been before remarked with reference to Italian asbestos, the better qualities are usually procured from deposits at considerable altitudes; these, however, are not so great in Canada as in the Italian Alps, the altitudes in Coleraine and Thetford ranging from 700 to 800 feet, although some of the unworked parts of Coleraine are higher even than this.

The probabilities also point to a continuation of the deposits to some considerable depth, though that important matter cannot at present be proved in the absence of deep workings. No trial borings have as yet been made anywhere, except on a limited scale, by Mr. Sheridan, at Thetford; but in one mine there a depth of about 200 feet has been reached without any indication of a cessation, or any diminution of the quality of the ore. The desirability of testing the lower portions of the serpentine have often been advocated in the Reports of the Geological Survey, but, as has been already observed, up to the present very little in this way has been attempted.

As a general rule the harder and darker-coloured serpentines are the most productive, the light-green rock being usually either sterile, or yielding only a brittle quality of ore, to which but little value is attached. An exception to this rule occurs at Broughton, where a pale rock is found accompanied by splendid fibre. Admixtures of hard and soft serpentine occasionally occur; but when this happens successful mining is always doubtful, whatever may be the nature of the surface indications. Should the serpentine be crossed by quartzose gneiss or transverse dykes of granulite, the prospects are much better, especially at the junction with diorite, the contact with granite being by no means so favourable.

The chrysotile found in the Eastern Townships may be roughly divided into three classes:—

a. A coarse, brittle, compact variety, plentiful, but of comparatively little value.

b. Ore possessing well-defined fibres, of a yellowish-brown colour, fragile, and containing much foreign body ; and

c. A pure, white, silky, fibrous quality, easily separable by the fingers, and much of it adapted to the manufacture of textile goods.

The last-named variety is that chiefly sought after, and this is graded at the mines into three classes, known commercially as Nos. 1, 2, and 3, according to quality of fibre; No. 1 commanding the highest price, as being considerably superior to the other two. This, when of a pure white colour, and free from silicic acid or metallic oxide, is rendered specially valuable by its native lubricating qualities, which last property is also possessed by one, at least, of the Italian varieties, and is owing to the presence of the large amount of magnesia in its composition. It is also said to constitute the chief value of a particular kind which occurs in parts of the United States.

Veins of six inches or more in width are often spoken of; but samples of such a width as that, when found, are usually preserved as specimens, being by no means of frequent occurrence, even at Thetford, where, as a rule, a narrower fibre prevails. A width of one and a half or two inches is as good as any that can be had. Some specimens of Thetford ore now before me are by no means wide, but are of singular beauty, and are certainly both broad enough and good enough for any purpose to which the fibre could possibly be put. On this point extraordinary ideas occasionally prevail among persons whose knowledge of the subject is limited, probably engendered by confounding Italian asbestos with Canadian chrysotile. An instance of this came to my knowledge quite recently. A gentleman who was commissioned to inquire for a good Canadian mine, for some parties in London, called upon me for my assistance in procuring one likely to suit the proposed buyer. Upon talking the matter over, he told me that unless the average of the fibre was about 12 or 14 inches it would not suit, and then passed on to the question of price. To his great surprise, I stopped him, by saying that it was useless to go into the question of price because, as a matter of fact, such a mine as he was desirous of purchasing had no existence in Canada, or, as far as I knew, anywhere else.

It must, however, be borne in mind, when discussing the width of veins, that the same rule holds good with many other things which is observed in the vegetable world, namely, that the largest specimens are not necessarily the best. Large crystals, for instance, seldom have the perfection and transparency of those of smaller size; the finest qualities of wool are comparatively short in staple; * the largest varieties of fruit are seldom the most succulent; † and so it is with asbestos. The broadest veins do not, as a rule, yield fibre of so fine a quality as those of a medium, or even of a comparatively small size. Moreover, the length of fibre cannot be determined with any certainty from the thickness of the vein. On the contrary, the broader veins are not seldom found to be separated at right angles to the length of fibre by minute bands of serpentine, chrome, or magnetite, sometimes even by a separation, without any perceptible layer of rock, the only indication of this being an irregular, scarcely visible line, readily detected by the expert. In many places the serpentine contains magnetic iron, disseminated in fine particles, the associated asbestos showing the same iron, not disseminated, but usually concentrated towards the middle of the vein. It seems evident, Mr. Donald remarks, that both the serpentine and iron oxide have been dissolved by percolating water, and redeposited in the crevices of the rock; the less soluble silicate first, and lastly, in the middle of the vein, the more soluble iron. ‡

Under the hammer the big veins, in which the separation exists, are at once divided into two, or it may be into three, lengths of fibre; but if the cotton be pure and clear, this is no

* "Wool is divided into two classes, known as short or carding wool, which seldom exceeds 3 or 4 inches in length, and long or combing wool, varying in length from 4 to 8 inches."—Dr. Bowman on "Wool Fibres."

† "The Russians are probably the possessors of the largest grown peach in the world; it is called the 'Venus,' and is of a magnificent colour. I have picked three peaches weighing 2¼lbs. They are better, however, to look at than to eat."—Barry's "Ivan at Home."

‡ "*Canadian Record of Science*," April, 1890.

very great detriment. Veins of an inch, or an inch and a half, extracted from compact rock, seldom have these intersections. The veins, moreover, are extremely irregular in character, a small vein at the surface frequently developing into one of considerable size lower down, or breaking off altogether. This is the special characteristic of the veins in the Coleraine district—notably at Black Lake—at the mines of the Anglo-Canadian Company, and at Danville. At Thetford, on the other hand, where the ground is of a more uniform character, fine veins are frequently met with just below the surface, which continue with very little change (unless crossed by bands of granulite, when the course is interrupted), for a considerable distance.

Another special point to be noted is that the probabilities of successful mining are much increased if the indications are found on the hill side, among the rugged rocks, where the surface is but sparsely clothed with soil. The serpentine, it is true, frequently underlies cultivated ground, but in such cases the rock, when reached, is generally found to be comparatively sterile. The harsh and rugged-looking Coleraine mountains, which the forest fires have denuded of trees, and on which little or no good land is found, offer every inducement to the explorer; while, on the other hand, a district like Danville, where good land abounds, cannot be nearly so profitably worked. In Thetford, again, where the land about the mines is somewhat flat, the best workings have been found on the hill or knoll where there was but little superincumbent soil, the colouring matter from which could, by capillary flow, or through the planes of cleavage, penetrate the loose or shattered and decomposing rock, and deteriorate the value of the fibre by discolouring it. One of the mines there could of course be cited to show that this rule is not of universal application; three out of the four were opened on the knoll, but in the case of the fourth, about 30 feet of overlying clay and gravel had to be removed before the rock was reached. When this was opened, however, veins of fine quality were disclosed which have since been successfully worked, although the lower level at which they occur causes difficulty with water.

Certain peculiar conditions, as already mentioned, possibly connected with the intrusive bands of granulite, appear to have prevailed in Thetford and the more northern part of Coleraine, which have led to the formation of asbestos in special abundance, the veins being found interlacing the rock in all directions.

This rock, except at Thetford, is usually so split up and seamed, in every direction, by the veins and stringers of asbestos that, excepting at Broughton, where the formation is peculiar, tunnelling, as carried on in Italy, cannot be adopted. Possibly when greater depth is reached, and the rock becomes more solid, means may be found to advance the work in this way; but at present open quarry working is the rule, the main disadvantage of which is that the work necessarily suffers in bad weather, and is of course considerably interrupted by heavy falls of snow in winter.

Chrome iron and magnetite, always found in association with the asbestos-bearing rocks, are frequently found, as at Thetford and Lake Nicolet, in large deposits close by the mines, and it has already been explained how the fine, threadlike veins of these metallic ores cut and destroy the continuity of the fibre. It is a curious thing that the asbestos seems to deal with these ores, in precisely the same way, for on examining the specimens of iron ores, brought by me from the neighbourhood of the asbestos mines, the stringers of asbestos, although very minute, are found intersecting them in a precisely similar manner.

The various distinguishing characteristics of the ore of the different mines are of so marked a nature that an expert can often determine the locality of the mine from which a sample has been taken, and occasionally name the mine itself from an inspection of the ore. This fact is worth noting, as it should effectually prevent the fraudulent substitution of one ore for another, which has been sometimes successfully practised.

The rock also varies considerably, and requires careful examination. In some places it is apparently still in the transition stage between the original rock, from which it is derived, and a true serpentine having almost the hardness of feldspar, while it yet retains the general aspect and colour of the serpentine in which it is found.

At nearly all the mines large quantities of so-called bastard asbestos (picrolite) are found. This is a woody, brittle variety of, apparently, as yet unformed mineral, for which at present no use seems to have been found; but, judging from its composition and the new applications of the mineral now being introduced, there can be little doubt that this inferior article will presently command its price in the market, a use being found for it in some of the many purposes for which coarse pulverised asbestos is applicable.

Occasionally very singular types of ore are also to be seen. Some of the pieces, of the nature of mountain wood, as they lie on the ground, after blasting, have so much the appearance of a wood-cutter's choppings (being in the coarse and peculiar grain of the fibre so like chips of wood) that, if placed side by side with actual chippings from rough timber exposed to the weather in the woods, the one could not be distinguished from the other, except by handling, when the weight and stony feeling of the asbestos would make the difference at once perceptible.

The characteristic colour of the ore largely depends upon the locality of the mine, and the nature of the rocky gangue. At Thetford it is of a greenish hue, being there found in the darker coloured serpentine; whilst at Broughton the ore is of a pearly yellowish green, the surrounding rock being mostly of a grey or pale green colour. This difference of colour in the ore, however, in no way affects the value of the mineral, as, when crushed out, the fibre is mostly of a uniform whiteness.

When treating of asbestos, serpentine must necessarily always be present in the mind, and whatever relates to that rock must consequently be interesting and worthy of note. It may, therefore, not be altogether out of place here to mention that serpentines of an ornamental character are abundant

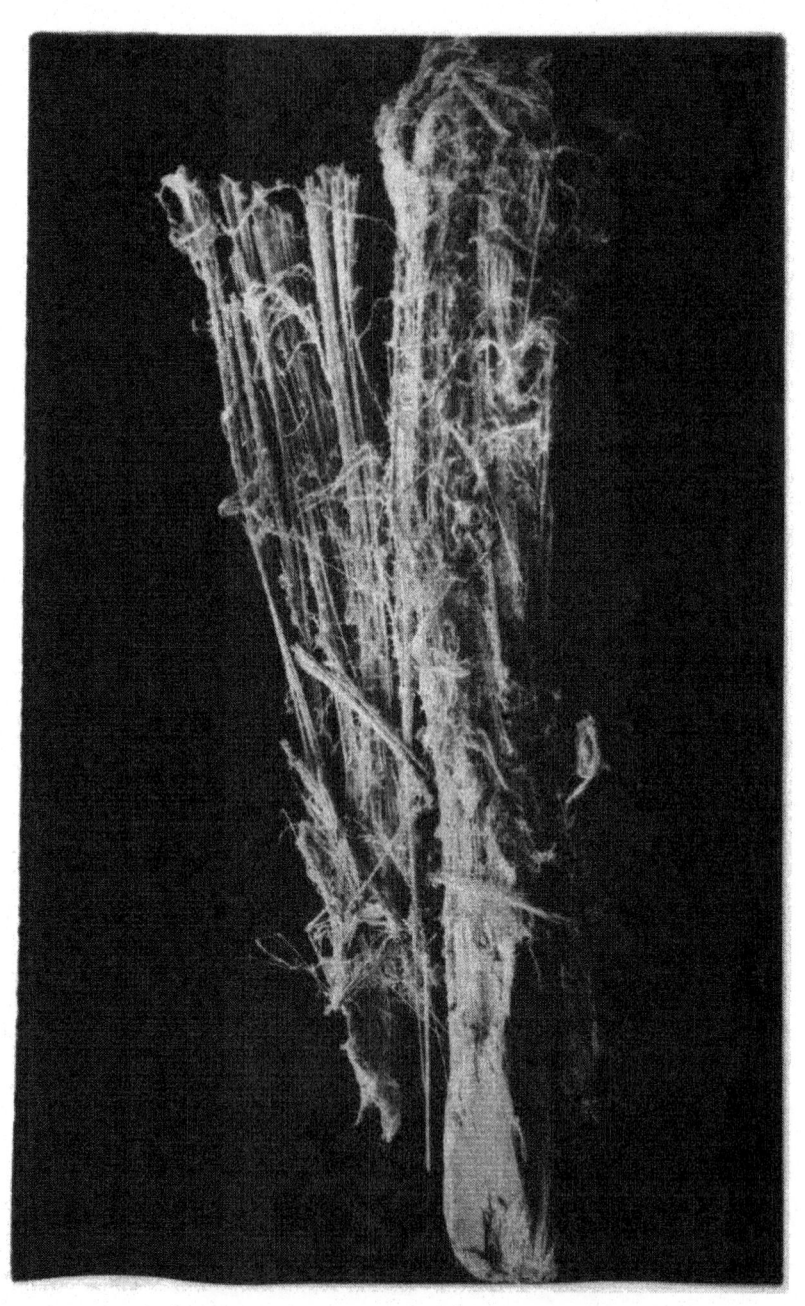

PICROLITE, "BASTARD ASBESTOS."

in Canada. Some very beautiful specimens were shown in London, at the late Colonial and Indian Exhibition at South Kensington. Many of these contain small quantities of chromium and nickel, and are associated with soapstone, potstone dolomite, and magnesite. A band of limestone also occurs at Templeton containing masses of a light-coloured translucent serpentine. These ornamental serpentines are exploited with some success by the Canadian Granite Company of Ottawa, and are used by them for monuments, mantelpieces, vases, and such like. One would certainly think that their importation into England would meet with success, seeing that there is always a demand here for fine marbles and stones for architectural and other purposes. Variegated serpentine marbles of great beauty are found at Gaspé also, especially about Mount Albert, where the mass of serpentine is about 1,000 feet thick, and is mixed with chloritic and epidotic gravel, covering a space exceeding 10 square miles. In this region, and in the Eastern Townships, whole mountains are formed of serpentine marbles, of which abundant use could be made both for ornamental and building purposes; but although, on account of their richness and varied colouring and their capability of taking a high polish, few stones surpass some of the varieties of serpentine for decorative purposes, yet they are more fitted for indoor than for outdoor decoration because, being easily acted on by hydrochloric and sulphuric acids, they are liable to decay and to speedily become tarnished superficially; consequently they are not to be recommended for outdoor use in the smoky gaseous atmosphere of cities.

Sir William Logan says: "Les serpentines, dans toute l'étendue de leur gisement, fournissent de très beaux marbres vert-de-mer souvent ressemblant au vert antique."

Jaspers of very brilllant colours, yellow, red and green, called Gaspé pebbles, are found in the Gaspé limestones.

CHAPTER V.

THE CANADIAN MINES OR QUARRIES.

THE THETFORD GROUP—Discovery—The Johnson Mine—Boston Packing Company—Bell's Asbestos Company—Ward's Mine—King's—Quality of Thetford Ore—Western Limit Theory Exploded—THE COLERAINE AND BLACK LAKE GROUP—Anglo-Canadian Company—Scottish Canadian Asbestos Company—Frechette's Mine, now the United Asbestos Company's—Bell's—Wertheim's—Megantic Mine—White's Asbestos Company—Broughton—Soapstone—Danville—South Ham—Antimony—Wolfestown—Profitable Nature of Asbestos Mining.

The Thetford Group.—Notwithstanding that the existence of asbestos in Canada, especially in the province of Quebec, had been known to scientists long before 1877, it was not until the autumn of that year that a mine of any importance was opened. The building of the line of the Quebec Central Railway, across the serpentine belt at Thetford and Coleraine, was the approximate cause of the discovery. It fell to the lot of an agriculturist, named Fecteau, to light upon the mineral which has since had such an important influence on the welfare of the district. The accidental knocking off of a fragment of rock, and the consequent exposure of a vein of chrysotile, would be sufficient to strike any man with wonderment, and set him on inquiry. When exhibited, experts at once pronounced the quality to be good, and their statement, that asbestos of so fine a quality had never yet been found anywhere in the country, was abundantly justified on further examination; and, true to its early reputation thus gained, Thetford has continued to be the headquarters of the industry and the main source of supply ever since. But if her reputation is to continue much longer, a better and more careful system of mining must soon be inaugurated, and means must be found of getting rid of the enormous piles of refuse now mounting up about the mines to dangerous heights.

Following on Fecteau's discovery, the first mine was opened here, by Messrs. Johnson & Ward. The demand for its produce was, at first, so limited that some difficulty was experienced in finding a market for the first year's output, which only amounted to 50 tons. The demand, however, rapidly increased, and the value of the mineral being soon recognised, active exploration was at once prosecuted in the immediate neighbourhood, and new companies quickly secured possession, at nominal prices, of the rocky tracts adjoining, and set to work opening up fresh mines. Asbestos of good quality was soon afterwards found to be distributed over a considerable area of the district. The four Thetford mines, which until very recently formed the Thetford group, were all located on a knoll, or mound, close by the line of railway, and rising 80 or 90 feet above the track. This knoll is now rapidly disappearing under pressure of work, and in its place enormous piles of refuse rock are daily mounting up on all sides, which disfigure the country, just like the hideous mounds of slag in the black country in England.

The Johnson Mine (*Johnson Asbestos Mining Company*) was the first mine opened on the knoll. This is situated on Lot 27 of the 6th Range of Thetford. Of this company the Hon. George Irvine, Q.C., of Quebec, is president, and Mr. Andrew Johnson, resident manager. In its main features this mine is very similar to the other three. The formation here consists of a massive serpentine, which varies in colour from a dark green to nearly white; this is intersected by numerous veins of asbestos, the fibre of which is singularly free from any admixture of foreign substances. When first opened, a trench about 50 yards long was cut, exposing a wedge-shaped mass of feldspathic rock in the serpentine. From the opening, the mine has been very successfully worked, and its produce has always been regarded as second to none in the district. The output, in 1886, was approximately 375 tons, and the total produce up to the end of that year amounted to 2,500 tons; since which time it has continued rapidly to increase, and the quality of the fibre to improve, nearly the whole of the latter now being classed as No. 1. The returns for 1889 were not sent in in time to be included in the Government Report, but it is well known that the result of the year's work was very satisfactory.

The Boston Company's Mine (*now Bell's*).—Alongside the last-named mine is one which formerly belonged to the Boston Asbestos Packing Company, but is now the property of the Bell's Asbestos Company, Limited, of London. Of this, Mr. Thomas Sheridan has long been the resident manager, and, under his skilful guidance, the mine has always borne a very high reputation, both on account of the manner in which the work is carried on, and of the excellent way in which the ore is prepared for sale. This mine is on the same level as the Johnson, and the produce is of a very similar character, some of the veins disclosed being of an exceptional width of fibre, and the whole of the produce remarkably good. In a pamphlet published some short time back by the Canadian Government on the Mineral Resources of Canada, it was stated that the yield of this, and the Johnson Mine, had been pronounced by European manufacturers to be the finest and strongest fibre known, and that there *was no question at all of the profitable nature of asbestos mining in this belt of country;* a fact which has never been disputed by anyone who has watched the operations carried on.

The Boston Mine is of about equal extent with the Johnson, covering about 100 acres. It changed hands in the spring of 1888, on the formation of the Bell's Asbestos Company, Limited, which was formed in London to acquire the option of purchasing this mine, with 100 acres of land at Coleraine, and Mr. Bell's property, of about 700 acres, at Belmina, Wolfestown. The prices paid for these properties, as given in the prospectus, are worth recording. These are stated to have been £41,300 for the Boston Mine, £8,000 for the 100 acres at Coleraine (part of the Reed & Hayden property), and £8,394 for the Belmina land. As soon as the purchase was completed, a steam plant was put down at Thetford, and very energetic work prosecuted, the difference effected by the change from hand labour to steam power being very quickly shown, by the increased output, which rose (for the season of 1888) to 1,350 tons. In 1889 the produce increased to 1,800 tons, of which the classification was as follows :—

No. 1	. . . . .	1,200 tons.
,, 2	. . . . .	200 ,,
,, 3	. . . . .	400 ,,
		1,800 tons.

The evil effects of the early dumping arrangements, and the want of technical or engineering knowledge displayed in laying out the mine, are here eminently conspicuous, although the same remark may, in some measure, be made as to all the mines laid out in the early days of the search for asbestos. The depth reached in the excavation here is greater than that at any of the other mines, and the practice has all along been to dump the waste rock on to the land immediately surrounding the opening. The consequence is that the surrounding hills of refuse are towering up higher and higher, in such a formidable way that it is much to be feared that, in the near future, the work will perforce be brought to a stand, unless means are devised of removing this waste.

The produce of this and of the adjoining mine, as already noted, is practically No. 1, which is a noteworthy feature of the Thetford mines. Occasionally there is a proportion of waste, but this is now waste only in name, as all of it can be sold. An attempt was made here recently by Mr. Sheridan to test the value of the rock at a lower depth, when the trial boring proved very successful, veins of a beautiful silky nature, some three inches in width, being brought up from about 30 feet below the present level; the expenses of the shaft being much more than repaid, according to Dr. Ells, by the quantity of asbestos removed.*

The Ward and Ross Mine (*Thetford Asbestos Mining Company*).—This mine, situate on the south half of Lot 27, 5th Range, is of more recent date than the last. It is worked by the Brothers Ward, being owned by them conjointly with the representative of the late Hon. James Ross, of Quebec. The property comprises a little over 100 acres, and is not quite so advantageously situated for work as those already described, being on a lower level; it, however, turns out very good material. The output for 1886 was returned at 150 tons, probably at that time a fair average of what was being done. The figures for 1888 and 1889 were not sent in in time for the Government Report, so cannot be given here, but there is no doubt that under the stimulus of the high prices lately ruling the output has been very considerably increased. The same gentlemen have recently opened ground on the other side of the railway, between the line and the river. Here also good ore has been found, and the operations are likely to be carried on with success, but being on a lower level it is probable they will be much troubled with water, and that continual pumping will be necessary. When last at Thetford I saw some good ore on this land, which appeared to be of a very promising character; and notwithstanding the low level of the ground, which must necessarily add to the cost of mining, the size and quality of the veins are in no degree inferior.

King's (*The Hampden Mine*).—The only other mine here is that owned and worked by Messrs. King. This is situate on Lot 26, in the 5th and 6th Ranges. It bears much the same character as those already described; its produce having a high reputation on account of the careful way in which the ore is cobbed and prepared for the market, which is in marked contrast with the work done at one of the mines in the adjoining township. The output for 1888 was given as 580 tons, being

* Second Report for 1889.

a considerable increase upon that of the previous year. This was classed as—

No. 1	170 tons.
,, 2	165 ,,
,, 3	245 ,,
	580 tons.

This large proportion of Nos. 2 and 3 was due to the opening up of fresh land, the general produce of the grading being in no way inferior to that of the other mines. The average number of men and boys employed to get out and prepare this quantity was 32 men and 20 boys, but as the number of working days is not given the information is not of much value.

In his Report for 1889, the Commissioner of Crown Lands states that "MM. King frères, en outre de leur mine du Lot 5, 26 de Thetford, ont travaillé avec succès sur les terrains bas du Lot 5, 28 (*Thetford Royal Mine*), où la même qualité d'amiante a été trouvée." These four mines at present form the Thetford group, and as they were the first opened, so they are now by far the most important.

Two other mines have since been opened here, one by Messrs. Lucke & Mitchell, of Sherbrooke, and the other by Messrs. Murphy & Co., Montreal, both of which are shortly expected to show good results, especially the first named, although the last has apparently struck some rich ground.

The Thetford mines are at a lower level, and are worked at a greater depth than those of Coleraine and Black Lake, and probably for this reason the general output is of a more uniform character, and does not require such close classification. Nos. 1 and 3 are the practical grades, most of the produce being available for No. 1. No. 3 is a very inferior kind, merely the refuse, which, until the recent rise in prices, was sold and shipped in bulk at $10 per ton; but this is now more carefully looked after, as it fetches a paying price, and is in considerable demand for cement and similar purposes. The low-lying ground between the railway and the river has been proved in various places, but, although good ore has been found here, it does not generally present so promising an appearance as that on the knoll.

In the summer of 1889, the belt of serpentine was uncovered by Dr. Reed on Lots 16, 17, and 18 (600 acres) in Range 4 of Thetford, and, although only a limited amount of work was done, a large number of veins of exceptionally good quality were disclosed. Indeed, all the mineral found in this locality is of excellent quality; the fibre is clear and fine and easily worked; the veins generally, especially those in the lower cuts, being comparatively free from chromic iron and other impurities, and of a width ranging from three-quarters of an inch to four and even six inches. Experience, however, has shown, as before stated, that veins ranging from one and a half to two inches give as good material as can be desired.

When the Thetford mines were first opened, the veins were often found to be cut or charged with grains and threads of chromic iron or of magnetite, the latter sometimes forming conspicuous masses between, and occasionally entirely replacing, the veins. But as the work progressed this intrusion of foreign matter gradually became less troublesome. As a general rule, however, the upper veins at Thetford have been found nearly as pure as those lying deeper in the rock.

Here as elsewhere faults are of frequent occurrence; and sometimes sheets of imperfect or immature asbestos, having a long, coarse, woody fibre, are to be met with lying all along the sides of the fault.

The Thetford mine owners are always ready to give every information about their work, and willing to facilitate an inspection of their mines by any one taking the trouble to visit them, a trouble I found very amply repaid by the courtesy with which I was always received, and the candour and obliging readiness with which all my inquiries were answered.

The workers are mostly resident on the spot, the proprietors appearing to act in a spirit of liberal consideration towards them, doubtless finding the advantage of looking after the welfare of their men by not running short of hands at critical times.

The Quebec Central Railway runs right through the town, where there is a commodious station facing the mines. On stepping out of the train the mines are seen all together in front of the platform, and as the train moves on, the rail has only to be crossed to reach them. At the rear, that is, divided from the mines by the line, are the dwellings of the workmen, at either end of the place being two houses of a superior class, belonging to two of the principal mine-owners, and in the remoter background the Thetford river rolls sluggishly along.

This river, until quite recently, was believed to mark the western limit of the asbestos-bearing serpentine, the rocks on either side being mostly altered slates and sandstones; but the existence of valuable deposits of the mineral on the further side has now been amply proved. To the east, or fronting the railway, the serpentine forms a knoll which has an elevation of 80 or 90 feet above the line of rails, and it is upon this knoll that the present mines are all being worked, and which they are rapidly cutting away. Until very recently but little had been done to ascertain the value of the ground between the rail and the river. Although the ground is low hereabouts, there are certainly good indications of asbestos; and as mentioned above, some very promising looking ground has recently been opened up by the Messrs. Ward, sufficiently proving the prolongation of the serpentine area between the present workings and the river. Further west, and nearer the river, both Messrs. King and the Johnson Company have since opened ground which has proved highly satisfactory as regards quality and quantity of fibre.

The uniform practice, at all the Thetford mines, hitherto, has been to close down entirely for the four winter months, it not having been found sufficiently lucrative to encounter the additional expense of winter work in the open, the difficulty being then materially enhanced by the rigorous weather and heavy snowfalls. Now, however, the great rise in the price of crude ore, and the increasing demand for it, have caused attempts to be made to carry on the work through the winter season on a reduced scale, but it is doubtful whether this can be done with more than a limited amount of success.

Chromic iron is found in this area, but the quality is not rich. Veins of a soft white mineral are also found here, which hardens on exposure to the air; but, unlike the soft serpentine found in the Megantic Mine (*post*, p. 102), this does not acquire a waxy lustre, but has much the appearance of unglazed white earthenware, and absorbs water with avidity.

On analysis its composition was found to be—

Silica	43·191
Alumina	1·463
Ferrous oxide	·293
Magnesia	41·520
Water	14·000
	100·467[*]

The fibre from the Thetford mines differs a good deal from that obtained elsewhere. That from Coleraine and Wolfe is to some extent affected by harshness and a want of elasticity which causes the percentage of No. 1 from these two districts to be less than at Thetford. The fibre is also mostly shorter in staple, and much of it is discoloured by the infiltration of water impregnated with iron.

As already mentioned, great mistakes were made, here as well as elsewhere, when the mines were first opened, arising mainly from inexperience and want of the knowledge now possessed, which will inevitably entail serious loss in the future, much valuable ground being now covered by the dumps which will unquestionably have to be moved when the land is wanted for working, the cost of which will be enormous. Moreover, these mines, being located on ground which, excepting the knoll now fast disappearing, forms a level plain, the clearing of the pits and the removal of the ore and waste rock will always be a troublesome and expensive task.

The same want of foresight in selecting proper dumping

[*] J. T. Donald, Esq, M A., Montreal.

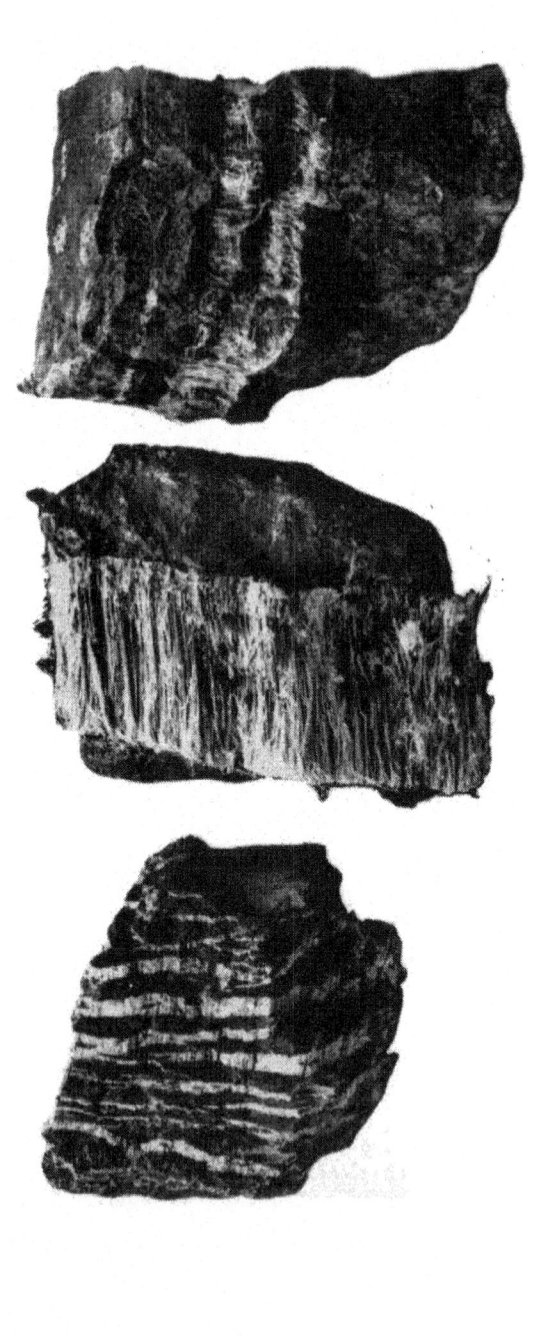

SURFACE VEINS AND OUTCROPPINGS.

ground, for which there was less excuse with the Thetford experience to guide them, will inevitably cause trouble in the near future at Black Lake, even to a more serious extent. The parties who first opened up the ground there evidently knew what they were about, but their immediate successors, being destitute of all practical mining knowledge, have, by their neglect of professional assistance, committed errors of judgment such as will presently occasion very serious expense. At one of the main pits many thousands of tons of waste rock have been dumped on to some of the richest of the ground, and this must be again moved before that ground can be worked. From the peculiarity of the work, there probably exists no class of mining which so absolutely necessitates the services of a practical mining engineer, to mark out the land in the first instance for mining and dumping, as that for asbestos does.

During the visit of the American Institute of Mining Engineers, in the autumn of 1889, these defects caused considerable remark, and many suggestions were made as to the desirability of putting matters on a different footing for the future working of the mines.

The cost of extraction of the ore varies in different localities, depending mainly on the mass of barren rock to be removed, which, owing to the action of faults, is greater in some places than in others. At Thetford it may be put at from $20 to $25 per ton, the latter being probably nearer the average, except at the Boston Mine, where the machinery employed reduces the cost to about $15.

The Coleraine and Black Lake Group.

The mines grouped about this district are next in importance to those last described; but, although the distance from Thetford is only four miles, there is a very perceptible change observable in the face of the country. The rock formation alters as the station is approached, and when Black Lake is reached you are at once face to face with the grim and rugged-looking hills which rise somewhat precipitously, from the shore of the Lake, to a height of 600 or 700 feet, and form the beginning of the bare and cheerless-looking district of Coleraine. There is but little soil here to cover the rocks, and often, as is quite apparent, after the first growth of timber which covered these hills when in a state of nature, had been cut, the undergrowth was destroyed by forest fires, and then the comparatively thin layer of soil having been washed away by the rains, the bare and sterile rocks are left exposed to view. This is a far more likely-looking country for the prospector than that about Thetford; but, although good ore is abundant throughout the district, it does not, as a rule, come up to the standard of the latter place. The quality of the ore is found to have perceptibly changed, becoming, especially in the upper veins, coarser and more brittle; in places also there is more depth of soil, and the rock is a good deal shattered and occasionally decomposed by weathering, offering more facility for the infiltration of surface water, which, being a good deal impregnated with metallic oxides, detrimentally affects the value of the fibre by discolouring it.

Owing to the destruction of the forest over the knolls of serpentine by bush fires, to the action of the weather, or to the intrusion of masses of granulite, the fibre here is frequently harsh and brittle, especially near the surface, changing, however, to greater silkiness as the veins are opened out deeper in the solid rock. This peculiarity has given rise to a good deal of speculation, and various causes have been surmised to account for it: difference of level, for instance, the forest fires, or the granulite, which is here abundant, and the heat from which on its eruption would have a tendency to dissipate a certain proportion of the contained water in the chrysotile, in the same way as the forest fires, though on a more extended scale. Mr. Donald has shown that harsh and brittle kinds of chrysotile contain less water than the softer kinds; in very flexible fibre he found 14·05 per cent., whilst in a harsh-fibred sample there was only 12·62. The same effect can be produced by placing a piece of the ore on a sufficiently heated surface, when the fibre will be found in a very short time to have lost its softness and flexibility, and to have become harsh and brittle,* and in this state it may often be crumbled between the fingers. The writer has frequently seen boxes of ore brought into the cobbing-shed after a wet night, when the men would at once set to work to pile it up round about the stove, so as to dry it somewhat before cobbing, when that which was placed nearest to the stove, or possibly kept there too long, would gradually become changed, and present the harsh and rough features mentioned.

If the aqueous origin of asbestos be admitted, it seems reasonable to suppose that all the fibre, when first deposited, was soft and flexible, containing a maximum amount of water, and that movements of the rocks, producing heat, have driven off a portion of the water of the contained asbestos and thereby destroyed the softness of the original fibre. Veins at considerable depths may have been subjected to the heat produced by these movements, and yet not deprived of any portion of their original water, because of the resistance of overlying rocks.†

The granulite referred to above is of a greyish-white colour, and mainly consists of orthoclase feldspar and quartz, which is thrown up after the manner of dykes. Near the contact with this, the serpentine is often considerably shattered, as though the presence of the granulite had exercised a marked effect on its condition. At Thetford, the intrusive rocks in the mines are limited to small and thin dyke-like veins, which do not appear to have produced any marked effect on the ore; but here the granulite forms masses of a much greater size, and these have produced a correspondingly greater effect. Dr. Ells, however, truly remarks that the stiff-fibred mineral is not in all cases confined to the vicinity of the granitic masses, and consequently it is just possible that other causes may have tended to produce a similar effect. It is scarcely likely that the difference in level can have anything to do with the change in quality of the ore, because the operations of the Scottish Canadian Com-

* Dr. Ells on the "Mining Industries of Eastern Quebec," 9.
† J. T. Donald, *Canadian Record of Science*, April, 1890.

pany are carried on 300 feet higher than the Thetford mines, and Dr. Reed's mine (now Wertheim's) is 300 feet higher still, and in both these mines excellent fibre is found. The most likely cause is that of dehydration, caused by the intrusion of the heated masses of granulite when forced up from below.

In one of the granitic dykes, on the Scottish Canadian Company's property, Mr. Donald found scolecite * occurring in transparent glassy needles, filling minute veins, and in masses of white, grey, and colourless radiating fibres. This is believed to be the first zeolite found in the dykes cutting the serpentine here, and the first known to occur in Canada. Enstatite, conspicuous because of its bronze lustre, is also found in the serpentine here.

The Anglo-Canadian Asbestos Company.—The pioneer of the mines in this district, the next in importance to Thetford, was Mr. Noel, of Richmond, in the same province, who in 1881 opened a mine here, which he afterwards sold to Mr. Lionais. This mine was called the "Eureka," and soon afterwards Mr. Lionais opened another, which he named the "Emelie." The property, on which these two mines are located, subsequently came into the possession of the late Mr. Sénécal, and was by him transferred to the Anglo-Canadian Company on its formation in London by Baron Grant in the autumn of 1885.

The estate comprises something over 300 acres. The output for 1886 was stated by Dr. Ells in his report to the Government to have amounted, according to information given him at the mines, to 550 tons. This was so manifestly exaggerated that, after the report was in type, the error was rectified by giving the correct figures obtained from Captain Evans, who certified the quantity to be 330 tons.

The output for 1889 was returned at 630 tons, with an improvement in quality, the percentage of No. 1, according to the manager's statement, having increased from 10 to nearly 20 per cent.; but even this large output proved of no benefit

* From σκωληξ, a worm, in allusion to its action when heated before the blowpipe, when it will curl up in worm-like fashion.

to the shareholders, as the company went into liquidation at the close of the season. It has since been reconstituted on the footing of a surrender of the old shares on which £2 per share had been paid, and the issue in exchange of £1 shares, on which 17s. 6d. was credited as paid, the remaining 2s. 6d. per share being paid up in cash.

The Scottish Canadian Asbestos Company.—A few minutes' walk across the hillside brings us to the property on which the Martin Mine is located. Here we find broad, well-made roads traversing the property, well-built premises, and the business of the place, when I last visited the spot, was proceeding with intelligent regularity. Unfortunately, this company has also, since then, gone into liquidation, but from altogether different causes, the whole of its capital having been expended, under previous management, in a too lavish outlay for machinery, railway tracks and buildings before work was properly established. The property is a good one, and will no doubt presently show adequate results. At the time of my visit the Martin Mine had only been recently acquired by the Scottish Company, with the intention of working it in conjunction with their property at Broughton.

This company's land lies in the form of a parallelogram, and covers somewhat more than 100 acres. Towards the north and along the northern boundary the ground rises to about 100 feet above the level of the railway, which is distant about a quarter of a mile. To the south-east the hills, mainly composed of talc and mica schists, increase in elevation until, at a distance of about 1,800 feet from the railway, it attains a height of 900 feet above the level of Black Lake. At this point the serpentine formation begins, forming a ridge 300 feet higher than the highest point of the shales. The serpentine belt crosses the company's property east and west, and is bounded along its northern margin by a mass of quartzose granulite, which is here separated from the serpentine by a narrow band of steatite. The mine is fully equipped with powerful machinery, and a new set of appliances for crushing and separating the lower grades of ore, which, as we have already seen, are very considerable in all the Black Lake mines, as well as to save the expense of hand cobbing. In 1888 the production here had risen to 400 tons, of which amount 40 tons were No. 1, 110 tons No. 2, and 250 tons No. 3. Since then the mines have much improved, and the output also, until the stoppage of work.

The developments of the Martin Mine consist of an excavation on the hillside 225 feet long by 100 wide. The lowest level of the quarry, at the time of my last visit, was about 80 or 100 feet below the highest point of the profile of the mountain (now much lower) and communicated with the dumping-ground by a cut through the granulite and soapstone.

Another quarry opened on the same property is called the "Bonanza." Both quarries are, from their position, well drained, and free from the water which is so great a trouble at the last-named works. The houses for the manager and workmen, stores, factories, stables, and workshops form groups on the hillside, and give a cheerful appearance to this part of the country.

The Frechette-Douville Mine is located on a narrow strip of land running up the hillside, and comprises about 95 acres. It is bounded throughout its whole length by the property of the Scottish Canadian Company on the one side, and that of the Anglo-Canadian Company on the other. Work has lately been very energetically prosecuted here, and some very good material obtained. The mine has now been sold to the United Asbestos Company, of London, who have placed it under the management of Mr. Penhale, Junior, formerly of the Scottish Company. A good steam plant has been laid down, consisting of two 70 horse-power boilers, duplex 7 by 10 inches Bacon hoist, and a 16 by 24 Rand compressor. The equipment of steam derricks, air compressors, drills, &c., was put in by the Tenckes Machine Company, of Sherbrooke. A force of about 35 men is employed and work will be very energetically pushed on this season. A new opening, now being worked, shows some very excellent fibre. The exports to the United States from this mine in 1889 were :—

No. 1	165½ tons.
,, 2	62 ,,
,, 3	132¼ ,,
Waste	20 ,,
	379¾ tons.

The Southwark Mine is opened on the northern halves of Lots 27 and 28 on Range A, part of what was formerly known as the "Reed & Hayden" property; it comprises 100 acres of land, and formed part of the purchase of the Bell's Asbestos Company, Limited, as previously mentioned. Until quite recently it was under the charge of Mr. Calvin Carter, late of Belmina. The output of this mine to 30th June, 1889, is returned as 198 tons, but the comparative grades are not given.

The Wertheim (American Asbestos Company's) Mine occupies the southern halves of the two lots last mentioned, and was bought at the beginning of 1889 from Dr. Reed by Mr. Wertheim, asbestos manufacturer, of Frankfort-on-the-Maine, and transferred by him to a company formed in Germany, called The American Asbestos Company. A good steam plant was at once put in, and the work has been carried on with such energy and success, that this mine bids fair to turn out the best in the district. It is situate on part of the high ridge south-east of the Black Lake Station, and is at present the most elevated in the district, being about 600 feet above the level of Black Lake. A good many houses have been put up for the workmen, and many Belgian miners and their families have been taken over and located there. The machinery was ready to run at the end of July, and notwithstanding that work was impeded by an epidemic which soon after broke out among the workpeople, the output for the year ending 30th November last reached the satisfactory total of 530 tons, sufficient to pay a good dividend on the capital employed. All the arrangements for working were good, the plant judiciously selected, and in the result fine veins of very soft and silky fibre were opened.

A new departure has been taken here; in order to facilitate the development of the mine, a tunnel was run in from below under the No. 2 and 3 pits, whence a shaft was cut for 100 feet to reach No. 2. This tunnel is 6 feet by 6, and both the tunnel and shaft run the whole distance through asbestos-bearing rock, all pumping being thus obviated, and a splendid working face formed.

During the first six months of the year hand labour only was employed, after which steam plant was put in operation. The mining figures for the first year are worth recording; these were :—

No. 1	79¼ tons.
,, 2	81¼ ,,
,, 3	357¾ ,,
Hornblende	12 ,,
	530¼ tons.

Reed's Mine.—On the north side of the Poudrier road, on Lots 27, 28, and 29, Range A, work has been commenced by Dr. Reed, by clearing the ground and opening up, so as to show the quality of the ore: some good veins have been disclosed and are now open to view. In the spring of 1890 active work was commenced here by the owner, about thirty men being employed on contract, with highly satisfactory results.

Between these properties and Cariboo Lake the serpentine extends in a continuous ridge, and shows at intervals very good indications of asbestos. This area, however, has not yet been sufficiently explored for much to be said, from actual observation, of its value as asbestos land, though it seems reasonable enough to suppose that this portion of the serpentine belt will presently be found equally valuable with that of the adjoining section.

Mr. Obalski, who has examined the ground, states that the

whole mountain is formed of rich asbestos rock, a careful inspection of the summit of the mountain, as well as its base below the road, giving the same indications, the asbestos everywhere showing at the surface in veins sometimes 2½ inches broad.

Megantic Mine.—On again entering the train and progressing towards Coleraine, serpentine is found to occur near the station, but the main ridge of the rock, extending south-west, keeps to the north-west for about a mile and a half, where it forms a conspicuous hill feature. An opening made on this south-west extremity some time ago, by Mr. Kennedy, disclosed a number of asbestos veins, one of which had a width of nearly four inches. In 1888 preparatory work only was carried on, but the result was sufficiently satisfactory to justify active operations. Dr. Ells reports for 1889 as follows:—"The rock here is very much shattered near the surface and the fibre is consequently discoloured. Veins up to one inch and a half are found and in the more solid portions the quality improves. The output from this place has been necessarily small, owing to the time spent in opening the mine, and the delays from bad weather, the quantity mined in four months, to October 1st, being 39 tons, of which one third may be classed as No. 2, the rest as No. 3. An average number of twelve men was employed."

In the immediate neighbourhood of this last mine, operations have been commenced by Messrs. Lambley & Co., of Inverness, some good veins being met with at the top of the hill.

Mining in this locality was commenced in 1886, when the four-inch vein was found not to be persistent for any depth, the rock being greatly shattered near the surface and for about 15 feet down, and though a great many veins were found, some of them in the solid rock, much of the fibre was discoloured. A peculiar feature here, which has not been observed in any other of the mines of this district, is the presence of irregular veins of mica, in scales of an inch or more in diameter, in a paste of decomposed serpentine or soapstone.*

* Dr. Ells, Second Report, 1888.

There is also a singular form of serpentine which occurs here in narrow seams, so soft that it may be compressed between thumb and finger, and varying in colour through white, blue, green, and yellow; when exposed to the air it becomes hard and assumes a waxy lustre.*

On the same ridge, but on the extreme west limits of Lots 24 and 25, Range 3, Ireland, Messrs. King Brothers have started two openings. The elevation of these by aneroid above the level of Black Lake is 500 feet. The asbestos found here is principally met with in two knolls lying about a quarter of a mile apart. Many of the veins show a selvage of white weathering serpentine, separated by a vein of asbestos from a quarter to three-quarters of an inch in width. The general aspect of the rock and veins strongly resembles those found at Belmina, but the quality of the ore is much better and successful mining far more likely.

White's Asbestos Company.—In the spring of 1889, a company was formed in London, under this title, for working two lots of land in Coleraine and two others in Garthby, containing in the whole 372 acres. It is much to be feared that the ground was not judiciously selected and that no beneficial result will ensue. The Commissioner for Crown Lands reports, for the past year, that the company has done some prospecting work without obtaining any appreciable result.

These are the only mines at present being worked in the district, but from indications on other properties lying on the same line, there can be little doubt that others will presently be opened up in this locality. Capital is all that is wanting at present; but, as the demand for the mineral increases, the necessary capital for producing it in larger quantities will no doubt be forthcoming.

The cost of mining, for the reasons already given, must of necessity be greater at Black Lake than at Thetford, and cannot be put at less than $28 a ton. After removal of the surface earth and rock, the proportion of refuse rock is about 25 tons to one of asbestos.

* J. T. Donald, Esq., M.A.

The following very interesting comparative analyses of some of the ores of this part of the country have been furnished by Professor Donald, of M'Gill College, Montreal, who is making a special study of the mineral:—

	No. 1 Asbestos	No. 2 Asbestos	No. 3 Asbestos	No. 4 Asbestos	No. 5 Serpentine	No. 6 Picrolite
Silica	39·22	41·90	41·84	42·64	40·34	43·70
Magnesia	40·27	42·50	41·99	39·54	43·32	40·68
Alumina	3·64	·89	—	—	1·32	—
Ferrous oxide	2·26	·69	2·23	3·66	1·23	3·51
Water	14·37	14·05	14·28	14·31	14·17	12·45

No. 1 is from the Southwark Mine, at Coleraine, the sample being classed as fair No. 1.

No. 2. Very fair quality ore from the Scottish Canadian Company's mine at Broughton.

Nos. 3 and 4. Asbestos from Mr. Jeffrey's mine, at Danville; analysis by Professor Smith, of Beloit College.

No. 5. Serpentine from Brompton Lake.

No. 6. Picrolite from Bolton; analysis by Dr. T. Sterry Hunt.

The special point to be noted here is the variation in alumina, ranging from 3.64 per cent. at Black Lake to none at all in Danville.

EAST BROUGHTON.

The Frazer Mine.—In order to visit this mine it is now necessary again to take the train and return through Coleraine, Black Lake, and Thetford, after which the East Broughton station is soon reached, whence it is only a short drive to the mine, the road passing through a much more cheerful-looking country than that previously traversed. Broughton, which marks the extreme eastward limit of the asbestos region, so far as yet opened up, is in Beauce County, just outside the boundary of the Eastern Townships, and here the land is of a more pastoral character, with pleasing stretches of woodland scenery.

The Frazer Mine was first opened and worked by Dr. Reed

some few years ago. The discovery here made a great stir at the time, as no mine in Canada had then, or indeed has since, produced asbestos of quite the same quality; but, to all appearance, the big vein (there was only one) was soon worked out, the ore exhausted, and work in consequence discontinued. When first worked the vein was nearly a foot thick, and remarkable for the silky softness of the fibre. It was found at the contact of the serpentine with blackish slates, which in places have a greyish or purple shade, containing bands of hard bluish-grey quartzite of the Cambrian series, thickly veined with quartz. It is overlaid in places with soapstone of good quality, from 10 to 14 inches thick, with which the asbestos seems to be intimately associated. The vein had the general aspect of a well-defined vein with, in some places, a hanging wall of soapstone, and was worked for a distance of several hundred yards to a depth of about 70 feet. In the lower workings it was found rapidly to decrease in size, and ultimately it split up into minute strings which rendered it worthless.*

Although at some little distance from the station, the mine lies close to the rail. It is now the property of the Scottish Canadian Asbestos Company, and comprises 116 acres of freehold land, supplemented by mining rights extending over about 2,000 acres more. Large sums have been expended in laying out this property, perhaps too lavishly, and in buildings, factories, machinery of all kinds, tram lines, &c., the extravagant outlay being, doubtless, the cause of the company going into liquidation, which was a great misfortune for the district.

When I visited the mine, in the autumn of 1886, I went all over the ground with the late Mr. Frazer, but we were quite unable to trace any part of the big vein. Our search, however, was a good deal impeded by the depth of water in the cut, which prevented our making so complete an investigation as I could have wished.

The vein here was from 8 to 10 inches thick near the sur-

* Dr. Ells, on the "Mining Industries of Eastern Quebec," Second Report, 1888.

face, but decreased at the bottom of the workings, some 62 feet down, to two or three inches, and then it became irregular, splitting at times into many fine strings disseminated through the serpentine, at others presenting a continuous fibre. Three shafts were sunk to a depth of 61, 62, and 75 feet, which followed generally the slope of the bed or vein at an angle of about 75°, the rock dipping S. 40° E. to true meridian. The mass of serpentine, which lies to the west, was carefully examined at several points, but only in one place, about 150 feet in rear of the openings, were small strings of asbestos, of one-fourth to half an inch, seen. Much of the fibre in the north slope appeared to be stiff and harsh, while other portions were beautifully silky. The serpentine resembles in character that near St. Sylvester and along the Chaudière.*

The belt just here is very narrow, contracting in places to not more than 15 feet in width, the veins of asbestos being found closely compressed together. This imparts a certain regularity to the deposit, which up to this time has been observed nowhere else. Schists, talc, and serpentine are interstratified to a depth of from 8 to 10 feet, and the asbestos veins in the serpentine connect with and join each other, forming distinct leads, from 14 to 16 inches wide, occurring as congeries of divided or partitioned-off seams. There is less waste here than usual, but the breaking out of the rock is more difficult.

The Broughton ore has a pale yellowish green hue, as distinguished from the darker greenish metallic lustre which distinguishes the finer samples from Thetford, which is another peculiarity of this ore, the light-coloured serpentines being almost always barren everywhere else. The colour of the ore, however, in no way affects the clear whiteness of the fibre when crushed out, although it affords a means of identifying the locality of production. There are, in fact, as I have already mentioned, certain peculiarities, even of colour, attaching to the ore of each locality of so marked a character that an expert can at once tell, on inspection, from whence it was obtained.

The cost of extraction is put by Mr. Obalski at $35 per

* Second Report, 1888.

ton, which is caused by the peculiarity of stratification and the greater than usual difficulty of mining, and he is of opinion that the output will be certainly limited.

Operations were going on here and also at Coleraine, previous to the stoppage, for the utilisation of waste; the narrow veins of only a few lines in thickness usually passing as such, and being thrown on the dumps. There is certainly no reason why this should be so, because, if properly treated, these thin veins would pay for the trouble bestowed on their separation. Thousands of tons are annually wasted, much of which is as much due to careless work as to inefficient machinery; but this will no doubt be presently remedied as the mineral becomes more valuable and improved machinery is employed in its preparation for market.

There is great abundance of soapstone at Broughton, much of it of good quality, some remarkably pure, and some of it curious. I brought away with me a fine specimen, having all the grain and fibrous markings of asbestos, but pure and unmistakeable steatite. No use is made of this at present, all attention being devoted to the production of the higher-priced chrysotile.

Danville.

At Shipton, about four miles from the village of Danville, there is another mine, lying contiguous to the Grand Trunk Railway, which has been worked, for some years, by Mr. Jeffrey. Time did not permit of a visit to this mine, consequently I can give no details of my own knowledge.

The property covers about 75 acres, the output of serpentine forming a knoll of somewhat limited extent, with steep sides all round it. Numerous veins of asbestos are found here, mostly of small size, seldom reaching two inches, but of good quality. Faults are numerous, which considerably affect the value of the mine; good veins of two inches being sometimes cut off completely at a distance of 50 feet from the surface. The output has, however, been considerable. For the year

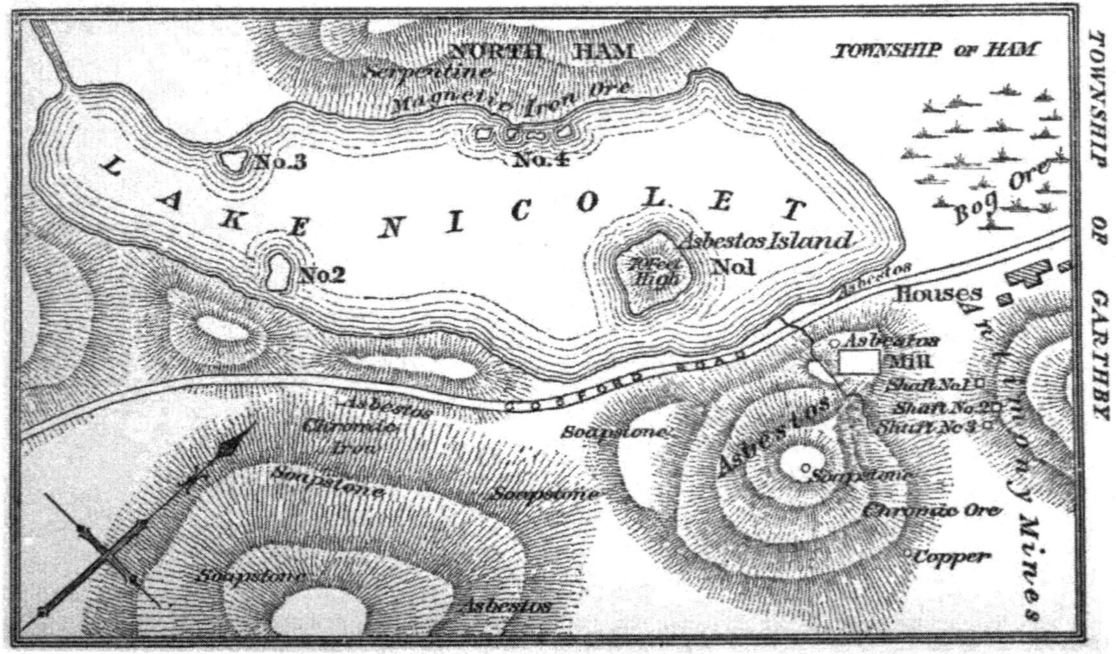

SKETCH MAP OF THE LAKE NICOLET ESTATE

ending 28th August, 1886, it was 455 tons; though, from some cause not explained, the output has since been less, the mine not being worked to its full capacity. The proportion of No. 1 grade here, according to Dr. Ells, is at present (1889) about 20 per cent., and of No. 2, 60 per cent., the remainder, of course, being No. 3 and waste, thus approximating closely to the output of the mines at Black Lake.*

Mr. Jeffrey has also found asbestos at Cleveland, where the mineral occurs in good massive serpentine, apparently forming a wide band, but not showing much on the surface.

South Ham.

The mines here, of which a rough sketch is shown, are situate on land known as the Nicolet Estate, in the township of South Ham, about $7\frac{1}{2}$ miles from the Garthby Station of the Quebec Central Railway.

It was on a brilliant morning in the latter part of October, 1886, that I started from Black Lake, where I was then residing, to visit Nicolet, on the invitation of the owner. There had been a sharp frost in the night, forerunner, as it proved, of an early and severe winter; but when the sun rose the air was delightfully crisp and invigorating. A quick run on the rails took us to Garthby, a characteristic Canadian settlement, pleasantly situated on the shores of Lake Weedon. The view over the lake, with its background of timber-clad hills, bathed in brilliant sunshine, was very charming; but as that was not what we had come out to see, we had to mount our buggy and start off at once, for a drive over a rough mountain road, in order to reach our destination before evening set in.

On arrival, we went straight on to examine the owner's antimony mines, to which he was then devoting his whole attention, he being satisfied with knowing that asbestos existed in abundance on the property, leaving its exploration for a

* Dr. Ells, "The Mining Industries of Eastern Quebec," October, 1889.

future day; but as it is that mineral only with which we are now concerned, we will reverse the operation.

The asbestos deposit here was first discovered on what is called Big Island, being the largest of seven islands ornamenting the sheet of water called Lake Nicolet. The serpentine rock which forms Big Island, rises very abruptly out of the water to the height of 70 feet, forming, on the western side precipitous cliffs, the whole of which is seamed with asbestos; recent exploration, however, has shown that the main body of the mineral, passing under the lake, occurs on the hillside, and is of such extent as altogether to eclipse that proved to exist on the island, which was at first thought to be the chief source of supply.

The mine on the island is not being worked, but has been fully proved by numerous openings which have been made at the most promising points, revealing in every case veins of asbestos of remarkably good quality and in great abundance. These pass under the lake, and can be seen cropping out in many places, off the shore and on the hillside.

The mineral as seen on the island presents many points of difference from that at Thetford and Coleraine; and in the Geological Survey of Canada, written many years ago, it is stated to consist of four varieties, viz. :—

1st. Small veins, rarely exceeding half an inch in width, the fibres not easily separable. This, however, does not detract from its commercial value.

2nd. Apparently occupying a position at right angles to the veins above noticed, is a coarse fibrous mineral, resembling rope, and evidently derived from the associated picrolite. The extreme length which these fibres may attain could not be determined, but judging from exposed portions, it cannot be less than three feet.

3rd. Veins somewhat resembling the latter in aspect, but much finer in texture. The fibre can be separated with great facility, though firmly attached at one end to the parent rock.

4th. A steatitic asbestos rock, resembling "Mountain leather," forming important masses, which enclose small concretionary pellets of asbestos, the centres of which contain a nucleus of serpentine.

Very little (the report says) has yet been done on the island to develop these asbestos veins, perhaps owing to the difficulty of transport across the lake. *This, however, would probably be more than counterbalanced by the magnificent returns which this locality promises to afford.**

There could, however, be no practical difficulty in arranging this question of transport; but when mining for asbestos is undertaken here, there will be but little temptation to commence operations on the island, as the deposits on the mainland (which were not known to exist, at the date of Mr. Willimott's visit) will furnish abundant scope for energetic work for many years to come.

The temptation to describe the scenery round the lake is very great, but as that does not fall within the scope of the present work, it must be sufficient to say that it is of a very charming character.

The estate itself might very justly be termed unique for mineral riches, for, comprised within its 2,000 acres, are found not only rich veins of antimony and asbestos, but enormous deposits of steatite, magnetic iron, chromic iron and bog-ore, as well as copper and sulphur, and it is believed both nickel and cobalt. Silver to the value of $4 a ton is found with the antimony, and reefs of auriferous quartz run through the entire property, a sample from which, on assay, gave $2\frac{1}{2}$ oz. gold to the ton.†

The Commissioner of Crown Lands in his report for 1889, says that the antimony mines have not recently been worked, except in the way of exploration, which has led to the discovery of many new veins. Since then a considerable amount of work has been done, an adit, from the bottom of the

* Willimott's Report (1882) on some of the mines in the province of Quebec.
† Report of the Committee appointed by the Dominion Government to investigate the Gold Fields of Canada.

hill, effectually drains the mines and some very fine veins have been disclosed, including much native antimony. Some fine crystals of Senarmontite* have also been found here. It is also worthy of note that Professor Dana, in his "Descriptive Mineralogy" (1877), instances these mines amongst the few places in the world where veins of antimony occur. Some singularly fine specimens of native antimony, kermesite, stibnite, and valentinite† from these mines, shown at the late Colonial and Indian Exhibition, for which a medal and diploma were awarded, are now in the charge of the Canadian authorities in London, having been presented by Dr. Reed to the Imperial Institute. These will be found specified in Dr. Selwyn's "Descriptive Catalogue of the Economic Minerals of Canada, 1886."

Everything necessary for the working of these valuable deposits already exists on the ground—unlimited water supply, and timber for building and mining purposes, as well as for charcoal for any furnaces that may presently be erected; sufficient, if judiciously managed according to the rules of forestry as practised in Germany, Austria, and Russia, to last until a new growth matures. In regard to transport, the roads are good, and a line of rail connecting the Grand Trunk with the Intercolonial will presently touch the property, and will, it is expected, have a station there just below the antimony mine. In regard to steatite, the quantity here is so enormous that an expert, lately sent to report on this property, speaking of the steatite, says, "All I can say is, there are mountains of it."

WOLFESTOWN.

The description of the asbestos area of Wolfestown is given by Dr. Ells. It is situate on the north-east extremity of a serpentine ridge which extends south-westerly, with many

* The isomorphous sesquioxide of antimony.

† Valentinite, with the same chemical composition as Senarmontite, differs from the latter in crystallisation.

interruptions, from the road leading from Coleraine Station to Wolfestown, in the vicinity of Lake Nicolet.

The Belmina Estate, distant about four miles from the railway station at Coleraine, comprises about 700 acres, and as already stated, was formerly the property of Mr. John Bell, and by him transferred to the Bell's Asbestos Company, on its formation in London, in 1888, for the sum of £8,394. The surface indications here are said not to be equal to those at Black Lake, but at several points numbers of veins are shown, some of which are from one and a half to two inches thick. A very fair showing of workable veins has been exposed on the upper part of a deep cut, which it is proposed to intersect at a considerably lower level. Should the same rule of increase which holds good at Thetford and Coleraine apply here, there should be good paying ground exposed when the lower level is driven in past the cap of barren rock, provided the veins already disclosed are not cut off by faults, whose presence is noted here as at other points.

Late in the autumn of 1889, operations were announced as about to be commenced by some capitalists of Montreal on property acquired by them near Brompton Lake, where deposits of asbestos exist; a very fine sample of which has just reached me.

The foregoing comprise all the Canadian mines now in work. There can be no doubt, however, that new mines will presently be opened. At this moment, supply by no means keeps pace with demand; manufacturers are consequently unable to obtain the ore they are perfectly willing to pay high prices for, the prices charged now closely approaching the prohibitive; active steps are therefore being taken all over the serpentine belt for the discovery of fresh mines, but until these are discovered and get to work it is abundantly clear there will be no drop in prices. *Long before this state of things had occurred it was conclusively proved that mining for asbestos, properly conducted, shows a more steady return for the money invested, with less elements of risk, than mining for any other known mineral.*

CHAPTER VI.

OUTPUT, COST OF PRODUCTION, WAGES, ETC.

RAPID ADVANCE OF THE INDUSTRY—Upward Tendency of Prices—Progressive Output—America the Largest Consumer—Commissioner's Report for 1889—Percentage of Output—Old Methods of Work discontinued—Cost of Cobbing—French Canadian Labour—Drink—Points for Consideration—Causes of Failure.

THE exploitation of asbestos in Canada has been making rapid strides from the date of the discovery of the Thetford deposits in 1877; but even now, more than twelve years later, viewed in the light of its possibilities, the manufacturing industry in England is but in its infancy. For the first ten years after the discovery, that is, down to 1887, the price of the crude ore had been gradually increasing in correspondence with the demand, with some, but by no means a proportionate, augmentation of the supply. In that year, however, several new quarries were opened, many buildings were erected, including two factories for the manipulation of the crude ore on the spot, and one of the companies built a branch line of railway to connect their works with the main line; the general result of the year's progress being such as to make it clear, that the industry was assuming such proportions that in the near future it would be the most important, as it already was the most remunerative, in the Province.

Satisfactory to the producers as was the result of 1887, still greater progress was made in 1888, and from the returns for 1889, just issued, it is seen that a yet greater leap forward has been taken. The extraordinary rise in prices which took place in the autumn of last year, and which still goes on, is a natural consequence of the fact that, notwithstanding every effort, the mine-owners find themselves unable to fulfil contracts; the supply for the past year, although considerably in excess of any previous output, not sufficing to keep pace with the ever-increasing demand.

Until, therefore, fresh mines are opened, or other discoveries made, it is clear that this upward tendency of prices must continue to go on; probably, this will not so much affect the manufacture of the higher class of spun goods, as it will materially limit that of such materials as felts, sheathings, and carpet or partition linings, &c. One unexpected result of the unusually high prices has, however, been to drive all the more important manufacturers into the market to buy mines for themselves, and so to turn producers as well as consumers, in order that, by employing more scientific methods of work and improved machinery, they may raise for themselves such supplies of ore as day by day it becomes more difficult for them to obtain through the ordinary trade channels. This, again, has the effect of driving prices up still higher, because the produce of the mines so purchased is practically withdrawn from the general market, the new mine-owners requiring for their own factories all the ore they can raise. Unusual efforts are, consequently, now being made over the whole of the productive areas to find and open up new mines, fresh capital is being continually brought in, whilst new developments of the industry are as constantly preparing the way for continued success.

The following may be taken as an authentic record of the progressive output of the mines, with the local value of the ore, since the commencement of the industry in Canada in 1878. It would have been more satisfactory to have been able to show the relative increase in price per ton in each year, but that could not be done without a knowledge of the proportions of the annual output, ranking as Nos. 1, 2, and 3. So far as possible, I have endeavoured to show this for 1889, and doubtless the importance of the industry will lead to greater particularization in future official returns. The advisability of this is practically recognised in Mr. Brumell's last Report (1889), which is a model of detailed accuracy :—

	Tons.	Value at the Mines.
1879	300	$19,500	£4,020
1880	380	24,700	5,093
1881	540	35,100	7,237
1882	810	52,650	10,856
1883	955	68,750	14,175
1884	1,141	75,079	15,480
1885	2,440	142,441	29,369
1886	3,458	206,251	42,526
1887	4,619	226,976	45,562
1888	4,404	255,007	52,578
1889	5,919*	—	—

The official Report for 1888 states that the price of first-class asbestos was then firm at an increase over previous years, the quality of the mineral shipped being correspondingly higher. During 1889, especially towards the close of the year, the prices of asbestos lands were considerably augmented, and the prices of crude ore advanced by "leaps and bounds."

It is not possible to give tabulated statements of production and prices, because this is the first year in which production and value has been authentically given for the full year. For the year 1888 a new system of returns was inaugurated by the Government officers, and from that time forward authentic figures will be tabulated.

Returns for this year (1888) were sent in by all the producers (11 mines, of which 9 only were productive), showing an output for the year of 4,404½ tons of all grades, valued at the mines at $255,007 (£52,578), an increase of 185 tons in quantity and $34,031 (£7,016) in value over the figures of the previous year.

The output from Ontario (actinolite returned as asbestos) for the previous year was 400 tons, value $6,000 (£1,237);

* This figure is that given by the Commissioner of Crown Lands for the year ending 30th June, and is consequently not the correct figure for comparison with those up to 1888, which are for the year ending 31st December, the official returns not being yet published.

OUTPUT, COST OF PRODUCTION, WAGES, ETC.

for 1888 it was nil. Consequently the production is shown as follows:—

From Thetford Mines	. . . .	3,067 tons.
,, Coleraine and Black Lake	. .	1,337½ ,,
		4,404½ tons.

These amounts were made up as follows:—

Thetford No. 1 .	. 1786 tons,	valued at	$157,040	=	£32,379	7	7¼
,, No. 2 .	. 519 ,,	,,	29,740		6,131	19	2¼
,, No. 3 .	. 762 ,,	,,	11,430		2,356	14	0
	3,067 tons.		$198,210		£40,868	0	9½

Coleraine and Black Lake No. 1	. 337 tons,	valued at	$25,040	=	£5,162	17	8¼
,, No. 2	. 601 ,,	,,	26,495		5,462	17	8¼
,, No. 3	. 399 ,,	,,	5,262		1,084	18	11½
	1,337 tons.		$56,597		£11,710	14	4

Totals—No. 1 .	. 2,123 tons,	valued at	$182,080	=	£37,542	5	4¼
No. 2 .	. 1,120 ,,	,,	56,235		11,594	16	10¾
No. 3 .	. 1,161 ,,	,,	16,692		3,441	12	11¾
	4,404 tons.		$255,007		£52,578	15	3

The quantity exported in the same year (1888) was as follows:—

No. 1	. . . 3,625 tons,	valued at	$262,552	=	£54,134	8	8
No. 2	. . . 110 ,,	,,	5,306		1,094	0	5
No. 3	. . . 201 ,,	,,	9,884		2,037	18	9
	3,936 tons.		$277,742		£57,266	7	10

Out of this total export no less than 3,612 tons, as already stated, was taken by the United States, the insignificant remainder being divided between Great Britain, France, Germany, Belgium, and Newfoundland.* The figures for 1889

* Brumell's Report on the Mining and Mineral Statistics of Canada for the year 1888.

and following years will show very different results, as the whole of the produce of three of the mines will now be sent to England direct, and of one other to Germany.

The Report of the Commissioner of Crown Lands for the Province of Quebec for 1889* gives important information as to the further working of the mines, but it is, unfortunately, useless for purposes of comparison, as, instead of dealing, like the former, with the whole year 1889, the Report makes the year end with the 30th of June, in the very height of the season, when facts and figures would be more difficult to arrive at accurately. For this reason, apparently, the figures are given as approximate only, and without any indication of classes or value. This question of date-discrepancy must be borne in mind, or the figures will be difficult to reconcile with known facts, especially in the general scale of prices, which are now much higher all round.

According to this last Report the output from the several mines for the twelve months ending 30th June, 1889, was as follows:—

THETFORD MINES.

Bell's Asbestos Company	1,800 tons.
King Brothers	700 ,,
Johnson Company	900 ,,
Ross and Ward	360 ,,
Thetford Asbestos Mining Company	80 ,,
Lucke and Mitchell (prospect)	10 ,,
	3,850 tons.

BLACK LAKE.

Anglo-Canadian Asbestos Company	618 tons.
United Asbestos Company (Frechette and Douville)	330 ,,
American Asbestos Company (Wertheim)	380 ,,
Bell's Asbestos Company	198 ,,
Scottish Canadian Asbestos Company	34 ,,
	1,560 tons.

* Rapport du Commissaire des Terres de la Couronne de la Province de Quebec pour les douze mois expirés le 30 Juin 1889.

COLERAINE.

Megantic Mining Company	100 tons.
Lambley & Co.	25 ,,
King Brothers (Ireland)	50 ,,
	175 tons.

DANVILLE AND BROUGHTON.

W. H. Jeffrey	328 tons.
Scottish Canadian Company	6 ,,
	334 tons.

TOTALS.

Thetford	3,850 tons.
Black Lake	1,560 ,,
Coleraine	175 ,,
Danville and Broughton	334 ,,
	5,919 tons.

In reference to which the Commissioner states that the Scottish Canadian Company and the Montreal Asbestos Company, of Black Lake, did no work during the year to which his report relates; and that the White's Asbestos Company, of Coleraine and Garthby, prospected only without any appreciable result.

"En resumé (the Commissioner concludes), l'industrie des mines d'amiantes est en pleine prosperité. Durant cette année, le prix a augmenté de 25 per cent., et la production 50 per cent. La demande continue d'être très grande, et les terrains miniers sont très recherchés."

The result of the twelve months' working ending 31st December, 1889, according to other (official) returns, are given as—

From Coleraine	124 tons.
,, Black Lake	1,725 ,,
,, Thetford	4,083 ,,
,, Broughton	8 ,,
,, Levis	16 ,,
	5,956 tons.

During 1889 the consumption of asbestos, in America especially, increased so rapidly that the demand was again greatly in excess of the supply. It is therefore manifest that, unless the production can be largely augmented, prices must still continue to rise. During the autumn, when the season was closing, none of the producers would venture to make contracts on any terms. Contracts for the previous season's delivery had in many cases to be deferred, and as a consequence of that it was found impossible to fix a price for the raw material even for a month in advance; nor was it practicable to obtain a guarantee for the delivery of the quantity which had been contracted for in the previous year.

The contracts entered into, at the close of 1888, were at prices unheard of before, and as the whole of the produce of 1889 was bespoken, although not contracted for, there appears but little prospect at present of a reaction. Owners confidently anticipated an advance of 40 or 50 per cent. upon the then current rates, refusing to bind themselves even at that; and subsequent experience has shown that their anticipations have been more than realized. It is quite clear, therefore, that no reduction in price is to be anticipated at present.

To give a general idea of the increased prices obtained it may be mentioned that, during the years 1881, 1882, and 1883, the prices of No. 1 crude were respectively $50, $60, and $70, rising by $10 each year; whilst in the autumn of 1889 they had risen to the following: No. 1, $125 to $130; No. 2, $75 to $80; No. 3, $35 to $40, and "waste," which had hitherto been unsaleable, $15 per ton, the ton being the short Canadian ton of 2,000 lbs. only; and the prices named being those obtainable at the mines. In the early part of 1890, $150 per ton was given for No. 1, and in the second week of April a parcel of 20 tons was bought in London at the rate of £43, or $208 per ton.

In June, 1890, the latest price received from New York was £53, with every prospect of its going still higher.

It must not, however, be forgotten that in the quoted prices there is a considerable variation, which is due to the fact that no uniform system of grading is adopted at the various mines. Thus, while at one mine No. 2 will be quoted at $75 per ton, at another the price of No. 1 will be very little more. Extra quality of No. 1, again, naturally commands a higher figure than the ordinary run of that grade.

It follows, therefore, that, when estimating the value of an asbestos property, the question of the relative percentage of output should be carefully considered ; since, while the number of tons produced by any two mines might be approximately equal, and to the uninitiated, therefore, the properties about equal in value, the one, from the large amount of No. 1 grade, would be capable of paying handsome dividends, while the other would require great economy of management and still yield far less satisfactory returns.* Again, if a mine be worked on the hillside it is obvious that it will be comparatively free from water, and the removal of the ore and waste rock a simple process, whilst if it be on the level ground, and the mine be worked by sinking, the water trouble becomes greater every day, and powerful pumping machinery and steam apparatus for raising ore and waste rock must add greatly to the working cost, and consequently to cost per ton of ore got out.

Wages run from $1 to $1.75 a day, according to the nature of the work performed, for men, and from 50 to 75 cents for lads and cobbers.

These rates do not much differ from those paid in the adjoining province of Ontario. There, surface men employed at the Bruce copper mines were paid about $1 a day, though of course some could get more. At Sault Ste. Marie ordinary labourers at the mines get from $1.25 to $1.50 a day. On this important question of wages we see by the Report of the Royal Commission just published,† that in the Sudbury district, outside men can get $1.40, and miners $1.75, but it is somewhat difficult to get labour at Sudbury on account of the

* Dr. Ells, Second Report for 1889.
† Report of the Royal Commission on the Mineral Resources of Ontario and the Measures for their Development, 1890 : p. 406.

isolated position of the mines. The following is the rate paid there in cash:—

Drill runners	$2.10 per day	Machinist	$2.25 per day
Miners	1.75 ,,	Pumpman	2.00 ,,
Labourers	1.60 ,,	Fitter	2.00 ,,
Foreman	2.00 ,,	Fireman	1.50 ,,
Watchman	1.75 ,,	Blacksmith	2.50 ,,
Engineer	2.00 ,,	Asstnt. Blacksmith	1.75 ,,

As to the mode of extraction of the ore, the method of work in all the chrysotile mines of Canada is simply open quarry work, except at Broughton, where the peculiar formation necessitates a mode more in the nature of regular mining; and at Mr. Wertheim's mine, at Coleraine, where a new departure has been taken, by driving a somewhat extensive tunnel from the foot of the hill, and then a shaft through the rock to reach the pits above; though, in this last case, the operation is simply performed to open out a fine working face.

All the old rule-of-thumb methods of opening and working are now being rapidly discontinued, these being found to be quite impracticable with large pits and constantly increasing production. Air compressors, steam derricks, and all the most improved labour-saving appliances are being everywhere introduced, and a rich reward awaits the inventor who shall enable the mine-owners to dispense with the tedious and costly process of cobbing, more especially of the lower grades, and at the same time help him to get rid of some of the enormous masses of piled-up waste rock, much of which contains short veins of fibre, which under the present system will not pay for extracting, but every particle of which will be turned to good account when some economical process is devised for extracting it.

Whether the drills are worked by compressed air, or by hand, in the old-fashioned way, the effect is the same. When a sufficient number of holes of the proper depth are drilled and duly charged with dynamite or powder, they are linked together, and fired by a battery in such a way that the face of rock shall be thrown outward, on to the floor of the pit. The asbestos is then picked out, the adhering rock roughly broken off, and the ore piled into boxes or tubs, which are loaded on to trolleys, and run off on tram-lines to the cobbing-sheds. The refuse rock, of which there is always an enormous quantity, (as much as twenty or twenty-five tons of rock to one of asbestos), is loaded into cars, run off and shot over on to the dumping-ground.

Boys are employed in the cobbing-sheds to chip, or cob, the rock cleanly from the ore, an operation which is much more troublesome with thin veins than with those of the better sort, to which the waste rock is less firmly adherent.

This cobbing is a very troublesome and expensive process, costing about $5 a ton. After cobbing, great care is required in sorting the ore into the respective grades of Nos. 1, 2, and 3. It is then put up in bags of 100 or 160 lbs. each, marked, and stacked away in the bins ready for shipment. All this is done in a very rough-and-ready style, and the waste is simply enormous; there is no doubt, however, that as the ore increases in value more scientific appliances will be adopted, and greater care used in the prevention of waste. At present thousands of tons of rock containing only thin veins of asbestos are dumped on the refuse heaps as waste which would all be crushed if a proper machine were at hand, and the valuable material consequently saved.

The sorting, or grading, of the ore is done by the cobbers simultaneously with the cobbing; the lads, whilst striking off the adhering rock, dividing the lumps of ore into Nos. 1, 2, or 3 class, and throwing them into their separate heaps, being guided in so doing by the colour and purity of the fibre, with a due regard to length. An investigation into the method and cost of this work, carried out by Mr. Obalski, showed that fourteen young lads in one day separated 4,000 lbs., or two Canadian tons, into graded and marketable material, their wages, at 70 cents each, reaching $9·08, or nearly $5 per ton; and he considered this below the general average cost of the work, which is probably nearer $6, bringing up the cost of production and preparation for market to about $25 per ton. This coincides pretty accurately with my personal experience. Taking, therefore, the prices at the mines at $125 only for No. 1, $75 for No. 2, and $35 for No. 3, and comparing these with the cost of production, it is evident there is a very large amount of profit in asbestos mining, and a considerable inducement for the employment of capital therein. And when it is stated that these calculations were made upon the old system of work by hand-labour, machinery being now the rule, whereby the cost of production is reduced to $15, and at old prices, it will be seen that the profit is very much larger than is shown above.

There is no scarcity of labour, a sufficient number of hands, mostly French-Canadians, being always forthcoming; but at those mines where there is an insufficiency of houses for married men, accommodation has to be found in a barrack-like building for single men: the married men, who cannot be accommodated, residing frequently at a long distance from their work, which causes them to be of a migratory disposition, and gives considerable additional trouble to the management. This remark, however, does not apply to Thetford, to Wertheim's, or, indeed, to any mine started on a business-like basis, as in such cases proper regard is paid to the welfare of the men by providing them with suitable accommodation.

A disadvantage in the employment of French-Canadian labour lies in the great number of festivals incident to their religion, with consequent loss of work at the mines, but apparently there is no remedy for this at present. The greatest curse of the place, however, is drink. The hip pockets in the men's pants form very convenient receptacles for bottles, and these are always pretty well filled after pay days and holidays. The liquor most in favour is a vile compound called gin. It is supplied in the regular square Dutch bottles from the familiar green-painted boxes in which "Hollands" is exported, and which are labelled "De Kuyper"; but the vile stuff is not much credit to that gentleman's manufacture if it be so, which is much to be doubted.

Although the district is under the Scott Act, and the sale of liquor consequently prohibited, like every other place where the sale is interdicted there is no difficulty, if you know how to go about it, and sometimes even if you don't,* in getting as much liquor as you please. At any rate I never yet was in any such place where I did not find it to be so, the only practical difference being that, in the absence of competition, the spirits obtainable are the vilest compounds imaginable.

According to my experience, no sooner is the sale of spirits interdicted anywhere than a craving for drink sets in like an epidemic, coupled with a determination to get it, and that unmitigated curse to any community, secret drinking, becomes rife. Practical experience soon taught me the comparative uselessness of alcohol when travelling in cold regions; the Russian fashion of tea-drinking is far and away the best. A tumbler of hot tea, flavoured with a slice of lemon, is not only palatable and comforting, but will carry a man twice as far as any concoction of alcohol.

In concluding this part of the subject, it may be well to point out that prior to the purchase of an unexplored asbestos property, it would be well to learn something of the surface indications, as well as the geological formation and surroundings of the property; and if the ground be opened, the

* Here is an instance: On one occasion I had been out driving in the pouring rain for several hours, had got drenched to the skin, and was bitterly cold. I pulled up, therefore, at a likely-looking house, went in and called for some brandy, but to my disgust was told that no liquors could be supplied, as it was against the law. As I turned to go out again, in no very cheerful mood, the man, seeing the state I was in, evidently took compassion on me, and said, "Better try some bitters"; so calling to mind the saying that all bitters are warm, barring a bitter cold day, which only proves the rule, I assented. He then pushed over a tumbler and a black bottle, when I at once poured out and swallowed a pretty strong dose, feeling when I had done so as if I had swallowed a streak of forked lightning. As soon as I had recovered my breath I muttered my thanks and paid up. "Have another?" says he, with a twinkle in his eye. "No, thanks," I replied. "Guess you'll remember our bitters," he then laughingly said, prefixing the name of the place, which I afterwards found was in a district where prohibition was very strictly enforced, and which I therefore purposely omit, his breach of the law having no doubt saved me from the dangerous effects of a chill.

direction and dip of the veins, the presence or absence of chromic iron ore, pyrites, or other minerals in association with the asbestos ore, the quantity and quality of the ore producible from the adjoining mines, and its analysis. Special regard must also be had to its tenacity, lubricity, flexibility, and infusibility. The most suitable method of extraction, the best arrangements for dumping, with the important questions of transport, cost and supply of labour, &c., and last, but not least (if the mine be at work), the relative proportions of grades producible, are important matters for consideration.

Upon this last point deception may easily be practised on the unwary; figures of prospective output and corresponding profit are sometimes put forward, which, if accepted without proper advice, are certain to lead to trouble, and perhaps to disaster. In one case of a mine put on the English market, it was boldly stated that the output for the first year might be taken at about 67 per cent. of No. 1, whereas the first year's production showed 67 per cent. and upwards of No. 3, which did not pay for working, some small amount of No. 2, and an almost infinitesimal amount of No. 1. In another case there had been no reliable expert's opinion obtained as to the quality of the land before purchase, and when work was commenced the ground bought proved to be barren. In both cases the money had better have been thrown into the Thames, as well in the interest of the shareholders as for the credit of Canadian enterprise.

When failures occur, they may almost certainly be traced to want of practical advice in the first instance, to incompetency or extravagance in the management, or to over-capitalisation; but with due care, economy, and honest and capable management, there are but few things which will pay better or with more regularity and certainty than mining for asbestos.

CHAPTER VII.

NEWFOUNDLAND AND NORWAY.

GENERAL RESEMBLANCE OF STRATA TO GASPÉ—Granite, Serpentine, Asbestos, and Picrolite — Pseudo-Chrysotile — Crocidolite — Coarse Asbestos—Minerals found in Norway.

So great a resemblance exists between some parts of the geological formation of Newfoundland and that of the Gaspé Peninsula, with parts of the Eastern Townships of Quebec, of which the former is doubtless a continuation, that it is naturally to be expected the same minerals would be found there, including asbestos. The Quebec group, a continuation of the Appalachian chain, is part of the great metalliferous formation of North America. In this group, as we have already seen, are found gold, silver, copper, asbestos, magnetic and chromic iron, cobalt, nickel, and some other minerals. These are associated with the ophiolites and other magnesian rocks, whilst they are apparently wanting in those of the same age in the Laurentian series. This fact was recognised by Dr. Sterry Hunt in 1881.* And Mr. Alexander Murray, then geologist of Newfoundland, when treating of the Lower Cambrian Rocks of Nova Scotia, compares them with the auriferous strata of his Intermediate series of Newfoundland. The resemblance in general character of the strata, with their included auriferous quartz veins, in Newfoundland to those of Nova Scotia, will occur to any one who has visited the two countries, and studied

* *American Journal of Science*, May, 1881.

their geological features, and I venture to say that the description given of the latter country might, in many respects, equally apply to the former; although the auriferous country of Nova Scotia is supposed to be of Lower Silurian age; whilst that of Newfoundland is undoubtedly unconformably below the Primordial.*

Gold has been found in many parts of this series, and asbestos also in the serpentine rocks of Newfoundland. The distribution of these latter is a matter of great importance to those interested in the discovery of metalliferous ores as well as of asbestos; the formation of which they are a part is largely developed in various parts of the island, and there is good reason to believe that, in course of time, the latter will become a great field of mining industry.

One day a friend of mine, while out shooting on the island, had to cross a mountain stream near the shore, and in passing over, saw a long-fibred white substance swaying about in the water, which he took for some kind of vegetation, but on pulling it out it proved to be asbestos. And on the banks of the stream he found it filling all the crevices in the rocks, which there and for some miles along the coast are all magnesian. Some specimens of the asbestos he gathered, and brought home with him to England. They were long, and of a fine white colour, in appearance exactly resembling that found in the Pyrenees, but brittle, and consequently of little value. From the description of the place where it was found there would appear to be little doubt that a seam of asbestos exists in the locality which would pay for working.

There are large developments of serpentine on other parts of the island, asbestos also being found in many places, notably on the north side of Hare Bay and between that place and Pistolet Bay. Some considerable extent of asbestos-bearing serpentine also occurs on the west side of the island; likewise at York Harbour, in the Bay of Islands, and running from the north arm of that bay to Bonne Bay.

* "Geological Survey of Newfoundland, 1880."

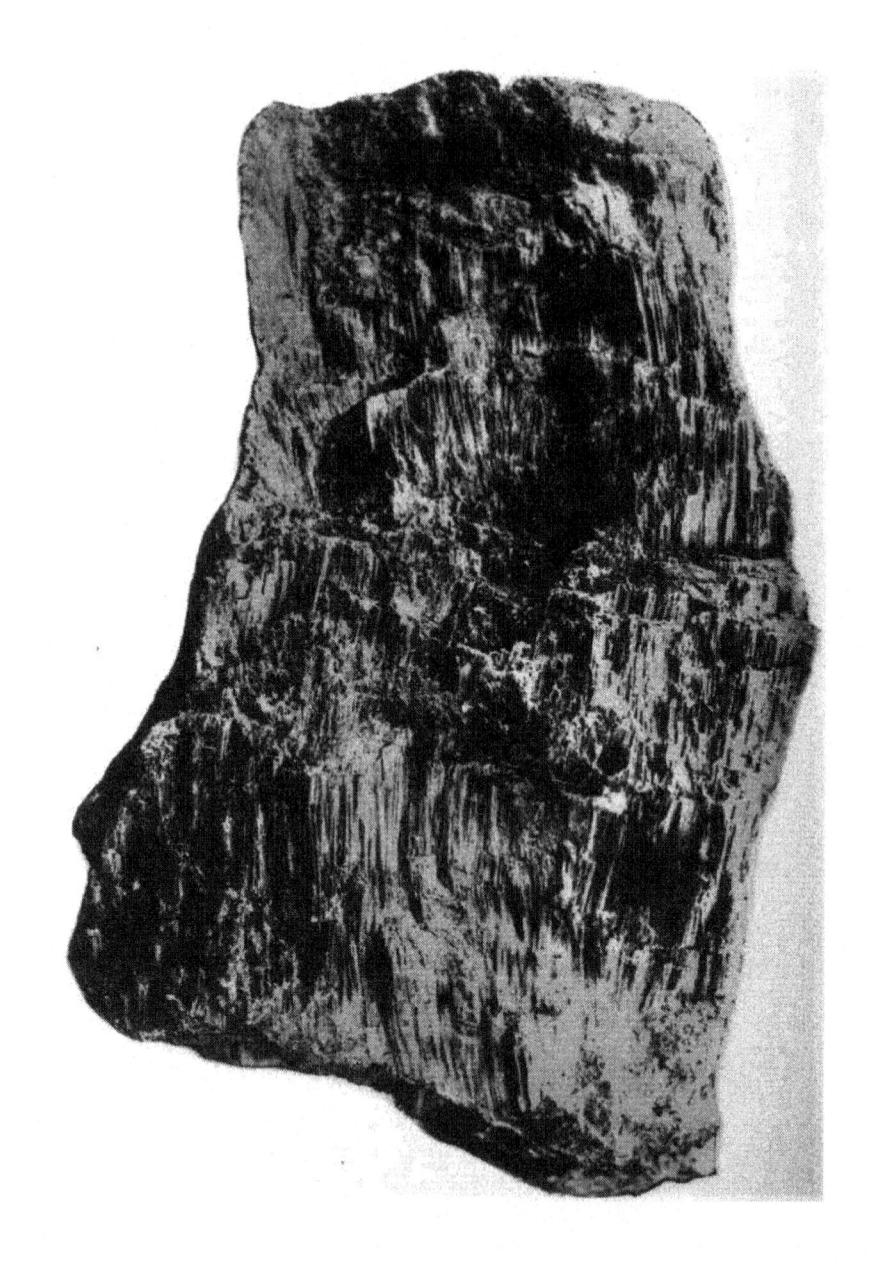

MOUNTAIN WOOD, HELGELAND, NORWAY.

At Tilt Cove great masses of serpentine and steatite occur, the magnesian rocks in that district being permeated throughout by magnetic and chromic iron in grains and crystals. In front of this, and overlying the mineralized lands, are masses of a hard, grey diorite, containing epidote in strings and patches. This is succeeded on the north-west by the great body of serpentine of the Castle Rock depression. A very soft and shaly serpentine containing asbestos is found here, the veins averaging at the surface a quarter of an inch in width.

On the west side of Tickle Harbour, north of Long Reach, is a group of altered rocks consisting of purple and variegated slates associated with serpentine and steatite, the veins of asbestos being intersected with layers of yellowish quartzite.

There is also a large development of picrolite towards the top of Sitdown Hill, which runs through the rocks and breaks out in long fibrous crystals, the surfaces of which are sometimes opalescent. Seams of asbestos are also frequent here; indeed it is manifest that there is abundance on the island, which is ripe for exploration.

Norway.

Norway is one of the oldest regions of Europe. A great part of it bears evidence of having been raised above the ocean level at a very remote period. Comparatively speaking, no other country exhibits such extensive areas of those primary or palæozoic rocks which form so large a part of the oldest crust of the earth.

The physical features of the whole of the Scandinavian peninsula are of a striking character. A chain of mountains runs from north to south nearly its entire length, which in a considerable part of its course forms the divide between Sweden and Norway. Nine-tenths of this latter country are of a bold, mountainous character, the valleys being mere rents or chasms, sometimes not more than a hundred feet wide, at the bottom of which runs a fjord, or a river winds its tortuous course as it rushes down to the sea, the enclosing mountains rising up in grim and bare sterility to an occasional height of about 4,000 feet. So strange, indeed, is the conformation of the country that Victor Hugo could only liken it to the skeleton of a great fish. Such a country as this is specially favourable for deposits of the economic minerals.

Granite, which is not generally favourable to asbestos, occurs everywhere; serpentine, nevertheless, abounds there as well as throughout the whole of Scandinavia. It occurs in massive form at Fahlun in Sweden, and crystallized massive at Snarum and many other parts of Norway, especially in the south. Precious serpentine occurs at Fahlun and Gulsjo, as well as a soft earthy variety, somewhat like meerschaum, with considerable quantities of picrolite.

Amphibole is an essential constituent of such rocks as syenite, diorite, and greenstone, and asbestos is frequently found associated with the greenish apatite rocks of South Norway, at Arendal, Snarum, and other places, where rutile, actinolite, chlorite, and epidote also occur. It is also found at Sundmoër, and a pseudo-chrysotile also occurs which has the following composition:—

Silica	42·92
Alumina	·87
Ferric oxide	2·28
Magnesia	41·66
Water	12·02
	99·75

There can be no doubt of the valuable character of this mineral; but, as a rule, most of the asbestos hitherto brought from Norway is coarse and hard, resembling mountain wood, mountain cork, and leather; in the limestone especially it partakes of the latter character. The whole of Norway has the appearance of a mighty upheaval of the primitive rocks, granite, gneiss, and syenite especially, varied, particularly on the coast line and along the fjords, by patches, in some cases miles in length, of serpentine and hornblende.

A variety of crocidolite is found at Stavern, which bears some resemblance to the African species.

At Helgeland, on one of the fjords, further to the north-west, beyond Trondheim, the serpentine, varied by masses of hornblende, runs for something like three miles in a heaped-up mammillated form, until suddenly cut off by a great upheaval of granite. Here, as might be expected, there is abundance of asbestos. That lying near the surface is of the usual Norske character—coarse and woody. Eight or ten small openings have been made between the boulders of serpentine and a few tons got out, which was sent to London and converted into cement, paint, and used up for other purposes to which pulverised asbestos is adapted. This was got out, shipped and delivered in London at something less than £6 per ton, at which price any quantity could be sold; the cost of extraction, transport, and delivery being about £3 10s.

A better quality, but still also partaking of the nature of mountain cork, occurs here and in the limestone region on the opposite side of the fjord. Still, with the fact before us of asbestos of fine quality occurring in this neighbourhood, we are fully warranted in expecting that when the time comes for exploration, the coarse, woody variety, supposed to be characteristic of the country, will be found to be merely the surface deposits, and that richer stores are to be had for searching, whilst even these inferior ones would well pay for working.

In the Report of the Royal Commission on the Mineral Resources of Ontario (1890) it is mentioned that Mr. Willimott has enumerated 61 species of minerals as distributed in the Upper Laurentian rocks of that Province; and these, almost without exception, are to be found in rocks of a similar character in Norway. Among these granite is everywhere conspicuous, in association with syenite, which abounds in zircon: pegmatite or graphic granite occurring in veins. In the north gabbro, greenstone, and granite are found among the eruptive rocks, whilst in central Norway the formation is mostly overlaid with clay slates and quartz.

CHAPTER VIII.

THE USES OF ASBESTOS: APPLICATION TO ENGINEERING PURPOSES.

EARLY EXPERIMENTS—Causes of Failure—Packings—Boiler Coverings—Fire-felt—Fire-felt with Superator Covering—Cement—Asbesto-Sponge—Joints of Hot-air Pipes.

ALTHOUGH many of the valuable properties of asbestos have been known, as we have already seen, for thousands of years, we are only now concerned with it in its modern adaptation to the industrial arts and practical mechanics. Its use, in this respect, dates from but a few years ago; nor can the first attempts to render it available be even then looked upon otherwise than as experiments, which were mostly of an unsuccessful character. One of the main causes of this failure was that the varied and dissimilar peculiarities of the different varieties were not, at that time, properly appreciated; nor was the requisite attention given to differences of composition. Even now, the economic value of the greater number of species is so far unknown that no use can be made of them; but as we know that there is nothing, in or under the earth, which cannot be made available for man's use, we may confidently expect that the rich deposits known to exist in various parts of the world, in America, in Africa and Servia especially, will presently be utilized. At this moment scarcely any but the fine silky and tenacious fibres of Italy and Canada find practical application; and as the value of these, for an infinite variety of purposes, day by day becomes more perceptible, the demand for them as rapidly increases, to a degree, so far as Canada is concerned, certainly far beyond the rate of supply. We can, therefore, only anticipate that these special varieties will become more and more valuable, until either fresh mines are discovered or means are found for bringing some of the, at present, unused varieties into competition with them for some at least of the commoner purposes to which they are applied.

The earliest modern application of the fibre to engineering purposes was the manufacture of an improved packing. This, at first, was mostly in the shape of millboard, but the various modifications of this special manufacture now in demand are so many that it would be useless to attempt to enumerate them here. It may be, however, that a general mention of some few of those

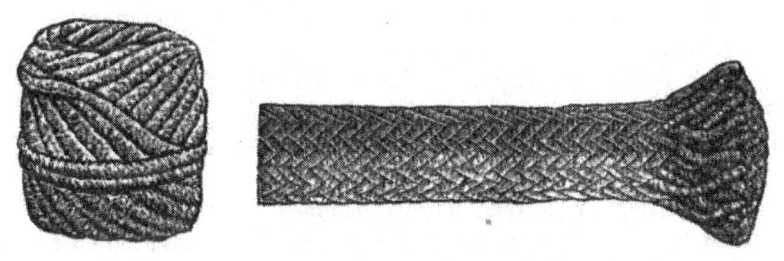

Asbestos Wick and Braided Packings. Chalmers-Spence Company, New York.

now in use in steam, hydraulic and electrical machinery may not be considered out of place. The utility of asbestos for such purposes as these, like that of every other material so used, depends a great deal upon its freedom from impurity. When the manufacture was first commenced, it was frequently found that the fibres were more or less charged with minute particles of pyrites, of magnetite, or other metallic impurity, which caused the piston-rods to be scored by the packing, and the damage thus occasioned was at first erroneously attributed to the action of the asbestos itself rather than to the impurities contained in it. As soon, however, as the real cause of this was properly appreciated, it became necessary, in order to prevent it, not only to select the most suitable kind of asbestos for this special purpose, but also to thoroughly cleanse it from all gritty matter before spinning; and in order effectually to accomplish this object, special machinery had to be devised, but as soon as this was done the yarn produced was pure and capable of being woven into any kind of fabric.

Whatever the material may be which is used for this purpose, it is a matter of the first necessity that, under the action of steam or heat, it shall not become hard in the gland; and its nature must be such that it shall remain unaltered, however high the pressure, or fast the steam, to which it may be subjected. The native qualities of asbestos admirably adapt it for such purposes as these, its inherent lubricity rendering it additionally valuable; and by its use a perfectly pure packing can now be produced, through which the rod slides with a minimum of friction. Another great point is that it does not require frequent renewing; regularity in the motion of the piston is preserved and all the machinery connected with it runs with perfect smoothness, its elastic nature keeping the joints tight, longer than any other kind manufactured.

Sometimes, it is true, more is claimed for these packings than they can accomplish, it being occasionally asserted that their self-lubricating qualities enable them to be used without oil. This is not so; they require a plentiful supply of oil and very careful attention as well: but these being given, they will last from five to ten times longer than any packing now in use. They possess many advantages over rubber, their weight is less, they last longer, and one half the thickness will generally suffice.

The various packings, in all the ordinary forms, made by the United Asbestos Company, of London, are too well known to need description here, and their Victor metallic packings are used wherever such goods are required.

As a special method of utilizing asbestos for packing, "Eastman's Asbestallicon" may be mentioned; and the combined asbestos and metallic packing of Messrs. Witty & Wyatt is also well spoken of. In this, soft metallic rings, of two forms are made, in two or three segments, with an asbestos ring attached to the segments, this last being only severed in one place. The segments are thus held together, and are put in place so as to break joint; the metal and asbestos press together, and are sufficiently free to follow any irregularity in the form of the piston-rod, and still remain quite steam-tight.

Dick's self-lubricating steam and hydraulic packing is made of native jute, which nearly approaches the texture of silk; each yarn, in the process of manufacture, being passed through

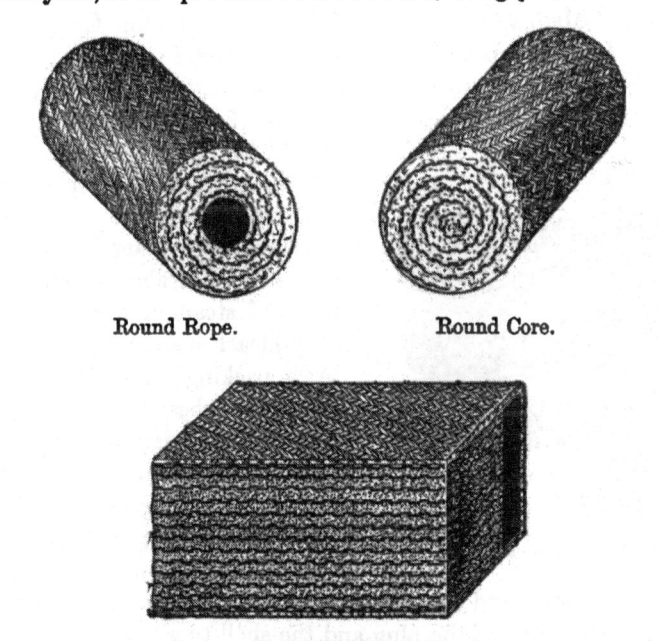

Round Rope.   Round Core.

The "Duriflex."

an asbestos compound, whereby a good all-round packing is formed.

Cresswell's "Special Marine Asbestos Packing" is manufactured for use in ocean-going steamers, fitted with triple-expansion engines, running at great and continuous speed.

The "Duriflex," of Messrs. Moseley & Sons, Manchester, is constructed of wire gauze and asbestos, so contrived as to combine the durability of a metallic with the flexibility of a fibrous packing, and this either with or without an indiarubber core, as shown on the previous page. The wire gauze is prepared, before insertion, by cutting or corrugating it diagonally, and then placing it between the layers of fibrous material with the corrugations diagonally arranged. By this means the rigidity of the wire gauze is entirely destroyed, and the packing has practically as great flexibility as one made entirely of fibrous material.

The "Manhattan," of the Manhattan Packing Company, New York, is a plumbago packing designed to prevent grooving and cutting. It is formed of a braided strip, either with or without a rubber centre, filled with fine floated plumbago, and with an oil of very high fire test, which cannot char or ignite, and is free from acids. It is specially useful in steam hammers, where it is desirable to avoid a leakage of steam or water, or on rotary bleach boilers.

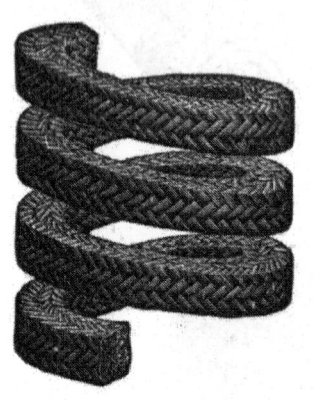

The "Manhattan."

As a packing for steam cocks, the use of asbestos is well-nigh universal for high-pressure fittings, the great heat of the steam speedily destroying any packing made from hemp; but as the joint in this case is made between a metal surface and one of asbestos, sufficient room is required to be left between the plug and the shell to allow for expansion. Dewrance's asbestos-packed cocks are too well known to engineers to need more than reference.

A durable joint can be made between rough cast-iron surfaces by the use of asbestos mixed with sufficient white lead to make a stiff putty.

The various coverings designed for the protection of boilers and pipes, for the preservation of the contained heat, and for the economy of fuel are specially numerous. Asbestos practically contains in itself every requisite for a perfect non-conducting covering, and consequently the most satisfactory results are obtained by using it in this way, in its pure and fibrous form, without any admixture of foreign material. One of the largest and most enterprising firms of asbestos manufacturers in the United States, the Chalmers-Spence Company of New York, has given to this department of manufacture considerable attention, and has designed a material for the purpose which they term Fire-Felt. In their construction of this covering, the mineral fibres are formed into cylinders, blocks, and sheets, according to the shape and size of the surfaces to be covered; and these being light in weight (1 lb. to the square foot, 1 inch thick), flexible, and easily handled, can

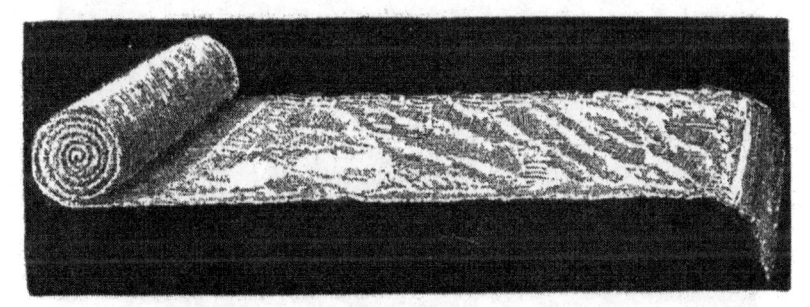

Fire-Felt. The Chalmers-Spence Company.

be readily adapted to a surface of any shape; whilst, being strong and tough on the exterior, and spongy and felt-like on the inner layer, they form a highly non-conducting material.

When tested with any of the various composition coverings produced, the superiority of the pure and fibrous asbestos, in this form, is quickly seen. It gives better non-conducting results, and possesses a guarantee of durability impossible to be otherwise obtained, inasmuch as it cannot char or burn out, because there are no organic or perishable materials included in its make-up.

Another form of this material is shown in the same firm's "Patent Roll Fire-Felt," which is made in rolls of about 3 feet in width, and of any required thickness. This is specially useful as a non-conducting fireproof lining under other coverings, or as a covering by itself, where great thickness is not desired, as in most kinds of steam-pipe work. In length each roll contains about 300 square feet. High pressure being now the rule, seldom less than 80 or 90 lbs. which means a body of heat of 300° Fahr., or over, contained in one quarter-inch thickness of iron, and rapidly conducting through the iron, it is of primary importance to prevent this heat from escaping,

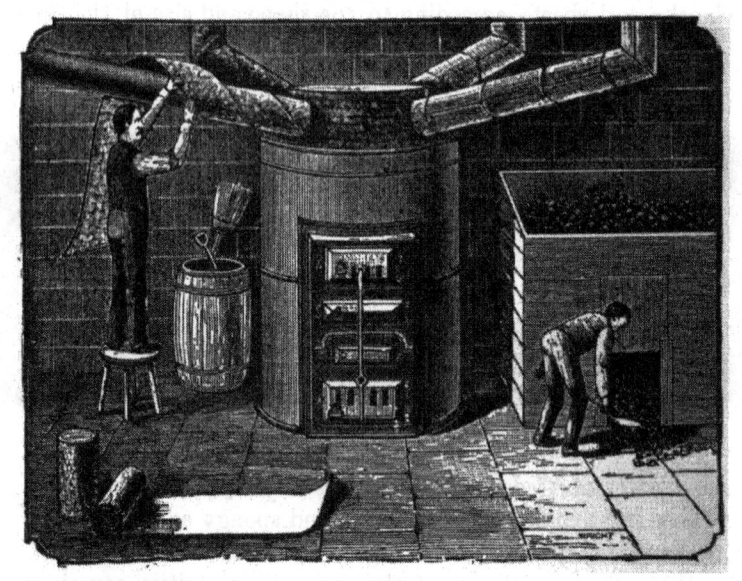

Patent Roll Fire-Felt. The Chalmers-Spence Company.

not only when the covering is first applied, but also during a term of years, and this requires a material of high non-conducting powers and great durability.

Fire-felt possesses these qualities in an eminent degree, as it is free from any ingredients that will cause it to disintegrate under heat or deteriorate through use. Its mode of application to house furnace pipes is shown in the diagram above.

A special boiler covering, manufactured by the same firm,

THE USES OF ASBESTOS. 139

and supplied by them under contract for several of the United States Government warships, is in the form of a quilting. These quiltings weigh about 2 lbs. per square foot, and can be removed without difficulty when required. The same firm also manufacture removable pipe coverings; some of these are made exclusively of pure asbestos fibre, and others of asbestos

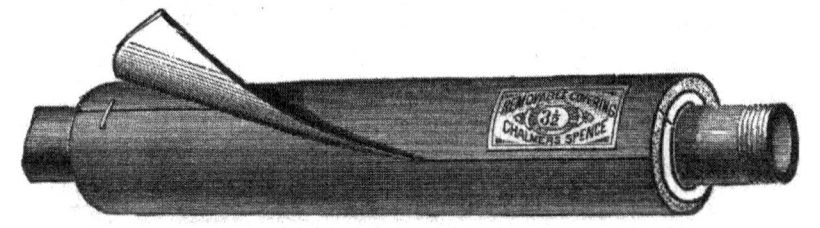

Patent Removable Covering.

combined with other materials, according to whether high or low pressure steam is used, or whether it be for the preservation of cold-water pipes from freezing.

These coverings are made in sections of three-foot lengths, of the exact size of the pipe to be covered, the asbestos fibres in the covering being so interlaced that the sections, whilst

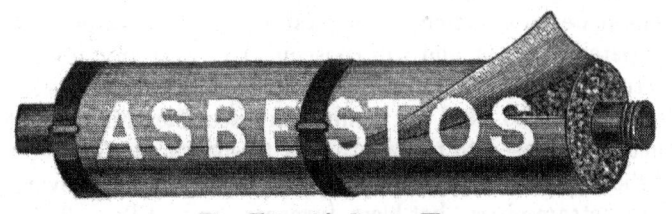

Fire-Felt with Canvas Flap.

combining strength with flexibility, afford so large a number of air-cells as to give this covering a very high non-conducting quality, whilst it is not liable to char or be otherwise injured by the most intense heat. It is occasionally found advisable to provide a heavy inner layer of asbestos fibre, with an outer layer of hair felt; but if a layer of asbestos fibre be substituted for the hair felt, greater durability is ensured. In whichever way the fibre is used, it is enclosed in a strong case or wrapper of non-porous sheathing, the inner section of which has a lining of asbestos to keep it from direct contact with the iron.

This patent Fire-felt is also furnished with a canvas flap cover, and when the pipes are to be used in wet places, out of doors, or in mines, a special class of "Superator" jacket is provided, thus :

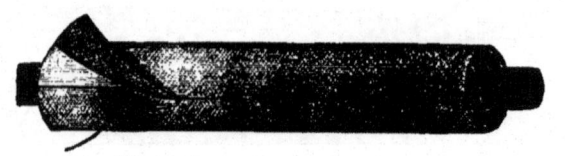

Fire-Felt with Superator Jacket.

The material which the patentee calls "Superator" is another speciality of the same house. This is a flexible sheet of asbestos, strengthened by an insertion of wire-netting. It is made of mineral substances only (mainly asbestos), with an admixture of some insoluble chemical ingredients, the asbestos rendering the jacket fireproof, and the wire netting giving it the necessary strength.

The material of which the Superator is made is waterproofed by a patent process, and will consequently resist any degree of moisture, thus forming a substantial protection to the covering. Superator is also used for roofing purposes, sheathing wooden structures exposed to the weather or to sparks, &c.

Asbestos cement is also very largely used for covering boilers, steam-pipes, hot-blast furnaces, and stills. This is made of pulverized asbestos, for which the inferior qualities will answer sufficiently well, it is worked up to about the consistency of mortar, and spread over the surfaces to be covered in precisely the same manner, with a trowel. In place of this cement, the Chalmers-Spence Company propose a substitution of sheet Fire-felt with Superator jacket, thus :

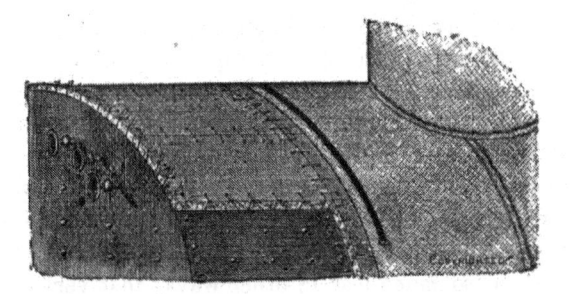

Sheet Fire-Felt with Superator Jacket.

Where the cement is preferred, in the preparation of it certain chemical ingredients have to be added which, while not injurious to the metal, cause the asbestos to adhere firmly to the plates, so that when dry it becomes quite hard and can be walked over without being injured. With a boiler carrying say 80 lbs. steam pressure, the application of from 1½ to 2 inches of this composition so well retains the heat in the boiler that a thermometer with the bulb held close to the outer surface of the covering will not indicate more than 80° to 85° Fahr., and when the boilers, steam-pipes, &c., are covered in this manner, a large saving of fuel is effected, as it is said, equivalent to 33 per cent. The non-conducting power of asbestos is twice as great as that of hair felt, which is believed to come next to it in value, but is soon destroyed by heat. When the steam pressure is not unusually high, one inch in thickness of the cement is sufficient; but the additional cost of an extra half-inch is amply compensated for by the larger proportionate saving of fuel and power effected by its use.

The cement, which is made from a cheap quality of asbestos, is now in common use in Canada and the States, where, as already shown, it is found to operate with a twofold effect, viz., by lowering the temperature of the boiler-house, to the great comfort of the engineers and firemen, and also, in a very marked degree, economising the expenditure for fuel. Unprotected pipes require a greater supply of fuel, and mean more wear and tear on grate bars, boilers, &c.; while in order to convey steam any distance through unprotected pipes requires a much larger pipe to furnish the requisite power.

It seems strange that the use of asbestos in this country, in this way, has as yet made so little headway. In one of the palatial buildings recently erected in London, where engines are required to be in constant work for pumping water for working the lifts and for general purposes, as well as for the dynamos, the heat from the boilers forms so great a nuisance, and occasions so much loss in other ways, that very considerable expense was lately about to be incurred with a view to lowering the temperature. When conversing with an expert, who had been sent for to devise a remedy for this, I asked whether the use of asbestos would not effect the desired object. Certainly it would, he replied, but it is too expensive.

In applying the cement the best results are obtained when it is put on with an air space left, as shown thus :

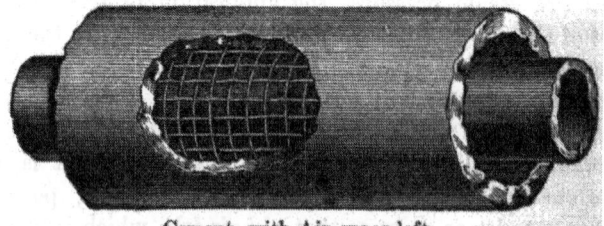

Cement, with Air-space left.

This is another patent of the Chalmers-Spence Company. A network of lathing or wire-cloth is formed round the boiler or pipes, at a distance therefrom of about an inch. On this framework the cement is applied, the material keying through the meshes of the wire, and thus obtaining a greater hold and consequently greater durability than if it were applied direct to the iron.

An asbestos cement felting is also manufactured in New York, for use in the same way as the ordinary asbestos cement. This is composed of fibrous asbestos, and a cementing compound forming a light porous covering, which is applied in much the same way.

Another material is a substance called asbesto-sponge. Recognising that in all non-conductors the manufacturer's endeavour is to provide as large a number of air cells in a given space as possible, the patentee considers that sponge, which is composed of fine, flexible, tenacious fibres, interwoven in the form of cells and meshes, constitutes the ideal structure of a perfect non-conductor. The tintack-like barbs of the sponge are so interwoven, in asbesto-sponge, with the fine, silky fibres of asbestos as to form an elastic, highly porous material, of so light a character that a barrelful in the form of filling will barely weigh 50 lbs., and this with so small a percentage of sponge that the material is practically fireproof.

In making the joints of hot-air pipes for blast furnaces, which are necessarily exposed to an exceedingly high temperature, asbestos in the form of a cord has been found very serviceable; the jointing piece consisting of an iron ring, wrapped round with cord, which is simply put in place and nipped between the two flanges. Previously to the manufacture of asbestos cord these rings were wrapped round with yarn, which gave incessant trouble.

A new material of a composite nature which the patentee calls "Randalite," is prepared and sold by Messrs. S. Minns & Co., of Trafalgar Road, Dalston, as an improved Millboard for washers, packing, &c. This is waterproof, incorrodible, and unaffected by heat, cold, or grease. It is sold in sheets at 8d. per lb.

It is by no means to be said that all the varied applications of asbestos to engineering purposes have here been noted, but merely a selection of some of the most prominent. Indeed, it would be difficult to say for what special engineering purpose asbestos cannot be made available; an enlargement on this head would probably be considered of too technical a character to be of general interest, and enough has doubtless been said to show the great importance of the mineral in an engineering point of view.

CHAPTER IX.

APPLICATIONS OF ASBESTOS TO MILITARY AND FIRE PREVENTIVE PURPOSES.

BIG GUNS—Miners' Safety Lamps—Torpedoes—Time Fuses—Dynamite Shells—Ironclads—Military Aeronautics—Safes and Deed Boxes—Carriage of Explosives—Lint—Building Operations—Bâches—Theatrical Curtains—Protection Shields—Fires in Theatres—Captain Shaw's Book—A Yankee Yarn—Fire Kings—Firemen's Clothing—Appareil Aldini—Barnum's Show.

THE bearings of asbestos on matters connected with the art of scientific warfare are numerous and important. We have the authority of Sir Frederick Abel for stating that asbestos is as effectual when used for closing the breeches of big guns so as to prevent the passage of gas, as it is for ensuring safety (in a more peaceful application) in the same way for miners' lamps. In these last it was for a long time found very difficult to get a good joint between the metallic and the glass parts of the safety-lamp, and a great many different materials were tried for filling these joints in such a way that air should not be able to pass through. In many cases the air was contaminated with a certain amount of gaseous material which would be likely to render the whole explosive, and if this got through the joint between the glass and the metal, there would be very serious risk of explosion. A great number of substances were tried but found unsatisfactory, and after some hundreds of experiments had been made by Sir Frederick Abel and Sir Warington Smyth, with asbestos washers, these were ultimately found to maintain their condition most admirably.

With regard to closing the breeches of big guns, we are

informed, also on the authority of Sir Frederick Abel, that the only contrivance which could be called an approach to a perfect arrangement, was one devised by a French artillery officer, M. Dubange, which consisted of a kind of pad of asbestos fibre attached to the breech-loading arrangement. This, from its mineral nature, was nearly indestructible, and consequently lasted without material deterioration for a great length of time, notwithstanding that it was subjected to the enormous pressures which are now developed in the bores of very heavy guns.

In connection with Whitehead torpedoes, we learn, from the same authority, that in these and other similar receptacles, within which charges of wet gun-cotton are enclosed, the use of asbestos is found to overcome a great difficulty. The vessels containing the damp cotton have to be soldered, in order to keep them perfectly air-tight, and thus prevent the water from escaping; and in order to do this with anything approaching safety the space between the gun-cotton and the metal surfaces which have to be soldered were formerly filled with damp felt wads or discs. This seemed to answer the purpose, but it was found after they had been stored for some time that the effect of the moisture on the felt was to cause it to undergo a kind of decay or fermentation, resulting in the formation of gas to such an extent that the vessels were distended, and threatened to burst, and sometimes actually did burst with considerable violence. Asbestos millboard was substituted for the felt, and the difficulty and danger were then removed; gas was no longer evolved, whilst the operation of soldering could be performed with safety, the material remaining perfectly unaltered.

In the manufacture of time-fuzes, again, asbestos washers are found most valuable. Washers of indiarubber and wash-leather were formerly used, but these in time became hard, and acted on the metal surfaces with which they came in contact in such a manner as to cement them together, instead of keeping them mobile, and it was not until the introduction of asbestos washers that difficulties, in connection with the proper action of these ingenious contrivances for the explosion of shells in a given time after their discharge, were removed.*

Experiments recently made with dynamite shells have revealed certain defects in their construction which have been overcome by the use of asbestos, and this terrible engine of warfare has been thereby in a great measure perfected.

One of the uses to which asbestos has been proposed to be applied in connection with warfare is as a coating for ironclads. It was alleged by the inventor of the process that if asbestos were packed between the armour-plates it would arrest, or certainly minimise, the inflow of water after the penetration of a ship's side below the water-line. This has already been tried by the Admiralty, and an interesting account of the trial may be found in the *Army and Navy Gazette* Supplement (August, 1887). Although this first trial was decided to have been very successful, it does not seem to have been followed up; but should further experiments in this direction confirm its success, it is obvious that confidence would be raised in our fighting ships, by practically insuring them from becoming waterlogged in action.

Some of the uses to which asbestos is proposed to be applied are sufficiently astonishing. Who, for instance, could have imagined that a substance of such specific gravity as crude asbestos could have been manufactured into a cloth, available for aeronautical purposes, in which absence of weight is of such primary importance? Yet here it appears to be the one thing wanting to give success to that despair of aeronauts, military ballooning. Many years have now passed since scientific military men first turned their attention to aeronautics, and it is long since the War Department of the Government first authorized experiments to be made, with the view of utilising balloons in warfare; yet, notwithstanding all the time and money which has been expended, the result in the way of practical success has been actually nil. No use of balloons was made even in the late Egyptian campaign, which is suffi-

* *Jour. Soc. Arts.*, No. 1743.

cient to show that, so recently as that, English military men had no great faith in their availability.

The difficulties to be encountered in this direction are doubtless sufficiently formidable. Gas, it is clear, could not be carried into a hostile country or into remote and nearly inaccessible districts. Even if procurable at all, near the battlefield, it could only be obtained by a long and difficult process of generation, at the very time when speed and simplicity would be the main factors of success. Gas, therefore, being practically out of the question, it seems to have occurred to Mr. Spencer, the well-known balloon manufacturer, that it would be better to revert to the original conception of Montgolfier. The old-fashioned fire-ball, which acquired its power of ascension from rarefied air, produced by burning straw or something similar, was of course of far too dangerous a character, and had been productive of too many fatal accidents. It was necessary, therefore, to construct a balloon of some uninflammable material, and with the assistance of his friend, Mr. Fisher, the General Manager and Secretary of the United Asbestos Company of London, Mr. Spencer ultimately succeeded in so doing. A balloon was constructed, the whole of the lower part of which was formed of fine asbestos cloth, the remainder being of canvas, covered with a fireproof solution. A trial took place in the grounds of the Welsh Harp, at Hendon, which was afterwards repeated at Chatham, under the inspection of the Royal Engineers' Committee, and on both occasions with success. The experimental balloon, about 30 feet high, was suspended between two uprights, from which it hung down like a limp rag. It was of a cylindrical shape, having a deep zone at the equator, and a containing capacity of about 30,000 feet. A copper spirit lamp was attached to the neck, and no sooner was a light put to the spirit than the inflation commenced, the balloon being fully distended in a space of about five minutes. These trials have since been successfully continued in India, and the Russian Government has adopted the balloons for use in their army.

The immense advantage gained, by this method of inflation, over the tedious and difficult process of inflation by gas is sufficiently obvious, whilst it is at the same time apparent that the quantity of spirit requisite for an endless number of ascents could be carried about with the greatest facility. Another advantage is that, whilst the large volume of gas required for an ordinary balloon is in itself both deleterious and a source of danger, the rarefied air in the new fireproof balloon is perfectly innocuous. The balloon can be raised or lowered at will simply by turning the lamp a little up or down.

In further continuance of this part of the subject, that is, the application of asbestos to matters connected with warfare, the particulars of a very interesting experiment, which may have an important bearing on the carriage of explosive material in time of war, was given by Mr. Boyd, the late Manager of the United Asbestos Company's works at Harefield, in the paper[*] before referred to. He was alluding to the value of asbestos millboard as a lining for fireproof cases and deed-boxes, so as to convert them into portable fireproof safes. The matter, he said, was put to a practical test thus: two iron rails were supported on brickwork at a height of about eighteen inches from the ground, and underneath them a strong fire of wood shavings and chips was made, and when this had well burnt up, a deed-box filled with papers was pushed along the rails to the centre of the fire, where it was completely enveloped in the flames, remaining there for a space of twenty minutes. On the box being withdrawn it unlocked easily, and the papers were found in perfect preservation, being neither charred nor discoloured.

On seeing this result, one of the gentlemen present asked if the boxes could not be used for transporting gunpowder, or other explosive substances. A quarter of a pound of powder was then put in a small bag, and placed inside another box, which was pushed along the rails into the centre of the fire, to which fresh fuel had been added; and after the box had been exposed to the fire for twenty minutes the question natu-

[*] *Jour. Soc. Arts*, No. 1743.

rally arose how was it to be got off again ? Mr. Boyd himself performed that operation, by means of a long iron rod and hook, after which the box was again opened and the powder found intact. The question was then asked by some one present who was not yet satisfied, " Why have the powder in a bag ? Let it be laid on the bottom of the box loose." This was done, and the fire ordeal repeated, again with the same result.

The Société Française des Amiantes, availing themselves of Mr. Boyd's idea, recently announced as one of their specialities, the manufacture of bâches, or awnings for military waggons. And the Chalmers-Spence Company have also secured a large contract for the supply of mail-bags made of asbestos cloth.

As yet another instance of its applicability to purposes connected with warfare, it may be interesting to mention that I have lately seen it stated that the fibre would be of great value for use as lint in hospitals and on the battle-field. Of the intrinsic value of asbestos in this form I am unable to speak, having no knowledge of the mode in which its non-absorbent character is proposed to be overcome ; but if it be a fact that it can be so used, in favourable comparison with the best lint, as stated, it is certain that its imperishable quality would be of great advantage, seeing that it could be used over and over again, only needing purification by fire after each time of using. Although, as has been recently remarked by the editor of the "*Engineer,*" we may never reach the time when our undergarments shall be purified by fire, instead of by the laundress's art; yet, short of this, many uses now fulfilled by materials, the thorough cleansing of which cannot be secured without their destruction, may possibly be better served by asbestos.

If we now turn from matters connected with warfare, to those relating to man's perpetual battle with fire, we shall find that here also asbestos stands him in good stead. Chemists are constantly bringing forward incombustible preparations of the various alkaline salts and other chemical combinations, calculated to render textile fabrics and other materials fireproof;

but most of these salts evaporate, and frequently damage the materials they are intended to preserve. It has, consequently, been imperative to find a material capable of opposing a negative action to the persistently devouring element, and up to the present time no substance has been found so efficacious in this respect as asbestos.

Probably its earliest use, for this purpose, in building operations was in regard to roofing. The utilization in Canada of the non-fibrous variety of asbestos has already been noticed; and we are informed by a New York manufacturer that the daily make at his works of a special fireproof coating for a roofing material exceeds two miles in length.

In America, where asbestos is used far more largely than it is here, it is brought into use in a variety of ways for building purposes. In the building laws of New York, Philadelphia, Boston, and other cities, special insistence is placed on its use, and very material and expensive alterations are sometimes required, by the authorities, to be made in the fittings of public buildings, in regard to its more extended use for the protection of the public. This is in many ways rendered compulsory on every one desirous of obtaining a licence, for the erection of a theatre, concert hall, library, or indeed any public building of a similar character. So carefully framed are these laws in the city of New York that, in regard to such places as these it is enacted that "all the shelving and cupboards in each and every dressing-room, property-room, and other storage-rooms, shall be constructed of metal, slate, or some fireproof material. All stage scenery, curtains, and decorations, made of combustible material, and all woodwork on or about the stage, shall be saturated with some incombustible material, or otherwise rendered safe against fire, to the satisfaction of the Commissioners of the Fire Department of the city. The proscenium curtain shall be placed at least three feet distant from the footlights, and the proscenium opening shall be provided with a fireproof metal curtain, or a curtain of asbestos, or similar fireproof material; and said fireproof curtain shall be raised at the commencement of each performance, and lowered at the close of said performance, and be operated by improved machinery for that purpose."

At the American Academy of Music, in Philadelphia, the underwriters offered a reduction of one per cent. per annum provided an asbestos curtain was placed in the house. The Fire Apparatus Committee then, it is reported, succeeded in perfecting "the only barrier of complete protection to an audience against fire in the world." This curtain, made of asbestos cloth (97 per cent. pure asbestos and 3 per cent. cotton), is 54 feet wide and 53 feet high. It is hung on wire lines, three-eighths of an inch thick, connected with a drum in the apex of the roof, and can be raised with ease by two men and lowered by one.

Again, after the disaster at the Ring Strasse Theatre, at Vienna, when attention was drawn to the great danger arising from the want of some certain and rapidly applicable means of separating the stage from the body of the theatre, the Roman Minister of Public Security issued an order that every theatre should be fitted with a fireproof curtain, capable of entirely isolating the stage from the theatre, and he indicated an asbestos cloth curtain as one that would meet the case. All the principal Roman theatres are now supplied with these curtains, the material having been furnished by the United Asbestos Company of London.

The same company make Booth & Fisher's patent asbestos double iron framed drop curtains, and Marius's patent asbestos double act drop; the former of these they have erected in Manchester, Birmingham, Edinburgh, and other places, and the latter at one or two theatres in London. These curtains have an air space between the two thicknesses of cloth, and are specially recommended by theatrical architects. The price of extra strong metallic cloth is 6s. per lb. Special precautionary measures are adopted by this company for preventing the iron frame from bulging in case of fire or sudden alteration of temperature. The asbestos cloth can also be used as an ordinary drop curtain, worked on rollers, and can be coated with asbestos paint, if desired, which effectually closes the pores of the cloth, rendering the passage of smoke absolutely impossible.

Asbestos fireproof curtains are also in use in most of the theatres in America, and are there made a speciality of by the Chalmers-Spence Company, who furnish the curtains all ready to hang, made from the best quality of cloth and yarn, both manufactured from pure asbestos fibre.

As further illustrating the great importance attached to the extended use of asbestos in New York, for the purpose of preventing the spread of conflagrations, a company was some time ago established there, with the object of extending the use of asbestos in the shape of protection shields, either to be kept permanently fixed, or hung in such a way as to be capable of being promptly applied on sudden emergency. One of these shields was exhibited at a firemen's convention held at Rochester, New York. It consisted of a sheet of pure asbestos cloth about 20 feet square, supported on an iron frame; and for the purpose of testing it, a pile of pinewood, saturated with petroleum and tar, was built up on its windward side, and then fired. The heat from this fire was so intense that spectators could not approach within 50 feet of it, on the exposed side; on the side protected by the shield, the heat was so little felt that a construction of wood and glass placed close beside it suffered no injury at all.

In France many of these shield curtains are now in use, and they are found to be as effectual in preventing asphyxiation, from the passage of the clouds of smoke, as in staying the spread of panic by a sight of the flames, which are not intercepted by the old-fashioned iron arrangements.

The terrible calamity which happened some time ago at the Opera Comique in Paris, followed by that at Exeter, set men's minds running in the direction of providing greater security from fire in theatres. Several kinds of curtain, all involving the use of asbestos, were then contrived, the motive power being so arranged as to fully guard against the destructive force of a too rapid or unexpected fall, such as happened at Toulon.

The curtain made for Terry's Theatre by the United Asbestos Company is similar to that made by them for the Queen's Theatre in Manchester, its special qualifications being lightness, strength, and ease of manipulation. A special method of preventing the iron frame from "bulging" or altering its shape in case of fire, or sudden variations of temperature, is employed. By using weights not quite sufficient to counterpoise the curtain, the work of raising and lowering is very light. Combustible ropes may be employed, which, on being released by the action of fire or otherwise, will allow the curtain to descend of itself. Pockets are provided to catch the counterbalance weight in case of the breakage of the chain, so as to prevent personal injury, and friction rollers are put on the balance weights to ensure their free action. Similar rollers are also fitted on the curtain frame, to give freedom of action in raising and lowering. The hinging of the lower part of the frame, so as to admit of its being raised to the top of the proscenium opening when there is not sufficient room for a curtain of the ordinary make to be raised above the proscenium opening, is a valuable addition. The asbestos cloth is specially strengthened by a fine wire running through each asbestos strand, and is stretched across the whole of the framework, and fastened thereto by means of hoop iron and bolts. A double thickness of asbestos cloth may be used, if thought necessary, one thickness on each side of the framework, with an air space between. This was accepted on all hands as far superior to the old-fashioned iron portcullis, which was an absolute nuisance from the harsh grating sound it made when wound slowly up or down. Queen's Theatre burned August, 1890.

Mr. Henry Irving, in bringing to the notice of the public his proposals for a "New Safety Theatre," laid special stress on the necessity of shutting off the stage from the auditorium by means of an asbestos curtain, so that in the event of fire, which generally originates on the stage, its perils should be confined to itself; with the further necessity of providing an outlet for the smoke, which is sometimes even more disastrous in its effects than the flames.

Experiments were also about this time publicly made by Captain Heath to prove the fire-resisting qualities of a new curtain invented by him, the proceedings taking place within a specially-built hoarding, in Oxford Street, within which was erected a large model of the Drury Lane proscenium. The curtain in this case was made of asbestos and canvas, and was rolled on a block of wood placed underneath the front part of the stage. The sides of the model were made of iron plates and the front of wood. When certain catches were released counterbalancing weights came into action, and the curtain was run rapidly up from below. On reaching the top, it pressed tightly and automatically against the back of the proscenium, turning on at the same time a supply of water from a perforated pipe, which ran along the whole length of the top of the curtain, so as to keep it constantly wet. The arrangement of the switch, for communicating action to the curtain, was such as to turn on the water and close the curtain at the sides at will. A very severe fire test was employed which was pronounced to be highly successful, the universal opinion of those present being that, in its construction, the curtain was as simple as it was effectual for the purpose intended.

Another novelty in this line was shown to the public on the opening night of the "Jodrell Theatre." In order to show their desire of doing everything possible for the safety of the audience, the lessees exhibited, after the evening's performance, a new "Niagara" or safety water curtain. On the drop being raised, an illuminated sheet of water was seen to be descending from the flies, in such a way as completely to shut off the stage from the audience.

Since then the Baquet Theatre in Oporto has come to the apparently natural end of all such structures, namely, by a fiery death. The calamity was caused by the wings catching fire from a gas jet, whereby the whole of the stage scenery was almost immediately afterwards enveloped in flames, the furious progress of which it was found impossible to arrest. Here, then, was a striking instance of a holocaust being caused by the want of such a curtain as has been described; for, had such a thing been available, the stage would have been at once shut off from the auditorium, and even if it had not been found possible to save the structure, the fire, at any rate, would have been localised for a sufficient length of time to have enabled the authorities to clear the building, and so have prevented the panic and horror which ensued.

And again, the Communal Theatre at Amsterdam has also succumbed to the devouring element. Here, notwithstanding that, as is reported, the major portion of the scenery "was painted with asbestos," everything was destroyed, including the costumes of the actors, and a library of 8,000 volumes.

It is worth while, perhaps, recording the foregoing, because there can be very little doubt that something of this kind will presently be made compulsory even in England, for use in theatres and music-halls generally. From the course matters are now taking in the United States, there is little doubt that the use of asbestos, in some form or other, will be made compulsory there for the shelvings and doors of public libraries and places for the custody of records, for sheathings between wooden floorings and below carpets, for hearthstones, for the linings of doors of elevators or lifts, for elevator shafts or stairways, and for the innumerable other places exposed to danger from flame or intense heat. The ease with which it can be applied, and the fact that it is absolutely impossible for flame to pass through it, makes it invaluable for purposes of this description. Where houses are constructed of wood, its non-conducting properties are found very useful, as it makes the house cooler in summer and warmer in winter than any other kind of sheathing.

In case of fire, in an adjoining house, it is quite possible the flames might destroy the outer covering; but, even then, the frame and interior would be as safe as if built of stone.

Before concluding this part of the subject, which is of such vital interest, it may be mentioned, as showing the extreme importance of the subject, that in Captain Shaw's book on "Fires in Theatres," a list is given of 112 theatres which had been destroyed by fire down to 1875. The loss of life is not mentioned in the aggregate, but, by the burning of only three of the buildings mentioned, no less than 800 lives were lost and 123 adjoining houses destroyed.

M. Mauret de Pourville, writing on the subject, says that in the years 1867 and 1868, fifteen theatres in Europe and America were destroyed by fire; the value of the property so destroyed, irrespective of loss of life, being valued at from £640,000 to £680,000; and this, Captain Shaw says, is well within the mark.

The following startling list will show what fearful calamities have taken place since 1876, by fires in theatres, and the imperious necessity which has constantly arisen of at once adopting effectual methods of protection:—

FIRES IN THEATRES, ORIGINATING PRINCIPALLY ON THE STAGE, SINCE 1876.

Place.	Dates.	Lives lost.
Theatre des Arts, Rouen	April 25th, 1876	8
Chinese Theatre, San Francisco	October 30th, 1876	19
Circus Theatre, Madrid	November 13th, 1876	2
Mrs. Conway's Theatre, Brooklyn	December 5th, 1876	283
Cronstradt Theatre	January 9th, 1881	8
Opera House, Nice	March 23rd, 1881	150
Ring Strasse Theatre, Vienna (iron curtain was not let down)	December 8th, 1881	794
Briggs' Theatre, Moscow	January 7th, 1883	300
Temporary Theatre, Dervio	June 24th, 1883	50
Theatre Govi Sanuke, Japan	August 28th, 1883	75
Tinhevelly, India	July 28th, 1886	100
Temple Theatre, Philadelphia	December 27th, 1886	2
Opera Comique, Paris (official report)	May 25th, 1887	77
Exeter Theatre	September 5th, 1887	188
Grand Theatre, Islington	January, 1888	—
Bolton Theatre	January, 1888	—
Varieties, Madrid	January, 1888	—
Theatre Royal, Blyth	February, 1888	—
Union Square Theatre, New York	February, 1888	—
Music Hall, Leith	March, 1888	—
Oporto Theatre	March, 1888	160
Total		2,216

APPLICATION TO MILITARY AND OTHER PURPOSES. 157

It is calculated that during the past eleven years 2,056 persons, or a yearly average of 184, have perished through fires in theatres, without taking into account the number of lives lost through panics.*

An extraordinary, or rather extreme, case of the use of asbestos as a protection from flames, has been recently reported from Canada, an account of which appeared in the London *New York Herald*, 25th August, 1889, which I give as narrated, being in no way responsible for the statements made. It appears that a gas well, at Ruthvan, having taken fire, the cap over the top of the pipe was so fixed that the escaping gas rushed out directly towards the ground, so as to make approach impossible, and consequently also the removal of the cap. All around the well the ground became so baked and heated that when cooling was attempted by a stream from a fire-engine, the water went up in a cloud of steam before it touched the ground. In this emergency the owners of the well offered a reward of $1,000 to any one who would remove the cap. A mining expert, named Marvin, undertook the job, and after many attempts to reach the well, made for himself a suit of asbestos clothing. In his first attempt, he had worn a heavy pair of cowhide boots, covered with wet cloths; but, before he got to the flames, the cloth had dried and burned away, and his boots were half burned off. So great was his hurry to escape that he dropped his cutting contrivance, and was dismayed to see it get red hot before his eyes. For his next trial he wore a pair of rubber boots, and inside these thrust his feet wound round with wet rags. Over these he put a heavy covering of asbestos. His asbestos coat was cone-shaped; his arms, sticking out through two holes in the cone, were wound round with several thicknesses of wet cloth, covered with a heavy coating of asbestos. His contrivance for cutting the pipe consisted of a very long and sharp chisel, fastened at right angles to an iron staff. His assistant, robed like himself, carried a long iron bar, on which was fastened a small farrier's hammer. His first stroke missed the chisel, and after two

* *Jour. Soc. Arts*, January, 1888.

where they extinguished the fire in a very short time, and so prevented what might have been a great calamity. The same course is now about to be taken in England, and the London firemen are to be protected in a similar manner; and there can be little doubt that this course will presently be universally adopted for the protection of the men engaged in saving life and property from destruction by fire. Nothing has yet been discovered that will equal asbestos for this purpose, as it will neither burn nor smoulder, and is as impervious to fire as well-made mackintosh is to water.

In a recent number of the *Canadian Mining Review* we are informed that, in the museum attached to the offices of that journal, there is to be seen a complete suit of clothing from helmet to shoes, such as is used by the firemen of Paris, dressed in which a man can walk into the hottest flame with comparative impunity. This suit was made and presented to the museum by Mr. Edward Wertheim, of the American Asbestos Company, Black Lake, and of Frankfort-on-the-Maine, Germany.

The following very interesting description of the "Appareil Aldini" is taken, by his kind permission, from Capt. Eyre M. Shaw's recent work on "Fire Protection," in which he gives it as his opinion that it is rather a matter of scientific interest than of practical usefulness. "In certain cases," Capt. Shaw says, "it may be indispensable to traverse the flames in order to reach some particular spot, and it was for the purpose of preserving persons who find themselves in such circumstances that the Chevalier Aldini, an Italian physician, thought of the apparatus which bears his name.

"This preservative apparatus consists of two vestments, one composed of a thick tissue of asbestos (amianthus), or woollen stuff, made incombustible by means of a saline solution, the other of a metallic cloth of iron wire, covering the first garment, and mounted with a helmet on the upper part.

"A person enveloped in these two garments can withstand the action of flames for some minutes without experiencing any dangerous effects, for on the one hand the external metallic tissue cools the flames, and on the other hand the internal former was protected by his skilfully made garments, from the heat to which he was exposed in appearance only, and by which the change of colour is fully explained.

The American Watch-Case Company, of Toronto, have their flooring protected by an asbestos covering, which recently saved their premises from destruction by fire. In connection with this part of the subject it may be added that various attempts have been made for the introduction of asbestos into the manufacture of lace curtains, dresses, &c., but I believe that the principal obstacle in the way of success, in this line, lies in the fact that in its present state, in the shape of curtains, for instance, it is found to be an obstinate holder of dust. This objection will, no doubt, be presently got rid of; and soon we may hope to have heard the last of those fearful scenes which have at times occurred from the firing of ladies' dresses at the footlights in theatres.

In regard to accidents from the footlights by reason of the dancers' dresses coming into contact with gas, it might be supposed that, by the substitution of the electric light, this danger would be obviated; but even the electric light, protected as the incandescence is, has its own especial source of danger, not the least singular of which may be noted in the following instance. At the Berlin Opera-House, one of the dancers, having inadvertently approached too near to a switch-board, her dress touched some metal parts between which a difference of potential existed. In the fabric of her dress metal threads had been interwoven which, bridging these metal parts, formed a short circuit and were heated by the current to such an extent as to set fire to the dress, whereby the dancer was much injured.[*]

The Chevalier Aldini's idea has been revived in Paris, the firemen there having been furnished with asbestos clothes. Immediately after this was done, it was reported in the papers that, on a conflagration occurring in the basement of a building there, the firemen arrived clad in their asbestos suits, and were thereby enabled to descend at once into the basement,

[*] "*Industries*," 2nd August, 1889.

out the child, who had in no way suffered; his skin was fresh, and his pulse, which beat 84 before the experiment, was only 96 after it. He could, without any doubt, have remained much longer in this wrapping were it not for the fear which seized him, and which was caused by one of the straps supporting the basket having slipped a little on the shoulder of the fireman who carried it. The child, at the sight of the flames which roared below them, thought he had been thrown into them. A few minutes after he was as merry as usual, and felt no uncomfortable sensation. The fireman who carried the child had before the experiment 92 pulsations a minute, and after it 116. The three others remained in the flames two minutes and forty-four seconds, and came out without having experienced anything except a sharp heat. The pulsations were before 88, 84, and 72 a minute; and after, 153, 138, and 124 a minute. The flame was continually fed with straw thrown upon that which was burning. There was very soon formed an enclosure of fire, in which the firemen were shut up, and as a portion of the straw scattered on the ground threw up a flame which at times enveloped their legs, it was certain that the bodies of the men were exposed to the direct action of the flames. At a distance of more than six yards from the focus of the fire, the heat was so intense that none of the numerous assembly could remain there. In other experiments the firemen were furnished with large shields, which they made use of to keep back the flames. It is obvious that such an apparatus as this could be of very little use for general work."

In concluding this part of the subject it may be worth remarking that in Barnum's recent Exhibition in London of the destruction of Rome by fire, surprise was constantly expressed at the wonderfully realistic way in which such apparently substantial buildings, as those erected in the representation of the Eternal City, were nightly destroyed in the conflagration. Here the whole secret lay in a liberal use of asbestos combined with skilful combination of chemical effects.

CHAPTER X.

MISCELLANEOUS APPLICATIONS OF ASBESTOS.

COLD STORAGE—Retention and Exclusion of Heat—Deck Cabins—Filtration—Filter Papers—Water Filters—Filtration of Sewage—Pipe Joints—Furnace and Kiln Linings—Crucibles—Gas Stoves—Open Fires—Fletcher's Stoves—The Leeds Stove—Plastic Stove Lining—Asbestos Paint—Insulation-Paper for Battery Plates—Gloves—Aprons—Stove Piping—Rope—Ladders—Rods in Dye-Houses—Lamp Wicks—Gas Shades—Wall Papers—Writing Paper—Cigarette Papers—Tobacco Paper—Pulp—Boards—Cork Soles—Moulds for Type—Silversmiths' and Jewellers' Moulds—Covering for Woodwork—Fireside Rugs.

FOR cold storage buildings and refrigerating chambers, the non-conducting properties of asbestos render it simply invaluable. For the preservation of meat, and all kinds of provisions brought from distant lands, specially-constructed ships containing the necessary refrigerating apparatus and chambers are in universal use; and buildings of considerable size are in existence in all populous places. These are mostly underground in London, but in New York and elsewhere many buildings are specially erected for the purpose, and these mostly have double walls surrounding the cold chambers with some kind of non-conducting material between, by way of lining, for which asbestos is largely used.

In order to show its value in the exclusion of heat, Mr. Boyd cites the case of a Channel steamer, the owners of which wished to have the boiler covered with asbestos composition. The engineer's berth, being quite close to the boiler, was unpleasantly warm even in winter; but, after the boiler had been covered in with an application of the composition, two inches thick, that functionary had a different tale to tell, the heat being so effectually confined to the boiler that the change made his berth unpleasantly cold. Again, in the case of the re-building of a seamen's floating chapel at Genoa, the old chapel, having been erected on the deck of a hulk, was found to be too expensive on account of the reparations frequently rendered necessary by the extremely high summer temperature. It was desired that the new chapel should be built of iron; but fears were expressed that, when exposed to the summer's sun, the roof and sides would get so hot as to make the temperature inside unbearable. Mr. Boyd, therefore, suggested that the space between the outer skin and the inner boarding should be filled with pulverized asbestos. Accordingly, this space, of about $1\frac{1}{4}$ inches, up the sides and over the ceiling, was tightly rammed with asbestos powder; and the result was that, while the outside temperature stood at 100°, the inside temperature, the doors and windows being kept shut, did not reach 70°, and was, therefore, in comparison, deliciously cool. Mr. Boyd consequently suggests that the deck cabins of steamers, passing through the Suez Canal, or navigating the Red Sea, should, by similar means, be made more comfortable for the passengers. Probably this object could be as easily attained by the use of "Superator," described in a previous chapter.

In the beetroot sugar refineries of France, Germany, and Austria, fine asbestos cloth is in universal use for filtering the saccharine juices. It is used also in chemical laboratories for straining and filtering acids and alkalies, which would quickly destroy any ordinary filtering paper; and it is specially useful when the liquid to be filtered is of a caustic or strongly acid nature, or where it may be desirable that the filter, with residue, should be ignited without consuming the filter, or where the residuum is to be dissolved off the filter by acids or other solvents. Asbestos filter bags are better fitted for this purpose than those made of any other material, they last longer, retain the heat better, and are more easily purified.

In many cases a very finely-divided asbestos is desirable. This is accomplished by a process recently patented in Germany by Fr. Breyer, of Vienna. The asbestos is first coarsely ground, and then mixed with some granular crystalline carbonate, which must be soluble in acids. The carbonate should possess a hardness between 3 and 4, 5, according to the mineralogical scale. The mixture is ultimately ground together in a mill, and then the mass is treated with an acid until the carbonate has been dissolved out. The escaping carbonic gas causes the asbestos fibres to be loosened and disintegrated from each other, so as to make the mass porous. It must be thoroughly washed with water before being used.

For filtration purposes generally, asbestos has proved to be so eminently adapted, by reason of its peculiar properties enabling it to resist the action of alkalies and acids, that, either in the form of cloth or finely carded fibre, which, when fouled, can be easily cleaned by hot water or steam, it forms a material adjunct to the filtering media in all the more important filters now used. All filters are modifications of the simple principle here shown, the object being the purification, by separation, of liquids from the substances held in suspension in them through the pores of the media used, which must be sufficiently fine to retain or keep back the solid matter. The filtering medium may be any substance of a sufficiently spongy or porous nature to allow of the free percolation of the liquid, the pores at the same time being sufficiently small to render it limpid or transparent.

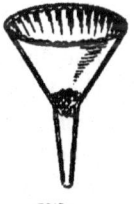

Filter.

If a large quantity of liquid has to be filtered, or if the substance is too viscid, or for acids or alkalies, a funnel of asbestos cloth suspended by a hook is found useful.

In other forms, rapidity of filtration is the point aimed at. To secure this, regard must be had to the porosity of the filtering medium, the extent of the filtering surface, the relative viscidity or mobility of the filtering liquid, the pressure or force by which the liquid is impelled through the pores of the filter, and the porosity and fineness of the substances it holds in suspension.

The various filtering media now commonly used, with the mode of applying the asbestos, will be sufficiently seen from the following examples:

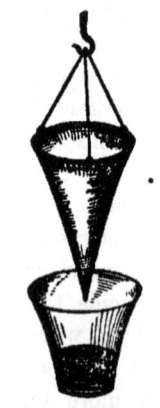

In M. Maignen's "Filtre Rapide," the apparatus consists of a hollow perforated cone of earthenware over which a specially woven asbestos cloth is stretched. Canvas or felt an inch thick was at first used for this purpose, but it was found that with soft rain water, containing ammonia, this felt became as rotten as wet blotting paper. Asbestos was accordingly suggested, but it was at first supposed that this would be too expensive, and it was some considerable time before a pure asbestos cloth could be made, of exactly the right porosity, to arrest the fine filtering medium which is used in this apparatus to purify the water chemically; but so successfully has this at length been accomplished, that Mr. Maignen anticipates that presently asbestos cloth will take the place of sand in the purification of the water supply of London. In this filter a layer of finely-powdered carbo-calcis is automatically deposited on the outside of the asbestos cloth (which is stretched over an earthenware cone), by being mixed with the water first put in; and to cleanse the filter all that is required is to deposit a fresh supply on the asbestos cloth.

Asbestos Cloth Filter Suspended.

In Judson's filter, the medium employed is said to give off minute particles of oxide of iron, which necessitates the use of a straining apparatus. To effect the required object, porous blocks or slabs of carbon, or silicates of various kinds, are used; but as these sooner or later get clogged, they have to be cleaned by brushing or scraping, or by replacing the block by a fresh one, in doing which it is difficult to prevent particles from passing round the joint. This difficulty is surmounted and perfect mechanical straining effected by substituting a layer of carded asbestos fibre for the block.

In Creswell's asbestos carbon filter (Parker's patent Niagara) the inside is quite plain, except for three or four projections, which are rounded below but shouldered on the top. These projections support a perforated stoneware tray, which carries the filter bed and unfiltered water; and any number of these trays may be used by placing them one above the other. The edges of the trays and the sides of the cistern are rendered waterproof by a flexible closely-fitting ring, so as to prevent the water, running between, carrying with it small particles of the filtering material. Whilst the upper bed detains the rougher particles of dirt and any organic matter, the water is effectually purified by the asbestos tray and the lower bed.

In Cheavin's "New Patent Removable Plater Filter," the construction is of so simple a character that the whole can be taken to pieces and the purifying medium renewed within a few minutes, whilst nothing comes in contact with the water but the stoneware, the "idiocathartes," and the asbestos cloth. The shape of this filter enables a large amount of the purifying medium to be used, over which is spread a screen of asbestos cloth, which arrests all the impurities before they are brought into contact with the idiocathartes.

Lipscombe's filter is noticeable for the simplicity with which the filtering material can be renewed. The construction is very simple, being one perforated earthenware cylinder within another, each covered with the United Asbestos Company's special asbestos cloth, with the filtering material in the intervening space.

In the filtration of sewage, and in the purification of foul gas in connection with sewer traps, and for ventilating and deodorizing manholes for cesspools and sewers, the asbestos fibre is saturated with deodorizing liquids which render the escaping gases harmless. The system of deodorizing sewer gas, formerly adopted, was to cause the gas to rise through charcoal, but the impurities soon clogged this up and prevented the passage of the gas. Messrs. Adams & Co., of York, suggested a new mode, by placing over the opening rising from the sewer a hood of galvanized wire interlaced with asbestos yarn, spun in such a way as to have good capillary action, the ends of the yarn being dipped into a liquid disinfectant. When the fibres are saturated, a disinfecting screen is formed, through the meshes of which the gases rise, and in their passage through they become purified and rendered innocuous.

For forming the joints of pipes exposed to the action of moisture, and for man and mudhole doors requiring frequent removal, asbestos woven cloth is very largely in demand. In these cases asbestos millboard, which is the cheapest form of jointing material, is comparatively worthless, if, indeed, it is not absolutely objectionable, from its permeability to water, which soaks through and attacks the iron of the bolts, and it was, therefore, necessary to devise a combination which would effectually resist the heat and damp. This is provided in what is known as Asbestos and India-rubber woven sheeting, which is made in any thickness, and is supplied either in sheets cut to the required shape, or in a tape 1 in. to 2 in. wide, which can be cut to length and bent to circle or oval without puckering. When all other materials have failed to give satisfaction, this has answered admirably, and in the case of manhole and mudhole doors and feed-water pipes the joint can be broken twenty times without requiring renewal of the strip.

The United Asbestos Co. supply "United asbestos rubber woven sheeting," which is now being superseded, for high pressures, by their asbestos-metallic "Victor" woven sheeting, in which a fine wire runs through the centre of each asbestos thread. Great durability is insured by the use of asbestos cloth, the requisite elasticity being imparted by a coating of india-rubber which fills the pores of the cloth and renders it waterproof. The "United asbestos rubber woven tape" is composed of the same materials, and being easily bent into position, without puckering, a joint can be quickly made without waste, and steam can be turned on as soon as the joint is screwed up. For manhole and mudhole doors, which have to be frequently opened, it is simply invaluable.

Being one of the most refractory substances known, asbestos is used in a variety of ways for the lining of furnaces. When the metal and fire are together, as in the cupola, or blast furnace, it constitutes a most enduring and heat-confining lining, and is particularly adapted for use where the metals or ores contain sulphides, as sulphides have no effect on asbestos. As linings for furnaces and kilns, and for use in the manufacture of crucibles, a patent has been granted for an improved refractory material composed of a mixture of the aluminous asbestos from Natal with fire clay, in the proportion of one part of asbestos to four of fire clay. Both are finely pulverized and formed into the desired shapes, while in a plastic state. The patentee states that if a material of greater fire-resisting properties is required, the worn out "saggers" are pulverised, and a fresh supply of fire clay equal to double the amount of powdered "sagger" is added. When this material is exposed to extraordinary heat it does not crack; but, on the other hand, it tends to fuse and bind its particles closer together. Another convenient property of the material is that it is capable of resisting the attacks of atmospheric and chemical substances, such as damp, sewage, &c. This special form of asbestos is stated to be additionally valuable both on account of its cheapness and the convenient form in which it is imported.

Perhaps the most popular conception of the use of asbestos is that where it figures in gas stoves; but there are so many varieties of these, and generally they are so well known, that little need be here said about them.

From an Englishman's point of view, engendered by long habit and the damp and chilly climate in which he lives, there is nothing to which he attaches so much importance as the luxury of a visible fire. The stoves and warming apparatus mostly in vogue elsewhere, excellent as they are in their way, are simply nothing to him in comparison with the comfort and cheerful appearance of his open fire, even when, as is only too frequently the case, the unscientific construction of his fire-place causes nine-tenths of the heat from the fuel to be lost in the chimney. When living in Canada, in rooms comfortably warmed by the stoves in use there, on re-entering from the keen air outside, I always felt an irresistible desire to kick open the stove door and revel in the cheerful blaze, and enjoy the sight of the flames rippling over the logs. It is only by very slow degrees that a more scientific manner of warming houses or rooms in England can make its way, such is the obstinate conservation of the people and their disinclination to move out of the old-fashioned ways of their fathers. For sometime past, however, practical men have been drawing attention to this subject, with the praiseworthy object of showing how to obtain the maximum of heat from a minimum of fuel, reserving at the same time the luxury of the visible fire. There is more than fancy in this, because heat, radiating directly from glowing coals, passes through the air without modifying its temperature in any important degree; consequently, coming in contact with the person it imparts warmth to the body, whilst leaving the air comparatively cool. For public rooms, or places which people simply pass through, warm air stoves are both economical and satisfactory, but for places where people remain seated for any length of time, the comparatively low temperature of the floor and walls, which always occurs when warm air alone is used, combined with the effect of the warm air on the lungs, causes an unpleasant feeling, which is not felt when moving about. Unless, therefore, the difference between radiant heat and warm air be taken into consideration it is not possible properly to appreciate the comparative value of the different systems. Registration by thermometer is no guide to comfort, and is useless in estimating the value of radiant heat. Acting on these principles Messrs. Fletcher, of Warrington, have produced an asbestos gas-fire respecting which the committee of the Gas Institute state, in a report issued by them, that in regard to floor temperature the highest recorded at the floor level, which may be taken as synonymous with comfort of body and warm feet, was obtained by it. Gas used in this way costs less than coal for making a room comfortably warm.

Another good stove is the "Leeds," which was shown at the Brussels Exhibition. Here the flame is made to impinge on an asbestos block, which it brings to a white heat, insuring complete combustion and the total absence of noxious vapours. In this case the heat is thrown, by direct radiation, on to the floor, which is undoubtedly the most hygienic way of heating rooms.

"Plastic stove lining" is composed of asbestos or other fireproof material prepared in the form of a cement, so that it can be used for the lining of cooking and heating stoves, as well as the fire doors of boiler furnaces, &c.

In regard to the fibre used in gas fires, the best long silky fibre is worth 10s. per lb.; 2nd quality, 3s. 6d.; and the asbestos fuel 6d. per lb., or 32s. 6d. per cwt.

The demand for asbestos paint is continually increasing. It is used largely in the Houses of Parliament and other public buildings, as it was at the several Exhibitions at South Kensington. The whole of the buildings at the "Healtheries" were coated with asbestos paint supplied by the United Asbestos Company; and, in his presidential address to the Institute of Civil Engineers, Sir Frederick Bramwell stated that these buildings owed their escape, during an outbreak of fire, to the fact that their walls were covered with asbestos paint. And at the "Fisheries" in 1883, the Prince of Wales, as Chairman of the general committee, announced that, owing to the use of asbestos paint, they had been enabled to insure the buildings and contents at fifty per cent. less than usual.

50 lbs. weight of asbestos paint is sufficient to coat about one hundred square yards of wrought timber primed in the usual way: for unwrought timber the quantity must be increased according to the condition of the wood. On rough wood one coat will offer great resistance to flame.

The woodwork in buildings constitutes, of course, the greatest danger from fire. Every one knows the difficulty of lighting a fire without wood; neither paper nor shavings are of any use, as these will only blaze up brightly and then burn out without firing the coal, though they will readily light up the wood which will inflame the coal. When, therefore, the woodwork of a building catches fire there is great danger, because the flame emitted is a clear flame of great penetrative power, which is the cause of the rapid spread of the fire from the starting point to staircases and passages affording communication from room to room. If all wooden fittings could be replaced by iron, many a fire would burn itself out, and ample time would be afforded for the engines to arrive before the conflagration could assume unmanageable proportions. But in the great majority of cases iron fittings are an impossibility, and there is no alternative to the use of wood.

Many attempts, consequently, have been made to render wood uninflammable. So long ago as July 1871, Mr. Frederick Ransome experimented in a wooden shed partly painted with siliceous paint, which was set on fire. The unpainted portion was completely destroyed, while that which was protected by the siliceous covering escaped ignition, and although deeply charred never took fire at all. The composition of the paint was analogous to that of Ransome's patent stone ; it consisted principally of a mixture of pure silex and soluble silica, converted into an insoluble siliceous covering by an outer coating of chloride of calcium. Although this invention promised well at the time it never came into extended use. But the idea of covering wood with a fire-resisting surface having been published, it was taken up and improved upon by others. The refractory quality of asbestos being well known, Mr. Thaddeus Hyatt, who had already spent much pains upon developing the industrial uses of asbestos, endeavoured to turn it to account in the protection of buildings against fire in the form of a coating of cement. He ground the shorter and less valuable fibres into a slip or paste, analogous to porcelain slip, and combined it with gelatinous silica, either alone or in conjunction with magnesia, baryta, alumina, or lime.

In 1881, Mr. E. G. Erichsen, of Copenhagen, who had been connected with the earlier experiments at the works of Mr. Ransome, brought out a new protective composition in which there is likewise a large percentage of asbestos. When intended for use as a paint or enamel it is composed of a siliceous solution, pulverised asbestos, metallic oxides and chalk, the asbestos forming 10 to 20 per cent. of the whole. Applied as a paint, it forms a fireproof enamel, capable of resisting a white heat. It is worked, upon brickwork and woodwork, with an iron trowel or wood plate covered with felt; it can be laid on in a thicker or thinner coat as may be desired, and can be cleaned from time to time with hot water.

The latest fireproof paint is the invention of Mr. C. J. Mountford, of Birmingham, whose patents have been acquired by the United Asbestos Company. This is simpler in its composition than the last, and consists of asbestos ground and re-ground in water, aluminate of potash or soda, and silicate of potash and soda. When it is to be exposed to the weather it is combined with oil, driers and gummy matters, and in some cases with zinc oxide or barytes. But by far the best material for a fireproof paint is steatite, which, like asbestos, is a silicate of magnesia.

For insulation purposes asbestos is much in use by electrical engineers in the form of millboard, in the construction of dynamos; and cables and leads, covered with plaited yarn, have been adopted in several installations. It is also made into tubes, fitted into sockets, for joining the lengths, and with elbows for turning corners. The advantage of an insulator, formed from a material unaffected by heat or damp, is plain enough. Cheapness of production, however, is very essential, as in this class of work asbestos is brought into competition with other materials, which though not possessing all its advantages, are more easily procurable and require less special adaptation in their manufacture.

A special quality of asbestos paper is made for wrapping battery plates in; and gloves are made of asbestos cloth for holding red-hot crucibles;[*] others of a lighter make, lined with rubber, enable the engineer to handle the wires with comparative impunity. Another non-conducting material is supplied for the wires, which, whilst preserving their perfect in-

[*] Watt's "Dic. Chem." Art. Asbestos.

sulation, guards them equally against risk from fire and damage from contact with water. Tubes are made for providing a non-conducting covering for electric wires, both fire and waterproof, which preserve a perfect insulation.

For the special class of work which relates to fuses and incandescent circuits there seems, at present, to be some difficulty, brought about by the contact of asbestos with copper; the former, for some unexplained reason, appearing to exercise an injurious effect upon the latter. The fuses for high tension currents used for transformers are made of copper wire, passed through sheets of asbestos, so as to break the arc when the fuse goes. In this application it may be that asbestos exerts some peculiar corrosive action on the copper wire, as, at the points of contact, the wire turns green and soon eats away.

Again, the non-conducting and fire-resisting properties of asbestos render it invaluable to iron and steel manufacturers for lining or covering the tubes employed to convey hot air from the stoves to the furnaces or cupola.

Its usefulness also for firemen's and stokers' aprons, or, indeed, for any one working in dangerous proximity to fire or sparks, as well as for salvage blankets, needs no comment.

In the United States an improved stove piping is made from asbestos, which in appearance exactly resembles cast iron. These have the additional valuable properties of extreme lightness, combined with great strength and a capability of ornamentation unobtainable with the cast-iron pipes mostly in use; paint, in the case of the asbestos pipes, not scaling off under heat as it will do in the case of ordinary iron pipes, nor will it even blister under the most trying circumstances. The manufacturers of these pipes claim for them that they combine the strength of steel with the lightness of paper.

Capability of ornamentation is a noteworthy feature in all similar cases, as well as in floor cloths, panellings, and such like goods which are all capable of being made ornamental and of being coloured and brought out in shades and patterns so as to harmonize with their surroundings. Composition mouldings, in imitation of stone, wood, metal, or bronze, old oak or

MISCELLANEOUS APPLICATIONS OF ASBESTOS. 175

other carvings in relief look remarkably well, and, if treated with dark distemper oakstain and oiled, singularly resemble the genuine carved oak, whilst possessing the additional advantage of being fireproof.

Possessing great tensile strength, and, as we have seen, being entirely unaffected by heat, asbestos rope at once asserts its applicability for a great variety of purposes, such as sash-lines and ropes for fire-escapes. Such a ladder as is here represented fitted with gun-metal heart thimbles, to attach to hooks or fasteners, will sustain the weight of two or three men with perfect impunity. The weight of a fifty-foot ladder of this description is about sixteen pounds only. It is related in the history of a man of fashion, a millionaire who died not long since, that he was accustomed to say when speaking of danger from fire, that he would never go to bed in a strange house without having an apparatus of knotted rope affixed to a ring in the wall, so that he might lower himself to the ground on an emergency. On one occasion when asserting this, he was asked, What if the rope itself took fire? Had he known of its existence, he might have replied, "Let it be an asbestos rope."

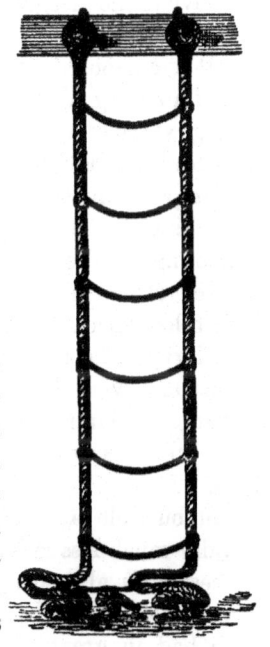

Asbestos Rope-ladder.

In dyeing and printing cloth it is frequently necessary to hang the fabric in loops from parallel rods for exposure to steam, air or ammonia. In order that it should hold upon the rods, without straining or slipping, rope or strips of cloth are usually wound around the poles, but this does not remove, although it mitigates, the difficulty, because the heat and corrosive action of the vapours will rot any covering, the first notice of the deterioration being generally the appearance of small pieces of rod-covering among the cloth which is in process of finishing. Asbestos rope and cloth are now largely manufactured and used for this purpose in the United States, with very beneficial results.

Indestructible wicks are used in some forms of safety lamps, their cost being slightly above that of ordinary wicks. These are specially useful to all who make use of mineral or heavy oils, as they obviate the disagreeable task of daily trimming: an asbestos wick can be used for twelve months without any trimming at all. It is composed of the finest asbestos fibre, made in the form of a strong soft wick, which can be used, if desired, as a packing, wound or packed round small steam or other valve stems, and for many other purposes.

A lamp which can be used as a night lamp, fire lighter, or for cooking, has been recently patented as "The Devonshire Everlasting Candle." It consists of an outer casing of metal, glass, or other material, with a perforated bottom; and is nearly filled with a porous earthy substance, which the inventor calls "Egyptian clay," by which the oil is absorbed. The indestructible wick is made of slag-wool and asbestos fibre. To charge the lamp it is placed on a saucer or plate containing the oil, which is drawn up and absorbed by the porous material within.

Incombustible and non-arsenical asbestos gas shades are naturally much less risky than the ordinary paper shades.

Asbestos is also manufactured into wall and ornamental papers; coloured wall papers, practically indestructible by fire, can be had in great variety. After severe heat tests, these retain their colourings and letterings as clearly impressed and as visible as before. They show up colours in a brighter fashion than ordinary paper, and are therefore specially useful for theatrical side scenes.

Jagnaux (p. 552) speaks of its use in a similar way in France, saying:—"On prépare avec les débris d'amiante, ainsi qu'avec une variété cotonneuse de cette matière, une pâte avec de l'eau et du silicate du soude, et cette mixtion peut remplacer la couleur à la céruse ou au blanc de Meudon pour la peinture des châssés employés pour les décors du théâtre."

Asbestos papers for writing and printing are a great desideratum. We have already noted Dr. Bruckmann's experiments in this direction; but actual successful experiment in the fabrication of paper has been greatly thwarted by the natural affinity of asbestos for water. Few kinds of asbestos are suited for paper making, and, even when the right quality is obtained, special treatment is necessary. A patent for asbestos papermaking was granted in 1853, and in this case the pulp was mixed with alum, with the object of producing a fairly indestructible paper. The low price of some descriptions of the mineral, coupled with its heat-resisting and low heat-conducting powers, have led to constant experiments in America for its use in paper-making. Most of the papers thus made contain only about one-third of their weight of asbestos. Some of them will burn with a flame, leaving a white residue which, if the sheet be carefully handled, will retain its shape, the writing, with common ink, being perceptible even after the organic substance of the paper is consumed.

A very good class of asbestos paper was some time ago manufactured in Paris, but the principal defect of all asbestos papers is the natural tendency to work up more like blotting paper than ordinary writing paper. It will be readily seen that, when the difficulties incident to its manufacture are successfully overcome, how invaluable such papers would be for bankers' and merchants' books, registers, deeds, and permanent records of all kinds. A good deal of the inherent difficulty has now been surmounted, but still the best writing paper produced is too tender, and any writing upon it is apt to disappear if the paper be subjected to a red heat.

Some time ago a firm in New York had its price lists printed on asbestos paper, and at the present time the Chalmers-Spence Company produce a class of paper as capable of receiving good impressions from type as any in use in modern books.

Cigarettes were recently sold in London having a case of asbestos paper, the object apparently being to get rid of the objectionable burnt paper in ordinary cigarettes. In this case the tobacco burnt out leaving the paper intact; but as these cigarettes have now disappeared it is presumed they met with no success.

The last new thing in this line is a "tobacco paper and compound tobacco asbestos mixture." The inventor makes paper from tobacco, rendering it more fibrous by adding a percentage of asbestos. The paper is cut up like cigarette paper, and a number of these leaflets are put up together in book form. To use it you take out a leaf and roll it up between your fingers, and it is then ready for smoking. As asbestos has neither taste nor smell, it does not interfere with the flavour of the tobacco, whilst the evil effects of smoking paper are obviated. The mixture is so made up that the asbestos is not observable in the mixture. It is very cool to smoke and consumes the nicotine in the tobacco, whilst it burns right down to the bottom of the pipe. A pipe smoked with this tobacco-asbestos is said to be always dry and to leave no filthy moisture in the stem.

In a recent number of *L'Industrie Moderne* there appeared an account of a new process invented by a Mr. Ladewig for manufacturing pulp and paper from asbestos fibre, which he asserts will not only resist the action of both fire and water, but will absorb no moisture; this pulp, he says, may also be used as a stuffing and for the joints of engines. He further proposes to use it, in the form of a solid cardboard, as a roofing material for light structures. The process of manufacture consists in mixing about 25 per cent. of asbestos fibre with about 25 or 35 per cent. of powdered sulphate of alumina. This mixture is moistened with an aqueous solution of chloride of zinc. The mixture is washed with water and then treated with an aqueous solution of ammoniacal gas. The mixture is again washed, and then treated with a solution composed of one part of resin soap and eight or ten parts of water mixed with an equal bulk of sulphate of alumina, which should be as pure as possible. The mixture thus obtained should have a slightly pulpy consistency. Finally, there is added to it 35 per cent. of powdered asbestos and 5 to 8 per cent. of white barytes. This pulp is treated with water in an ordinary paper machine, and worked just like paper pulp. (*Vide post*, p. 209.)

In order to manufacture a solid cardboard from asbestos which shall be proof against fire and water, and capable of serving as a roofing material, sheets of common cardboard, tarred or otherwise prepared, are covered with the pulp. The application is made in a paper machine, the pulp being allowed to flow over the cardboard.

Boards can be made in any thickness from that of the thinnest card to heavy shelving, fit either for partitions in safes, or for use in large libraries. I have been informed by a Canadian manufacturer that, in his early attempts to manufacture millboard, he could not get it stiff enough and tried a mixture of cotton fibre; but, after exposure to fire, the board again became limp, and that he was ultimately successful by the use of potato starch, (mixed to about the consistency used by laundresses,) stirred up with the pulp, and that then, after the application of fire to the finished board, it remained firm and stiff.

Asbestos has also been proposed to be used as an inner sole or lining for boots and shoes, with the object of keeping the feet warm in winter and cool in summer, the material possessing the double advantage of being at once a preserver of heat and a protector from cold. A patent has recently been taken out for this, and I have now a pair of asbestos socks in my possession. They are formed of a thin sheet of asbestos paper enclosed in a calico cover, and are intended to be used by slipping the so-called sock into the boot, like an ordinary cork sole.*

Respecting the use of asbestos in type foundries in France, Jagnaux says (p. 552): "On se serte dans l'imprimerie du

---

* The Laplanders gather what is called the "Lapp Shoegrass," of which there are two varieties, the *Carex ampullarea* and the *Carex vesicarea*, both of which grow near pools. This they place and wear in their shoes, it having the peculiarity of retaining heat, and keeping the feet so warm that cold can be defied.

papier d'amiante pour la confection de certaines moules dans lesquelles on coule les caractères typographiques. Ces moules ou flans se font tout simplement en encrustant le cliché dans un papier compressible. Lorsqu'on emploie le papier d'amiante on peut se servir une vingtaine de fois du même moule, tandisque ceux qui sont faits en papier ordinaire sont carbonisées après la deuxième ou troisième opération. Le papier d'amiante sert aussi à doubler les decors de théatre (marouflage) qu'il met aussi à l'abri de l'incendie. On emploi également l'amiante pour envelopper les cables télégraphiques; en effet, il presente sur la gutta percha l'avantage d'être infusible, tandisque cette dernière substance commence à fondre vers 50°, c'est-à-dire à une température qu'on observe frequemment dans le sol, en Algérie par example; aussi notre armée d'Afrique a-t-elle adopté ces enveloppes d'amiante."

Special asbestos moulds are manufactured for a variety of purposes by the Chalmers-Spence Company, such as for silversmiths' and jewellers' soldering work; a few of which are mentioned here, as specimens of the adaptation of asbestos to this particular class of manufacture. One of them is a patent watch case and jewellery soldering block.

This block is a homogeneous body of porous asbestos, which will neither break, crack, nor disintegrate under the most intense blowpipe heat, and is at the same time of such a refractory nature that the block may be held in the hand with perfect safety while one end is in the blowpipe flame. It is of so porous a character that binding wires or pins can be readily inserted, whereby small objects of jewellery can be easily and quickly secured to its surface; whilst being indestructible, the block can be used over and over again.

The block specially made for watch-case manufacturers is in cup form and of the proper size to hold a watch case. With the cup, but separate from it, is a handle provided with a metal frame or socket, on which the cup is placed when ready for use; and with each block a box of asbestos paste is furnished for protecting the delicate parts of fine work, in using which the fibre is moistened, and the jewel or case embedded in the paste. Another block, made for a similar purpose, is shown thus:

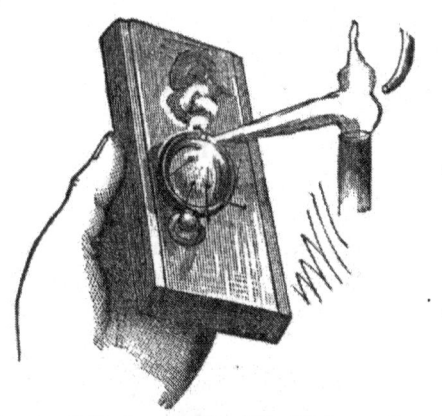

Asbestos Watch-case Soldering-block. (The Chalmers-Spence Company.)

Professor Tyndall explains that the transmission of heat is powerfully influenced by the mechanical state of the body through which it passes. Pure silica, in the state of hard rock crystal, is a better conductor than bismuth or lead, but if the crystal be reduced to powder, the propagation of heat is exceedingly slow. Through transparent rock-salt, heat is copiously conducted, but through common table salt very feebly. Asbestos, he explains, is composed of certain silicates in a fibrous condition; and he could place some asbestos in his hand, and in it a red hot iron ball, which he could hold without inconvenience. That the division of the substance should interfere with the transmission might be reasonably inferred, for heat being motion, anything which disturbs the continuity of the molecular chain, along which the motion is conveyed, must affect the transmission. In the case of asbestos, the fibres are separated from each other by spaces of air; the motion has, therefore, to pass from solid to air, and from air to solid, and it is easy, consequently, to see that the transmission of vibratory motion through this composite texture must be very imperfect.*

* Tyndall on "Heat."

182 ASBESTOS.

Another of the Chalmers-Spence moulds is a patent ingot block for soldering, melting, and moulding ingots; this is provided with a basin and mould, and the metal being placed in the mould and covered with a piece of charcoal to confine the heat, is quickly melted. An asbestos lid is held over the block and the melted metal allowed to run from the channel into the mould where the ingot is formed.

There are many other blocks of various descriptions manufactured by them, all of an exceedingly useful character; the patent ring block, for instance, for soldering stone set rings, is manufactured in cup form containing an asbestos paste. The ring being partially buried, with its

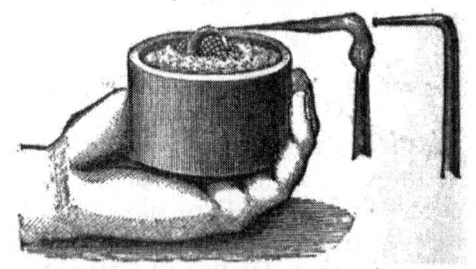

Patent Ring-block for Soldering Stone-set Rings.
(The Chalmers-Spence Company.)

stone embedded in the paste, an asbestos braid is passed through the ring as a shield, and the exposed portion can then be soldered without the slightest danger of injury to the stone. Spectacle and eye-glass blocks as shown on opposite page are formed for use in much the same way, so as to be of great assistance to the makers of these things.

A kind of tapestry is manufactured in France out of pulverized asbestos. The asbestos is reduced to powder in such a way as to preserve the short fibres, which are bound together by means of a cement. This product, which is about one-half asbestos, is stretched over a wire gauze, and when finished will take a fine polish. Woodwork covered by this material is thus rendered fireproof, and can be used for the interior lining of safes or wooden cupboards containing deeds or other articles necessary to be preserved. Chloride of zinc, which is used in the manufacture of a certain class of incombustible cloths, is volatile at a high temperature, and its vapours then become so dangerous that it is impossible to enter a room the woodwork of which has been protected by this salt, when exposed to a temperature at which ordinary wood will take fire.

Asbestos is also used in America in the manufacture of fireside rugs, which are woven in plain colours for after decoration.

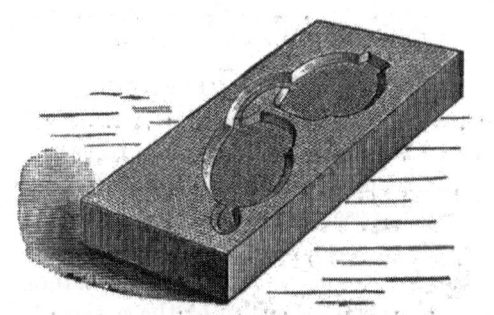

Spectacle-block. (The Chalmers-Spence Company.)

The foregoing comprise some only of the very numerous and diverse applications of asbestos which might be referred to or described; and this part of the subject must necessarily be far from complete; indeed, it would be impossible to make it so, without adding to it day by day as the constantly increasing items of special usefulness are brought forward. The writer trusts, however, that the matters described are sufficient not only to indicate the almost universal use of this singular mineral, but to confirm the statement with which he started, that asbestos is one of Nature's most marvellous productions.

CHAPTER XI.

SUBSTITUTES AND SIMILARITIES.

Slag Wool—Origin of—Pele's Hair—Properties of Slag Wool—Defects
—Rock Wool—Patent Fire and Sound Proof Plastering—Infusorial-
earth or Fossil-meal—Woodite—Whaleite—Wood Wool.

Among the numerous materials and compounds put forward as substitutes for asbestos, slag wool possesses very high qualifications as a non-conductor and a fire resister; it is applicable to many similar uses, and as to some of the purposes to which it is applied, it presents by no means insignificant qualities as a competitor.

Its history is singular. That curious natural production of the lava beds of Hawaii, called by the natives Pele's hair, (Pele being the name of the goddess who is supposed to dwell in the crater of Kilauea), doubtless originally suggested the manufacture.

Pele's hair is a basic glass, a filamentary variety of obsidian, containing long cylindrical cavities. Its production is brought about by gusts of wind crossing the viscid lava at the moment of its projection into the air by the steam escaping from the surface of the lava lake, its action in this way forming a kind of natural spun glass.* Miss Gordon Cumming † describes it as a silky volcanic hair, comparing it to the byssus of certain shells, and says that handfuls of it can occasionally be collected from the rocks to which it has drifted, most of it having a sort

---

* " Some very fine glutinous lavas are drawn out into fine filaments as portions are tossed into the air by the escaping steam."—Geikie, " Geol."
† " Fire Fountains of Hawaii."

of pear-shaped drop attached to one end. It is brittle to handle, yet the birds collect it for lining their nests. Its composition, which is as follows, will sufficiently account for the brittleness :—

Silica	51·19
Magnesia	18·16
Peroxide of iron	30·26
	99·61

The formation of this volcanic hair was very carefully watched by Professor Dana, the celebrated American geologist, who was one of the scientific party sent out by the United States Government in 1836-42, as a Government Exploring Expedition, and he has given the following interesting account of the process, as it was carried out under his eyes.*

At one of the pools of the crater by which he stood, the formation of this capillary volcanic glass was going on; and, as it was carried away by the wind, it thickly covered the surface of the rocks to leeward, where it lay like mown grass, its threads lying parallel, and pointing away from the pool. It soon became apparent, as he watched the operation, that it proceeded from jets of liquid lava, thrown up by the process of boiling. The currents of air blowing across these jets, bore off small points and drew out a glassy fibre, such as is produced in the common mode of working glass. This delicate fibre floated on till the heavier end brought it down, and then the wind carried over the lighter capillary extremity. Each fibre was usually ballasted with the small knob which was borne off from the lava jet by the wind. Mark Twain, who witnessed the scene by night, says that through their glasses the little fountains scattered about looked very beautiful. "They boiled and coughed and spluttered, and discharged sprays of stringy red fire, of about the consistency of mush, from ten to fifteen feet in the air, along with a shower of brilliant white

* "U.S. Geological Exploring Expedition," 179.

sparks—a quaint and unnatural mingling of gouts of blood and snowflakes."*

The scoria from which the fibre is made, or rather the lava that would have constituted scoria, had it cooled upon a floating stream, is mostly glassy in texture, a kind of ferruginous basaltic obsidian, the result of rapid cooling. This scoria has the following composition :—

Silica	50·00
Protoxide of iron	28·72
Lime	7·40
Alumina	6·16
Potash	6·00
Soda	2·00
	100·28

Professor Dana's description was very suggestive, but the time was not yet ripe for any practical result. A year or two passed on, and then Percy, the metallurgist, whilst on a visit to Dowlais, was struck by the formation of a hair-like form of slag, bearing a strongly marked semblance to Pele's hair, which he thus describes.† A little slag was seen to be leaking out through the clay-stopping, which was placed round one of the twyers at the back of the hot-blast furnace, and as it was in the act of escaping it was caught by the regurgitating blast, and blown out into fine threads, intermingled with minute adherent globules of glassy slag, which so exactly resembles Pele's hair that one cannot be distinguished from the other.

The mode of manufacture of this slag fibre, and its usefulness for a variety of purposes, was now very quickly seen; it was not to be supposed that the method of production having once been pointed out, it would long remain without some attempt at utilization. The form was singularly suggestive, especially when the composition of the slags produced in metallurgical operations is considered; these being essentially

* "The Innocents at Home."
† Percy on "Metallurgy," art., "Slags."

compounds of silica with earths, chiefly lime, magnesia and alumina, or with metallic oxides, such as protoxides of iron or manganese;[*] the three principal constituents being silica, lime, and alumina, the silica being the acid which neutralises the other two bases.

The way was now clear for the introduction of a new material to compete with asbestos which, although rapidly growing in favour, especially for engineering purposes, was dear. The brittleness and glassy texture of the slag fibre was certainly against it, as were also the small metallic pellicles, which it was found could not be entirely eliminated; still, if birds could utilize it for lining their nests, it was manifest that there were many useful purposes to which it could be applied; and these have, on continued experience of its qualities, so multiplied, that the material is now in considerable demand.

Attention was early directed to this substance by Mr. Charles Wood, of Middlesbrough, in a paper read by him before the Society of Arts, some time back, and to whom we are indebted for so many improved methods of dealing with slag that he is termed by Mr. Gilbert Redgrave "the pioneer of slag utilization."

Commonly spoken of as "slag-wool," this refuse production of the blast-furnace, which has hitherto so detrimentally encumbered the ground, and disfigured the country round about all the seats of the iron industry, offers a notable example of the utilization of waste products. If we take Mr. Redgrave's estimate of the annual production of cast iron in the United Kingdom alone at 13,600,000 tons, and the weight of the refuse slag at 1¾ tons per ton of pig iron, it will be seen that the vast heaps of this refuse by-product are increasing at the rate of upwards of 18,000,000 tons annually. This enormous mass of refuse, therefore, encumbers the ground to such an extent that, irrespective of any profit to be derived from its utilization, it is manifest what enormous advantages would be gained by its dispersion.

[*] "The Useful Metals and their Alloys," Pickett, 623.

In America slag wool, which is there termed "mineral wool," is manufactured by the "Western Mineral Wool Company," of Cleveland, in the State of Ohio. In England it goes by the name of "silicate cotton," and although the use of it here does not progress in anything like an equal ratio with its advance in estimation in the States, it is manufactured on a considerable scale at Middlesbrough for Messrs. Frederick Jones & Co., of Kentish Town, and their agents, Messrs. D. Anderson & Co., of Bow.

The process of manufacture consists in subjecting a small stream of molten slag to the impelling force of a jet of steam or compressed air, which divides it into innumerable small spherules, forming a spray of spark-like objects; the slag being dispersed, or broken up, by the jet of steam into countless small bead-like particles, each of which, as it is blown away, carries behind it a thread of finely drawn-out slag in extremely delicate filaments. This process is aptly compared by Mr. Redgrave to that of the production of the threads which are drawn out from sealing-wax when the latter is hastily withdrawn from the paper. These fine threads are sometimes two or three feet in length, and occasionally much longer; these readily break up into much smaller ones, which, in bulk, look like a mass of cotton of a somewhat dingy white colour, the length and fineness of the threads being dependent upon the fluidity and composition of the material under treatment. When the slag is of the proper consistency the shot are small at the outset, and to some extent are absorbed into the fibre; but in no case will they entirely disappear; it accordingly becomes necessary either to separate the two by strong currents while still in mid-air, or else to put the bulk through a riddling machine. The finer and lighter threads are carried away from the shot, the heavier fibres making a gradual separation between the extreme fine and the coarse. In order to collect the fibres and separate them from the beads, or heavier portion of the slag, the jet is now arranged at the open mouth of a cylinder of sheet iron, in which a strong air current is induced by means of additional jets of steam. This tube or shaft is furnished with a shield or striking plate, which detains the heavier particles, the lighter slag wool being carried by the draught upwards and onwards into a large chamber, constructed like a gigantic meat safe, having its walls formed of wire netting with about sixteen meshes to the square inch. Here the steam condenses and escapes, and the slag wool, which may be aptly compared to flakes of snow, is deposited on the floor and round the sides, the lighter portions being carried to the greater distances, some flakes even attaching themselves to the ironwork of the roof. The filaments of slag formed in this way, though of considerable length, are of such delicacy and fineness that they are broken up into numberless fragments and felted together into a substance much resembling cotton wool.*

The product of the blast is divided into two classes :—

The Ordinary, which includes all the fibre weighing over 14 lbs. and less than 24 lbs. to the foot cube ; and

The Extraordinary, which comprises all that comes under 14 lbs. to the foot cube.

Mr. Charles Wood found the product to possess the following valuable qualities :—

1. Extreme lightness and absolute fire-proofness (to which the American manufacturers add that it is also frost-proof, vermin-proof, sound-proof, indestructible, and odourless).

2. Marvellous powers as a non-conductor of heat and sound.

3. So great an amount of porosity that it will absorb large quantities of water, and readily retain it for a considerable time.

Although the resemblance of this material, so far as its outward appearance is concerned, to wool and cotton is so close as to have given rise to the names mineral wool and silicate cotton, by which it is known in America and England respectively, yet this is as far as the comparison can be followed. The hollow-jointed structure of the organic fibre, which gives it its flexibility and spinning and felting qualities, is altogether wanting in slag wool ; which, as already shown, is simply spun-glass of irregular thickness, without elasticity or any such

* See Mr. Gilbert Redgrave's description, *Jour. Soc. Arts*, No. 1,941.

features as the imbrications or spicules of wool or cotton necessary for facilitating the weaving process. There are, indeed, certain rough surfaces and markings on the fibre incident to its make, but these are only visible under a strong lens. The drawing out of the fibres is a purely mechanical operation, and is a remarkable illustration of some of the various forms mineral substances will assume under different conditions of cooling.

One cubic foot of slag will weigh 192 lbs., and the same weight of ordinary mineral wool measures 8 cubic feet; the wool fibres, therefore, encase eight times the quantity of air which is contained in the slag. In other words, the cubic foot before conversion contains 100 per cent. of material and after conversion only 12 per cent.; the product consequently contains 88 per cent. of its volume of air. The extra grade has 92 per cent. of its volume of air, and is consequently much superior to the ordinary as a non-conductor; but even in the finest product there is a great dissimilarity in the shape and thickness of the fibres. Slag wool, therefore, consists essentially of fine interlocking mineral fibres forming a mass of minute air-cells which give it its property of a non-conductor; air, when unconfined, being so subtle and rapid in movement, and so slow to convey heat, except by its own motion, that mineral wool forms a good distributor of heat, and at the same time presents the greatest barrier to its transmission, according to whether it has or has not freedom to circulate. If the air-confining substance is not very loose and porous it will be found to transmit heat, and the reduction of the percentage of volume of air, by making the material more compact, develops its capacity for conducting heat.

As illustrating this view, the following tables have been published by the Western Mineral Wool Company, which are worth quoting here for several reasons applicable to the subject. No. 1 was prepared by Mr. J. J. Coleman, and was read by him before the Philadelphia Society of Glasgow, and No. 2 was compiled in order to show the non-conducting properties of different materials at even thickness:—

SUBSTITUTES AND SIMILARITIES.

No. 1. Relative heat-conducting power of various materials used as boiler coverings :—

Mineral wool	100
Hair felt	117
Cotton wool	122
Sheep's wool	136
Infusorial earth	136
Charcoal	140
Sawdust	163
Gasworks breeze	230
Wood and air space	280

No. 2. Non-conducting property of various materials at even thickness :—

Black slate	100
Sandstone	71-95
Fire brick	61-70
Asphaltum and soft chalk	45-56
Oak, pine, and wood and plaster	25-66
Sulphate of lime and sand	18-70
Sawdust and tan bark	17-20
Asbestos cemented	18-20
Fine asbestos in thread	13-15
Extra mineral wool, ordinary mineral wool, raw silk	8-13
Ice	0

Among the many comparative tests that have been from time to time made with the view of determining the most efficient covering for boilers, steam pipes, &c., the following may be instanced as authentic and suggestive :—

At the Paris Exhibition, 1878, some experiments were made to determine the relative value of different kinds of pipe-covering materials. The experiments were made by MM. Geneste, Herscher & Co., with twelve vertical steam pipes, all of the same dimensions, and charged simultaneously from one boiler, so that the action of the steam was precisely the same in each case. Some of the tubes were bare, and the others were covered with different non-conducting materials. The following are some of the results arrived at, as published in the "*Moniteur des Fils et Tissus*" :—

Description of the covering, or the state of the surface of the pipes.	Thickness of covering.	Pressure of steam absolute.	Temperature of the air around the pipes.	Quantity of water condensed per hour per sq. ft.
	Inches.	lbs.		lbs.
Pipe of polished brass (bare)	—	54	77·9	0·50
Pipe of galvanised iron (bare)	—	54	78·2	0·81
Covered with plaited straw	2·00	54	76·7	0·37
Composition A	1·58	54	77·0	0·41
Composition B	1·58	54	77·3	0·41
Composition C	1·58	54	77·3	0·54
Asbestos	1·38	54	76·0	0·37
Asbestos	3·15	54	77·9	0·31
Silicate cotton	2·36	54	76·7	0·27
Wood	0·71	54	76·7	0·35
Felt	2 thicknesses	54	76·8	0·37

The materials, A, B, and C, representing three approved boiler cement or non-conducting compositions, ranked last, showing a result very little better than that of a bare tube, polished. Taking into consideration its incombustible and indestructible properties, the silicate cotton proved to be by far the most preferable substance as a non-conductor; whilst its cost is much less than asbestos.*

A wrought-iron tank 6 feet in diameter and 12 feet high, containing steam under 35 lbs. pressure, condensed 146 lbs. of steam per hour. Now 146 lbs. of steam represent, at the rate of 7½ lbs. to 1 lb. of coal, the combustion of 19¾ lbs. of coal per hour, or 460 lbs. per day of twenty-four hours. Allowing $3.00 per ton for coal 460 ÷ 2000 × 300 = 69, which is the loss in cents per day from condensation; in a year of 309 days the loss would be $213.21; the exposed surface of the tank was 225 square feet. Figuring from this data, together with the known value of mineral wool, it may be stated that at a cost of 15 cents per square foot, or $33.75 for the whole job, this tank can be so protected by a covering of mineral wool that the loss will only be 10 per cent. of the above, or, say, $21.32 per year.†

* *The Engineer*, March 12th, 1880.
† *The American Engineer*, November 19th, 1885.

For ordinary fireproofing purposes the slag wool is enclosed between two thicknesses of galvanized wire netting, which netting is kept at proper distance apart by loops of wire passing from front to back, and the layer of slag wool of a suitable thickness (an inch has been found sufficient for any purpose) is compactly felted between these two sheets of netting. Prepared in this way, very tough, light, and flexible sheets of "silicate cotton wire-net felting" are obtained. It has been found that in the thickness of an inch one ton of slag wool will cover 1,800 square feet, say $1\frac{1}{4}$ lb. to the square foot. It is employed, therefore, in this form under joists, instead of pugging, as a lining for corrugated iron buildings, sheds, &c., and for many other structural purposes.

As a non-radiator of heat and cold, it appears to be well adapted as a lining for temporary buildings either in extremely hot or very cold climates. It can also be advantageously employed as a lining for refrigerating chambers. In 1885 Mr. T. B. Lightfoot, C.E., tested it thus:—Two blocks of ice, weighing 30 lbs. each, were placed in separate boxes, one of them being surrounded by two inches of slag wool and the other with six inches of charcoal. Three days afterwards these boxes were opened and the unmelted ice weighed: the ice block in the box surrounded by slag wool was then found to weigh 13 lbs., and the other $5\frac{1}{4}$ lbs. only; showing that two inches of slag wool form a better non-conducting lining than six inches of charcoal.

As an insulator it takes high rank. It is said to be liable to become pulverized, if used on board ship, on account of the incessant vibration and the motion of the vessel at sea. Yet it does not seem to be so objectionable on locomotives, although the vibration in that case is necessarily severe. It has been used for many years by the Chicago, Milwaukee, and St. Paul Railway Company for jacketing locomotives, and the passenger cars of the Pennsylvanian Railway are lined with it.[*]

It also forms a good filling material, where the object is to

---

[*] *Canadian Mining Review*, vol. i., no. 4.

prevent the transmission of sound, on account of the vast number of minute air-cells distributed through it.

The result of practical experiments with slag wool, packed round joists, or employed in a loose state as a backing for fire grates, shows that the heating power of a fire is greatly enhanced by compelling the radiation from a stove to take an outward direction, and the combustion of the fuel is so thorough when a grate is packed all round with it, that, as soon as the fire gets under weigh, little or no smoke will rise, and, even

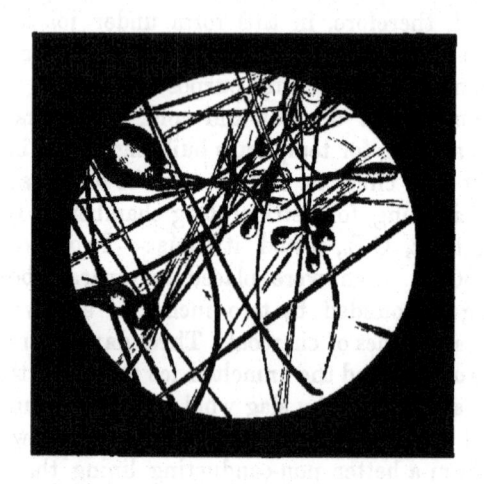

English make. $\frac{1}{2}$-inch objective.

after burning all day, if the fire be allowed to go out gradually, the residuum of ash will be surprisingly small.

It is now used largely for covering boilers, steam and water pipes. For boiler and pipe coverings slag wool mainly relies, in its competition with asbestos, on its comparative cheapness, and, as asserted by the manufacturers, on the fact of its being a better non-conductor. But, however that may be, its most manifest inferiority in this respect lies in its want of elasticity and lubricity. Even when most carefully prepared it has a harsh, gritty, metlliac feel, when crushed between the fingers,

SUBSTITUTES AND SIMILARITIES. 195

altogether unlike the soft silkiness and unctuosity of asbestos. The cause of this is at once apparent even on examination with the naked eye, but, when placed under the lens, its sharp, acicular fibres, studded with minute metallic grains or pellicles, are brought out into strong relief, these last being globules or pear-shaped drops of basic glass, precisely such as are seen in Pele's hair, being the points first blown off from the liquid slag. In the two first diagrams these pellicles are exaggerated in size, by manipulation of the fibre, so as to bring out clearly their peculiar form.

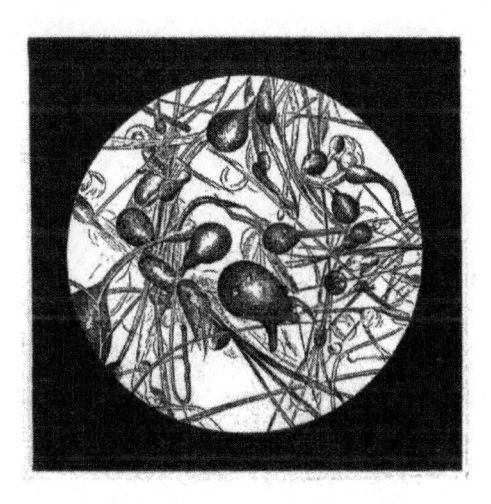

American make. ¼-inch objective.

From the peculiar formation of the material as it comes from the factory, it is very difficult to obtain a satisfactory microphotograph of it; the fibres are so crushed and closely compacted that it is not practicable to draw out a clear fibre, as can be done with some amount of care with asbestos: but the two following diagrams will give a general idea of the construction.

In regard to these, Mr. Eady, who kindly furnished the photos, says, as to No. 1, "the brittle, glassy filaments in this are exceedingly fine, and the bulbs are both small in size and few in number. Owing to the transparency of the filaments this was difficult to photograph; its extreme fineness can be best judged by comparing this with the equally magnified sample of American make"; respecting which last he says, " the irregular character of the glassy fibre shows the artificial nature of the wool; the filaments are much coarser and the bulbous ends larger." It is quite possible, however, that an injustice has been inadvertently done to the American make by difference of sample, that of No. 1 being a fine, picked

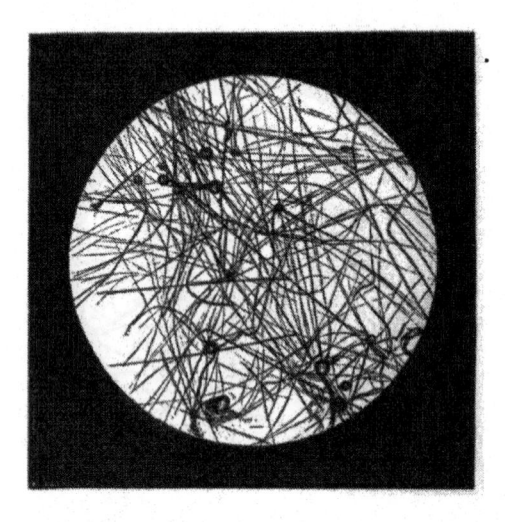

No. 1.—Silicate Cotton.   Manufactured by Frederick Jones & Co., Kentish Town.

specimen, and No. 2 being the ordinary first quality sample, sent over from the works at Cleveland.

Another very important property of slag wool is its power of absorption, which makes it capable of holding water to the extent of its own volume. Thus, when water is pumped into a burning building, instead of running through into the street and being wasted, as in the case of an ordinary iron and concrete construction, the water is held by the slag wool, as in a vast sponge, and will, owing to the surrounding heat, evolve sufficient steam to extinguish the flames, or at any rate to powerfully assist in so doing.

Being vermin-proof it is additionally valuable as a lining for wainscots, passages, pantries, dining-rooms, and ceilings; its glass-like fibres causing great irritation to rats and other vermin, as well as insect pests coming in contact with it.

It is also said to be an antiseptic, and this property, taken in conjunction with its great porosity, adapts it to some medical

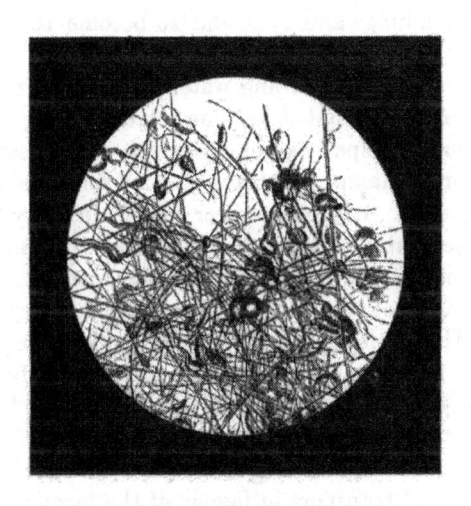

No. 2.—Mineral Wool. Manufactured by the Western Mineral Wool Company, Cleveland, Ohio.

purposes; for cholera belts, for use in hot climates, chest protectors, &c. Moreover, these antiseptic qualities can be specially utilized in the construction of hospitals, infirmaries, &c.

There are many other uses which might be enumerated, all tending to show the value of slag wool for certain purposes, and the many points in which it can compete with asbestos.

Its main feature is, of course, its comparative cheapness; but it is to be remarked that there is scarcely one point of value cited which does not carry with it a corresponding disadvantage. For instance, when its vermin-proof character is mentioned, the warnings of Percy and Bloxam at once occur to the mind. The former* specially cautions his readers that these slag fibres have to be handled with care, because the fine short threads, being very brittle, easily penetrate the skin and cause irritation; and Bloxam says, the fine filaments, being so exceedingly brittle, and the material itself so light, the needle-like particles are liable to become diffused in the air of a room, and pass into the lungs and eyes, and so become the source of serious mischief.†

Again, its power of absorbing water is doubtless a valuable quality in case of fire, but it has one corresponding disadvantage, as a boiler and pipe coverer, inasmuch as if a leak should occur, or exterior damp penetrate it, it at once becomes the cause of corrosion. Although water is the primary cause of rusting, the percentage of sulphur contained in the slag becomes dissolved in the water, and, in the form of sulphuric acid, will attack the surfaces, unless they are kept dry by radiated heat. This defect, however, is now in some measure overcome by entirely manufacturing the article from non-sulphur-bearing rocks, so as to render it absolutely free from sulphur and its compounds. It is then called *rock wool*, and although more costly than slag wool, the difference in weight reduces the cost of transport in favour of the former.

Practically the main objections to its use are its glass-like texture and the grittiness caused by the minute pellicles, which cannot be entirely eliminated, together with its liability to pulverise under vibration, and its water retention.

In its normal condition a cubic foot weighs 12 lbs., and its cost, as applied to steam-pipes, is 2d. per square foot for each inch in thickness.

The Patent Fire and Sound Proof Plasterings (Mr. W.

---

* Percy on "Metallurgy"; art., "Slags."
† Bloxam on "Metals."

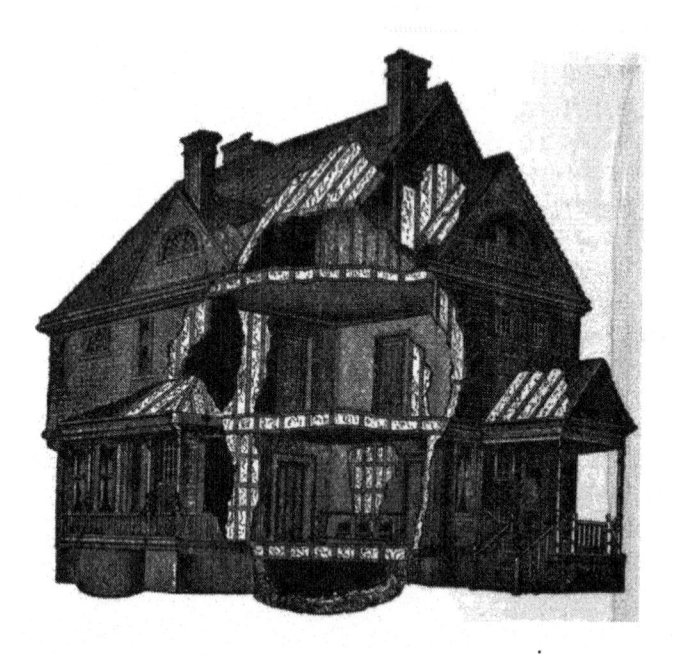

COTTAGE RESIDENCE

Designed by Messrs. Frederick Jones & Co., of Kentish Town, showing walls, ceilings, roof, and flooring protected by Silicate Cotton.

Hitchins' patents), recently purchased by Messrs. F. Jones & Co., made in many ingenious ways with a backing of silicate cotton, have proved their value repeatedly. The same manufacturers furnish a variety of fibrous wire netting, and fibre-ligneous slabs and compounds, which are rapidly making their way in the estimation of architects and builders, and all others who are desirous (as who are not ?) of ensuring perfect immunity in their habitations from damp, for preventing the transmission of sound, and the spread of fire in the case of conflagration. In this plastering, no lathing, lime or hair is required; there is no annoyance from dirt or rubbish, and the walls and ceilings can be painted or decorated the same day that they are put up. Cornices and enrichments, prepared in long lengths, are fixed dry, and buildings thus treated are rendered fit for habitation or decoration at once. The same firm's Salamander compound is composed of silicate cotton and prepared plaster, and when set this is not only a fire-proof non-conductor, but it possesses sufficient elasticity to prevent cracking under even extreme heat.

The illustration on opposite page represents a cottage residence specially designed by Messrs. Frederick Jones & Co., to illustrate their method of isolating such a structure, with a view to rendering it at the same time fire, frost, sound, and vermin proof, perfectly cool in summer and comparatively warm in winter. The ceilings and walls can be fitted with Hitchins' patent fire- and sound-proof plaister slabs, which have a lining of slag wool between the plaister and the wall or ceiling. These slabs are made specially to suit the building; they can be of any size and ornamented in any way desired, either by moulding, painting, or gilding; they can be fitted with the greatest ease and simplicity and without dirt or mess of any kind.

The cut on next page shows one of the same firm's patent portable anti-thermal and anti-septic huts, which they claim to be impervious to external climatic influences and to be so constructed that it can be readily put together or taken to pieces by any ordinary workman in a couple of hours. As these huts are not only fire, heat, frost, and sound proof, but give absolute freedom from insect pests, they are undoubtedly a great step in advance. Soldiers' huts, gentlemen's fishing boxes, and other buildings of a similar or temporary character can be fitted in a precisely similar way if constructed of wood or any other material. Apparently this would be a great boon to troops in camp, who, in such huts as these, would enjoy complete immunity from the annoyances caused by the all too friendly disposition of the insect inhabitants of the present huts, whilst they could at the same time depend on a tolerably equable temperature, cooler in summer

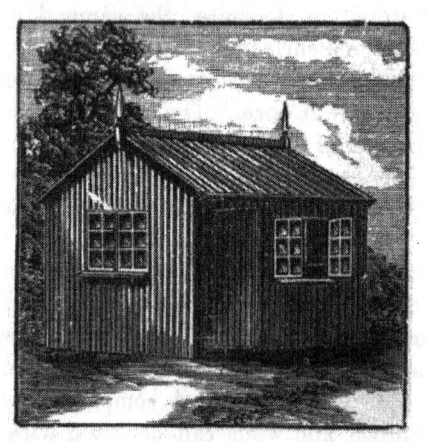

Portable Anti-thermal and Anti-septic Hut. (Frederick Jones & Co.)

and warmer in winter than that offered by any other system at present devised for ordinary camp-dwellings. In the wooden houses of Canada and Norway it is a common practice to ram in sawdust between the outer timbers and the matchboard lining; and although this makes the house undoubtedly warm, it forms a delightful harbourage and breeding ground for all insect pests. In Russia, where things in this respect are much worse, but much less regarded, it is almost needless to say that the Government has at once adopted the idea, and it is anticipated that a large order will be at once given for these portable huts for housing the troops in camp.

Soapstone.—This soft magnesian mineral frequently occurs in association with serpentine, and possesses many of the valuable properties of asbestos. Mainly composed of two of the most durable substances known for exposure to fire or atmospheric influences, it is often used in competition with asbestos, or enlisted as a valuable auxiliary, in certain forms of manufacture.

Technically called Steatite (Ger., Speckstein), it is also occasionally termed Synophite, as being an associate of ophite. The word *Steatitis* is used by Pliny as the name of a stone resembling fat. Like asbestos, soapstone is a hydrated silicate of magnesia, a more or less pure and compact talc, generally of a grey or greyish-green colour; it occurs in massive form, crystalline, granular, or impalpable, and is very greasy to the touch. Sometimes it is found in a fine granular, or cryptocrystalline form, of a milk-white colour and pearly lustre, soft enough to be used as chalk (craie de Briançon); it is then called Venetian or French chalk, and is the substance used by tailors and others for marking cloth and removing grease and other stains.

Analyses of two samples give the following :—

Silica	62·8	63·49
Magnesia	33·5	31·75
Water	3·7	4·76
	100·00	100.00

A little iron is occasionally found replacing magnesia. Sometimes it appears as a pseudomorph, taking the form of apatite at St. Just, Cornwall; or of arragonite in Bohemia.

Lapis ollaris (potstone, Ger., Topfstein) is an impure steatite of a greyish-green colour and slaty structure.

Soapstone occurs abundantly in many parts of the world. In the United States and in Canada it can be had in large quantities, and sometimes of remarkably pure quality. Large deposits have been found in several districts in California. In Arkansas a fine quality occurs in Saline County, where it is worked by the Arkansas Soapstone Manufacturing Company. The deposits here are mixed up in an unusual way with slates and serpentine, but are very pure, averaging 62 per cent. of silica and 34 magnesia.

In the Eastern Townships of Quebec it is abundant: the quality is not always good, but a good deal can be had in a comparatively pure state. Deposits exist at East Broughton, Lake Nicolet, Hatley, Potton, and Wolfestown. At the last-named place it is found in a bed from one to two feet thick in black and grey talcose schist; this is mostly pure and occasionally translucent. Excepting at Wolfestown, where a factory has been established for working it, and where slabs of a fine quality can be had, not much use is made of it in Canada. Possibly the high prices now realized for asbestos will cause greater attention to be given to the valuable properties of this refractory mineral.

In England, a company, operating at Newcastle-on-Tyne, imports it in bulk from China, mostly for use in the manufacture of pigments; the peculiarity of the Chinese soapstone consisting in the large proportion of potash it contains, amounting occasionally to as much as 60 per cent.

The following are some of its most important properties, which serve to explain the estimation in which it is held for manufacturing purposes. It is not liable to corrosion, is without expansion or contraction, and is unaffected by moisture, atmospheric influences, or chemical fumes. It will not discolour with age, and is a better radiator than any metal. When pure, and of a hard nature, it may be sawn into slabs, or made into knife-edged bricks, and, being a non-absorbent, may be washed without injurious effect. It can be used for almost any ornamental purpose, offering a fine surface for painting with oil or water colours; will take the richest tint, and when retaining its own, exhibiting a pure transparent white. Its refractory nature adapts it for use as firestones, and as a lining for furnaces and fireplaces, especially those designed for anthracite, as well as for the manufacture of crucibles. When highly heated it loses the small proportion of contained water, and then, becoming much harder, assumes a dark green colour, and is susceptible of a fine polish; in this state it is used by the Chinese for the manufacture of images, especially of their household gods: hence its name of figure-stone. The minerals pagodite and lardite * also are simply soapstone.

Possessing unusual powers of withstanding atmospheric and chemical influences, it has long been used, in China and Japan, as a preserving medium for woodwork, and buildings or monuments erected with any stone liable to disintegration.

In the manufacture of pigments it is simply invaluable. When it is remembered that one of the main causes affecting the durability of iron bridges, and metallic structures generally, is the tendency to oxidation, arising from the humidity of the atmosphere, it will be at once understood that if proper precautions were not taken to obviate this element of danger, by finding some means of lessening the corrosion constantly taking place, very serious results might ensue. And this liability to corrosion is still more persistent in ships both of iron and steel, in the latter especially, because of the difficulty of finding some kind of pigment capable of taking a firm hold of the fine fibres of the steel plates. Many modes of overcoming this difficulty, such as rough-rolling the steel, have from time to time been tried, and experiments are constantly being made in this direction, but these have mostly been without successful result. Some time ago, Mr. Goodall, Surveyor of Shipping to the Trinity House, spent a considerable time in the endeavour to find some material possessed of the necessary power of taking hold of the fine fibres of steel, and in the end gave the result of his experiments to the public. In doing this he strongly urged on paint manufacturers the desirability of trying soapstone as an ingredient in any paint designed to be employed in the protection of iron and steel ships, especially in the coal bunkers, as he had found nothing so suitable for accomplishing this object. The chief difficulty met with in carry-

* "C'est à la steatite que doivent être rapportées une partie des substances pagodite, lardite, &c., avec lesquelles les chinois sculptent des figurines."—De Lapparent, 376.

ing out his ideas was that steatite when mixed as an ordinary paint, that is, with raw or boiled linseed oil, driers, turpentine, terebine, &c., the steatite forming the basis, would neither mix properly nor dry hard, and was quite useless as a protective paint; but with quick drying varnish it was a success.

When ground into an impalpable powder, the grain of soapstone is of such extreme fineness as to be all but infinitesimal, and this quality, coupled with its imperishability, endows it with extraordinary qualities. It is, moreover, lighter than any metallic pigment, is not liable to be thrown off by vibration, and will cover a much larger surface than zinc white, red lead, or oxide of iron; all of which, especially the latter, are very difficult to obtain free from adulteration. The red oxide of iron being the pigment generally in use for iron structures can, according to Professor Lewes, be easily tested for soluble sulphates, by warming a little of it with pure water, filtering, and then adding to the clear solution a few drops of pure hydrochloric acid, with a little chloride of barium solution. If a white sediment is then formed in the solution, the sample should be at once rejected.

Oxide paints mixed with boiled oil are now regarded as failures; naphtha is a far better combination, corrosion resulting from the oxygen contained in the oil.

When soapstone, reduced to a fine impalpable powder, is mixed with a quick-drying, hard-setting varnish, it furnishes a paint superior to asbestos, not only of great covering capacity and firmness, but of an even, enamel-like surface. When ground by itself pure soapstone is transparent, the added colour alone therefore, is shown in the pigment. Its remarkable smoothness is due to the extreme minuteness of the atoms of which it is composed, and to which it may be reduced. Its extraordinary fineness and adhesive nature is shown by the fact that you may write with it on plate glass, the steatite finding a ready hold on its highly-polished surface. It consequently finds perfect and permanent adhesion to the surface of the smoothest steel.

The causes of rusting in ships are contact with sea water and the various acids it may contain, atmospheric influences, or electric or galvanic actions. The first two can be cured by preventing the sea water and the atmosphere from coming into contact with the steel, but in order to do this it is necessary to have a paint which will adhere to the fibre of the steel, which will be perfectly air and water tight, and which will have sufficient elasticity not to crack with the vibration of the vessel or the slight contraction and expansion of the steel. This elasticity, Mr. Goodall says, may be obtained in steatite by using a suitable varnish to convey it to the steel in the form of paint, which varnish should contain evaporating spirits, combined with a certain proportion of slow-drying oils, in order that the paint may dry and at the same time keep its elasticity. Varnish alone is porous, and admits the atmosphere and moisture to the body coated with it, but when mixed with steatite, owing to the minute atoms of which that mineral is composed, the fine pores are completely closed, and the paint becomes air and water tight. The third cause of rusting is due to electric or galvanic actions. The gums of which varnishes are made are, like steatite, isolators of electricity or galvanism; consequently, if a vessel's iron or steel plates inside and out, together with all iron or steel attached thereto, are properly coated with steatite paint they are completely isolated, and unable to set up electricity or galvanism from the atmosphere, sea water, &c., as they certainly will do if coated with paint made from metallic pigments.[*]

Infusorial-earth or Fossil-meal is also now much brought into use, either as a composition in conjunction with asbestos, or in competition with it. It is a siliceous mealy earth, composed of the flinty shields or skeletons of infusorial animalculæ; the infusoria found in the mineral called tripoli and in bog iron ore being mostly of vegetable origin.

Fossil-meal is a white, greyish white, or brown chalk-like earth, which occurs in deposits, often many miles in extent,

[*] *Invention*, May 10, 1890.

and either uncompacted as a fine earth, or compacted and moderately hard. The infusoria of which it is composed abound in moist earth, in which they have been found alive at 60 feet below the surface, in both fresh and salt water, often covering leagues of the ocean and giving a beautiful tinge to it from their vivid hue, from the mud of which they have been brought up from a depth of 1,600 feet; and occasionally under peat. The infusorial beds of Virginia, a vast accumulation of these microscopic organisms, are of tertiary age. In some parts of northern Germany deposits occur of more than 60 feet thick; the minute organised specks of matter requiring the aid of a microscope even to discover the fact of their existence, many of them being less than the three-thousandth part of an inch in length, of which it would require thirty-five thousand millions to fill the space of a cubic inch.

Near the mouths of the great rivers which flow into the Baltic Sea large banks, islands, and very broad tracts on the coast are known to be derived from this source. They are discovered in all climes, and have been found in almost infinite abundance in flint and opal, in the latter of which they encase the solid and translucent interior.

The composition of this fossil earth was first made known by Ehrenberg, who discovered 100 different species of diatoms in the beds of Richmond, U.S.A.

A large manufactory is carried on by the company owning the United Kieselguhr mines at Chelle, who claim to be the largest producers of the meal; the English agent is Mr. F. E. Clotten, of 23, Leadenhall Street, London.

The non-conducting qualities of the meal indicate its usefulness for the coverings of boilers and steam pipes, for the isolation of engine rooms, for protection against heat and cold, for refrigerating rooms and ice manufactories, for rendering floors, walls, and ceilings fire-proof and rot-proof, as a filling material for use in the manufacture of fire-proof safes, strong rooms, and ice boxes, for the protection in transit of dangerous, explosive, or easily damaged goods, and for a variety of other purposes.

It is sold in many forms, such as pure fossil-meal, fossil-meal composition (containing a mixture of asbestos), patent removable fossil-meal plates, specially adapted for isolating engine rooms and for roofing for use in tropical climates, removable coverings, packing and boiler coverings, and for other purposes for which asbestos is generally used. As an indication of its value, as a boiler and steam-pipe covering, it is now used for that purpose on some of the vessels of the Peninsula and Oriental, White Star, Inman, and Orient lines. It is also used in the manufacture of firebricks, and as a polishing powder, and when mixed with nitroglycerine it makes dynamite.

Asbestonit is a patent compound of asbestos and some other material, manufactured by Messrs. Ladewig & Co.,* of Rathenow. It is a form of millboard recommended for packing, jointing, roofing, and many other purposes for which similar substances are available and useful. The same firm also make an asbestonit sheeting and wire-wove cloth, which is used for a great variety of purposes, including the protection of timber or wooden posts when such are required to be fixed below ground or in water.

Spun Glass.—Mr. Reed, an American citizen, has recently applied this to the insulation of copper wires for electrical purposes. The wire is first wound round with woollen or cotton yarn, twisted slackly, and this is then overlaid with longitudinal strands of spun glass; above which another strand of silk and spun glass is wound in close spiral form, over which is then placed a braid of either cotton, hemp, flax, or silk. The whole covering is then well saturated with paraffin or varnish to exclude damp.

Woodite is a patented article which takes its name from that of the patentee, and not from the substance of which it is composed. It is an elastic rubber compound, said to possess properties which enable it to compete with goods formed of rubber, gutta-percha, leather, &c., owing to its being able to resist the action of heat, oil, steam, and some acids. An asbestos and woodite packing is made to supersede the asbestos

* *Ante*, p. 179.

packing with indiarubber core, which, under high-pressure steam and heat, has a tendency to become viscous and to lose its elasticity; to obviate which the asbestos woodite packing is formed of asbestos with a woodite core. It is also put forward as a competitor with asbestos for protecting the sides of war-ships, and on precisely similar grounds, the inventor claiming that if the blocks of woodite fixed on the sides of war-vessels were to be riddled by projectiles, the only effect would be that the perforations would instantly close up again and prevent the influx of water.*

Whaleite is another form of the same material, in which whalebone cuttings are intermixed with woodite, in order to give it the rough, frictional quality requisite in waterproof mats, floor coverings, &c.

With **wood wool** we have here nothing to do, its manufacture being for sanitary purposes only. It may, however, be mentioned that a German manufacturer has recently patented a wood fibre for spinning purposes. Here the wood is first boiled in a chemical solution, as sulphurous acid or bisulphide of carbon, the fibres being afterwards dried and softened in water, and then subjected to repeated mechanical pinchings.

In addition to the foregoing there are many combinations of asbestos and rubber, and similar compounds, which are used as packings, many of them possessing good qualities of their own, to supplement the main feature of cheapness.

* *Army and Navy Gazette*, October, 1886.

CHAPTER XII.

FIBRE SPINNING.

ORGANIC AND INORGANIC FIBRES—Powers Employed—Wool—Cotton—Silk—Spider Web—Spun glass—Quartz—Chrysotile—Italian Asbestos—Delicacy and Strength of some Mineral Fibres.

THE difficulty experienced in the early attempts to spin and weave asbestos fibre was purely structural, and in order to explain this we will contrast the peculiar form of some mineral fibres with others of animal origin. These structural differences between organic and inorganic fibres can be at once perceived when such fibres are placed under a lens. For ordinary purposes of examination and comparison their distinguishing characteristics can be sufficiently well seen with a moderate power, but very high powers are sometimes employed in investigations of a scientific character. Dr. Bowman, for instance, when engaged in the examination of the structural peculiarities of wool fibres for his well-known series of lectures on the subject[*] occasionally employed powers as high as 8,000 diameters, or such as would magnify 64,000,000 times. A power such as this would give to a single fibre of Leicester wool the appearance of a tube 2,000 ft. long and 10 in. in diameter, the dimension of which will be better understood when it is stated that if this represented an actual metal tube, such as a gas main, for instance, its size would be sufficiently large to supply all the gas requirements for a small town.

Wool.—The first fibre selected for examination is a hair

[*] "Lectures on the Structure of Wool Fibres," by Dr. Bowman.

212   ASBESTOS.

of sheep's wool, as this affords the aptest illustration of a spinning or felting fibre. In the cut this is magnified 600 diameters only, that power being amply sufficient to show its peculiar notched or serrated character, or what is technically termed its imbrications,* those irregularly shaped cylindrical scales, or plates, which form its outer structure. These overlap each other after the manner of house tiles, the effect being to give rise to very minute projections all along the surface or line of the fibre, which act like spikes or teeth, and so cause wool fibres to cling together when twisted. The imbrications thus being the cause of the felting property inherent in wool, it follows that the more numerous these imbrications are in the fibre of any particular wool, the more valuable that special variety becomes in the eyes of the manufacturer. In fine Saxon wool there are no less than 2,720 of these imbrications within the length of an inch, in Southdown there are 2,080, whilst in Leicester we find only 1,850. Thus we have no difficulty (other circumstances being identical) in assigning to each variety its relative value for manufacturing purposes. It must not be forgotten, however, that wool, being a part of the skin of the animal on which it grows, is capable of being modified to a very great extent by change of climate, food, and other surroundings, as well as by judicious breeding; but there can be no doubt that practically we now possess the best breeds of sheep possible both for wool-producing and food-producing purposes.†

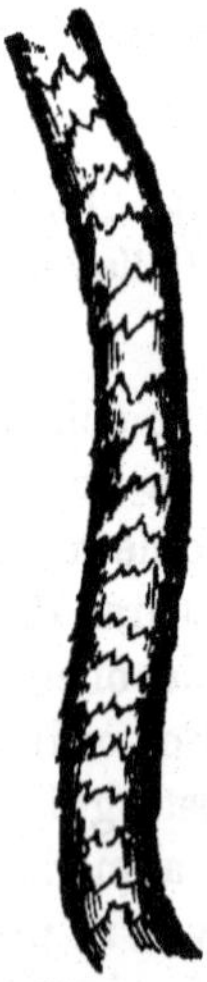

Fig. 1.
Fibre of Sheep's Wool. Magnified 600 diameters.

Cotton.—In cotton the fibre becomes twisted during its growth, and although not so strong as linen or silk, its irregular surfaces adapt it for being spun into a strong yarn, from which

* Deriv.: *imber, imbris,* rain; *imbrex, imbricis,* a tile; *imbrico,* I cover with tiles.
† Dr. Bowman's "Lectures," *ubi supra.*

all cotton fabrics are made. Its peculiarity as a fibre has been thus described by Mr. Thompson: *—"The filaments of cotton are transparent glassy tubes, flattened and twisted round their own axis. A section of the filament resembles a figure of 8, the tube, originally cylindrical, having collapsed most in the middle, forming semi-tubes on each side, which give to the fibre when viewed in certain lights the appearance of a flat ribbon with a hem or border on each side. The twisted and corkscrew form of the filament of cotton distinguishes it from all other vegetable fibres." When it is important to know from what material a fabric has been constructed, it can sometimes only be discovered by the use of a microscope. It was by this means that the discovery was made that the cere-cloths in which the Egyptian mummies are wrapped were made of linen, the Peruvians using cotton alone for this purpose. Much has been said about the "parallelism" of cotton fibre in manufactured goods, but if a bit of one of the best grades of cotton cloth be examined under the lens, it will be seen that there is no such thing as parallelism among them. In a lecture on cotton fibres delivered before the Franklin Institute, Mr. Thomas Gray, jun., suggested that the usual method of determining the quality of cotton fibre, by feeling it with the fingers, was an exceedingly crude one, inasmuch as these fibres vary from $\frac{1}{500}$ of an inch in thickness for the coarsest "upland" quality, to $\frac{1}{5000}$ for the best sea island.† The finest cotton

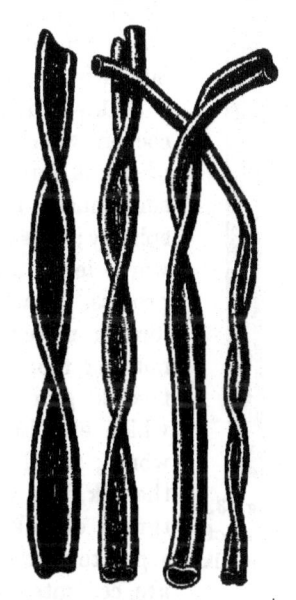

Fig. 2.
Filaments of Raw Cotton.

* James Thompson, Esq., F.R.S., on "Mummy Cloths."
† *Popular Science Monthly* (New York), vol. xxxvi., no. 4.

raised from any of the cotton-fields of the world comes from the Mississippi delta. Under the microscope this presents a beautiful structure and a perfect development; it is seen to be full of oil deposit, and has nearly 400 spirals to an inch. The form of the spiral is seen on page 213.

The actual length of the fibres shown in the drawing was $\frac{1}{100}$ of an inch; the thickness of cotton fibres varies from $\frac{1}{800}$ to $\frac{1}{3800}$ of an inch. There are in an inch in length of cotton fibre from 300 to 800 twists of the cylindrical tubes.

Silk.—Then if a fibre be drawn out from the cocoon, we shall see (Fig. 3) that the construction of silk is entirely different. Whilst not of a perfect smoothness, it is in no sense imbricated or twisted spirally; consequently although the fibre of the silk-worm lends itself readily enough to the spinning process, it cannot be felted unless mixed wtih some foreign material. The fibre of silk is, in reality, nothing more than a slender rod of consolidated flexible gum, secreted from a pair of long tubes which end in a pore of the underlip of the silk-worm; which explains the peculiar appearance of the silk fibre when examined under the lens. Each thread of silk is then seen to be composed of two separate filaments. These issue from the pores, and are cemented together longitudinally by the secretion from a small gland situated near the pores, the quality of the silk being dependent on the character and difference of the two secretions. The form of the fibre, as disclosed by the microscope, shows no sign whatever of structural markings; on the contrary, it bears some resemblance to a polished metal rod, the line of junction being made perceptible by a slight grove, which gives it the appearance of two somewhat irregular lines, longitudinally attached together by the glutinous matter; each of the lines being about the two-thousandth part of an inch in diameter.

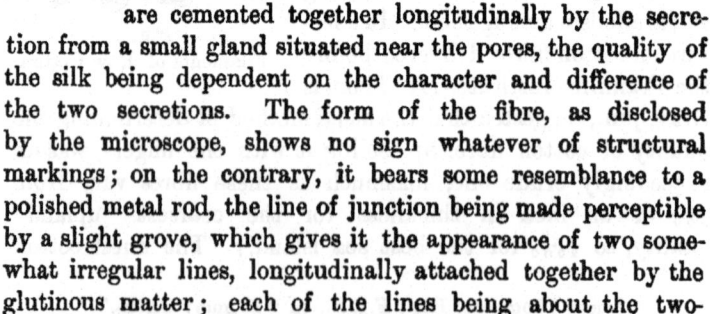

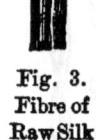

Fig. 3. Fibre of Raw Silk

The enormous comparative tensile strength possessed by silk fibre was shown by Mr. C. V. Boys, in a paper read by him at the Royal Institution in June, 1889,* in which he states that, when the two filaments had been separated and washed they were each capable of sustaining a weight of 60 grains before breaking, and each could be safely loaded with 15 grains; the carrying power, therefore, being equivalent to from 10 to 20 tons per square inch.

Spider's Web.—Now, if we turn to the somewhat analogous case of the delicate radial thread of the common garden spider, which is of so fine a quality as frequently to be invisible to the naked eye until washed with dew or exposed by a shower, we shall be better able to understand how this great tensile strength is obtained. The filamentary secretions exist in the spider's body in a semi-fluid state, and are secreted by glands which end in four or six teat-like organs called spinnerets, minute conical projections situated near the abdomen of the insect, towards the posterior end, where, when at rest, they present a bluntly conical appearance.

Each of these is composed of a multitude of fine hair-like tubes opening at the top of the spinneret, which thus forms the spinning apparatus. The narrow space which intervenes between the basis of the anterior spinnerets is filled by a tongue-like process. The silky matter, or secretion, so long as it remains in the spider's body, is in a semi-fluid state, and issues thence by a sieve-like apparatus; each sieve, according to Bonnet, containing more than 1,000 punctured holes. When the filaments are projected from these holes they agglutinate together in such a manner that each thread is composed of from 4,000 to 6,000 fibres, but yet it is of so slender a character that, according to Leuwenhoek, it would take 4,000,000 of them to make a thread as thick as a hair from a man's beard; the thread holes being so fine and so crowded together that 1,000 of them would be covered by the point of a needle; but after the thread is woven, Meckel could not recognise it as consisting of more than 8 to 10 strands. When this silky fluid

* "Quartz Fibres," by Mr. C. V. Boys, F.R.S.

216 ASBESTOS.

is exposed to the air it congeals rapidly, becoming of a tenacious consistence, and is then capable of being drawn out into a fine thread. This will be better understood by thrusting a piece of stick into a glue-pot and drawing it out again, when it will be seen that the adhering glue, so long as it retains sufficient heat, will remain fluid, but no sooner does it cool than it will harden, and then it can be drawn out into a fine hair-like thread, precisely as in the case of the sealing-wax referred to in the previous chapter. The single threads, therefore, with which the spinning is accomplished are in reality, each of them, composed of a multitude of strands issuing from the spinnerets and consolidated into a single fibre; so that actually the fine gossamer thread, which has become typical of the utmost tenuity, is composed of a vast number of different threads invisible to the naked eye, and even when magnified, as we see it in Fig. 4 representing only a single line.* Enormous strength in the fibre is necessary, as not only must the orb web be able to sustain the weight of the evening dews but also of summer showers, which occasionally fall heavily, and are also sometimes driven before a strong wind.

Fig. 4.
Radial Thread of
Garden Spider.

An interesting example of the use of the spider web by scientists is the following:—Professor Mitchell, wanting a clock to record its beat telegraphically as well as to perform in a perfect manner its work as a time-keeper, found the required makes and breaks in the battery could be effected by means of a cross of delicate wire and a mercury cup, the difficulty arising of procuring a fibre sufficiently minute and elastic to constitute the physical union between the top stem of the cross and the clock pendulum. A fine human hair was found to be too coarse and stiff, and, after many fruitless

* C. V. Boys, *ubi supra.* Wilson's "Science Jottings."

attempts, the assistance of a spider was invoked and his web, perfectly elastic and pliable, proved to be exactly what was required.*

Now, if we turn to inorganic fibres, it is well known that physicists, in their endeavour to find a really delicate torsion thread, have usually turned their attention to spun

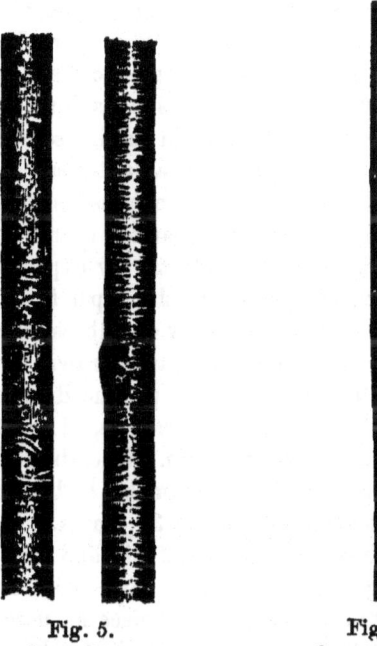

Fig. 5.
Spun Glass.

Fig. 6.
Quartz Fibre.

glass, which is about the thousandth part of an inch in diameter, and would appear to be an ideal torsion thread, its great strength enabling it to carry heavier loads than would be expected of it; but Mr. Boys confesses that he used it only to be disappointed, although apparently possessing every good quality, it is deficient in the important one of elasticity. So great had been his difficulty in finding a fine torsion thread that

* *Popular Science Monthly*, May, 1890

the attempt had practically been given up, and in all the more exact instruments he had been compelled to use silk. The torsion of silk, however, though exceedingly small, he found to be quite sufficient to upset the working of any delicate instrument, for the simple reason that it is never constant; at one time the fibre twists in one way and at another in another, this evil effect being only capable of mitigation by using large apparatus in which strong forces are developed, the result usually being that the smallness, the length of period, and therefore delicacy, of the instruments at the physicist's disposal had, until lately, been simply limited to this behaviour of silk. When, therefore, Mr. Boys was engaged in making some improvements in an instrument for measuring radiant heat, his experiment came to a deadlock; he would not use silk and could find nothing else. Spun glass being far too coarse and a thousand times too stiff, he was driven to try by experiment to find a new material, and he explains in the paper from which we are quoting, how he managed to draw out fibres from a fine rod of quartz which had been melted and drawn out in the oxyhydrogen jet. In this way he produced threads of great length, of almost any degree of fineness, of extraordinary uniformity, and of enormous strength. One fibre, of the five thousandth part of an inch in diameter, he had in constant use in an instrument loaded with about 30 grains. It had a section of only one-sixth of a single line of silk and was just as strong, while, not being organic, it was in no way affected by changes of moisture or temperature. The piece he used in the instrument was about 16 inches long, and had it been necessary for him, he says, to have used spun glass, which was generally considered to be the finest torsion material known, he would have required, instead of 16 inches, a piece about 1,000 feet long, and an instrument as high as the Eiffel Tower to put it in.

Turning now to the fibre of asbestos, after repeatedly subjecting some of them, especially of chrysotile, to test under high powers, which satisfied me of the nature of their structural form, I applied to my friend, Mr. Eady, of Southampton, who is experienced in micro-photography, to send me a micro-pho-

FIBRE SPINNING. 219

tograph of a fibre magnified in such a way as would best exhibit its structure. This he very readily did, and in those marked Nos. 1 and 2 we see a few fibres from a piece of ore, brought by myself from the Johnson Mine, highly magnified.

The first attempts were scarcely satisfactory, considerable difficulty being experienced in drawing out a couple of clean fibres entirely free from fluffiness. This would seem a very simple matter, and, judging by the naked eye, is easily accom-

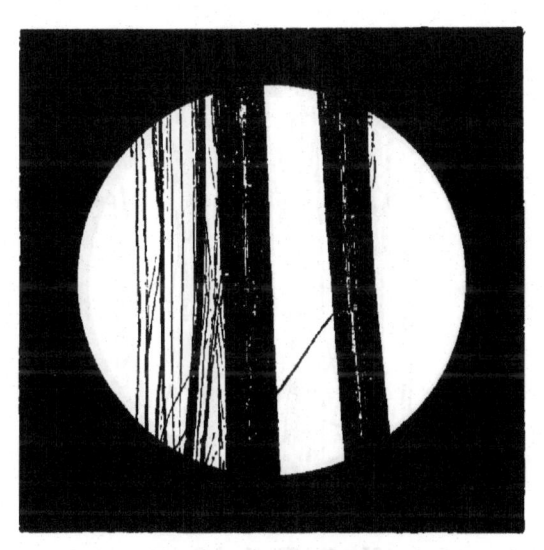

No. 1.—Thetford Ore.

plished, but when under the lens, the fluffiness is quickly apparent, and a couple of clean fibres seem as hard to get as they are difficult to place in parallel lines when successfully obtained.

When this difficulty was overcome the clear, rod-like metallic nature of the fibre as seen under the lens at once explains the stubborn obstinacy with which it so long resisted all attempts to subject it to the spinning or weaving process. Under the microscope this fibre shows up as clear and distinct as a polished steel rod, and in the photograph the rounded glass-

220　　　　　　　　ASBESTOS.

like nature of it is distinctly seen; but, in the coarseness of wood engraving the beauty of the fibre is entirely lost, though the practical idea is conveyed. No. 1 shows the formation distinctly. In Nos. 2 and 3, although the objective is somewhat crowded and the fibre not so clearly drawn out, its composite character, and the constant rounding off, or "silking out," of still more minute filaments from what appears to the naked eye to be but a single line, is very plainly shown. Some of the fibres, on examination, seem to show long cylindrical

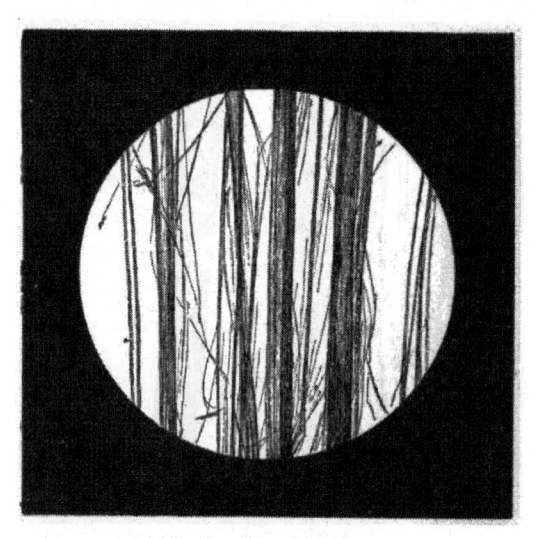

No. 2.—Thetford Ore.

cavities, but on closer inspection these seeming cavities are found to be merely the interstices between the minute longitudinal filaments, as will be better seen in the fibre of the Italian varieties which follow.

These fibres are of great beauty; when drawn out as finely as it is possible to do with the fingers, their extreme tenuity can be best realised by comparing them with some of the coarser kinds. Under the lens they look like glass or steel rods of the most precise and regular form, and in these also their com-

FIBRE SPINNING. 221

pound nature can be seen from the exquisitely fine lines slightly separated from the thicker fibre. The Flossy are more greasy to the touch than the Silky, and although not so brilliantly beautiful as the latter, are exceedingly soft and ductile. The nature of the asbestos fibre is thus so far identical in structure with the organic fibres already considered, that each apparently single fibre is actually composed of other still finer lines, ranged side by side, and these more minute fibres can be distinctly seen to be composed of other lines yet finer still, when higher

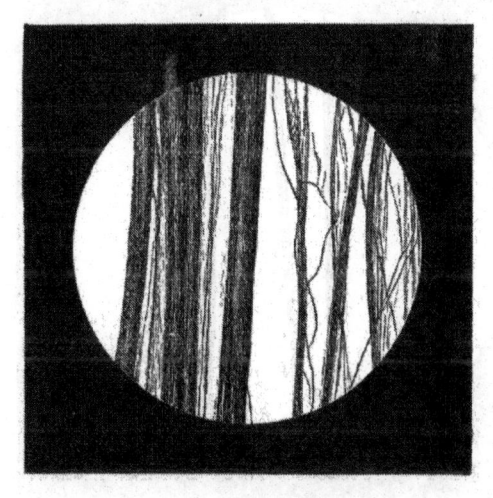

No. 3. Thetford Ore.

powers are used. So beautifully clear and fine are these lines when carefully drawn out that, at the suggestion of Professor Wallace, Mr. Troughton successfully employed them for micrometrical purposes, fibres of $\frac{1}{3000}$ of an inch in diameter giving an even line, and being considerably opaque.

The single fibre would not appear to possess any great degree of strength; but, in its natural form of a combination of fibres, its comparative tensile strength is in reality, like that of silk, very great indeed, and the cause of this is easily understood. But in whatever manner the fibre is examined, its rod-like smoothness of surface, and total absence of imbrications, irregularities, or twisting, at once explains the difficulty first experienced in spinning it, without the accompaniment of some foreign substance, such as a fine thread of flax, to give it the necessary clinging power. Under polarized light there would seem to be some slight approach to knots or irregularities, but it is quite clear that, even if these in any way detract from its

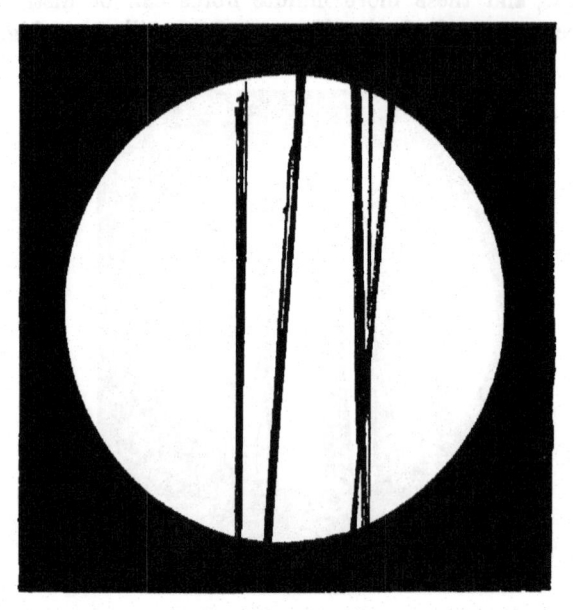

Italian "Silky" Fibre.

smoothness, they in reality add little, if anything at all, to its spinning qualifications.

The Italian "Grey" variety, as seen on page 224, is a coarser and altogether different fibre from any of the preceding. This, doubtless, was the kind selected by Madame Perpenti for her manufacturing experiments.

The fibres of the fine quality of Corsican asbestos, magnified like the foregoing, have a far more rod-like structure even than chrysotile, and look much like spun glass, which, in fact, they nearly resemble in appearance; consequently they are but little adapted for spinning, but are excellently fitted for interlacement so as to lead up the flame in gas-stove fires. The colour is of a soft, delicate brown, shading off to a pearly white. The coarser quality is of a greenish white colour, and consists of bundles of shortish twists of fibres, which have a soft and greasy feel and a fair amount of tenacity.

The South African variety, from Griqualand West, although

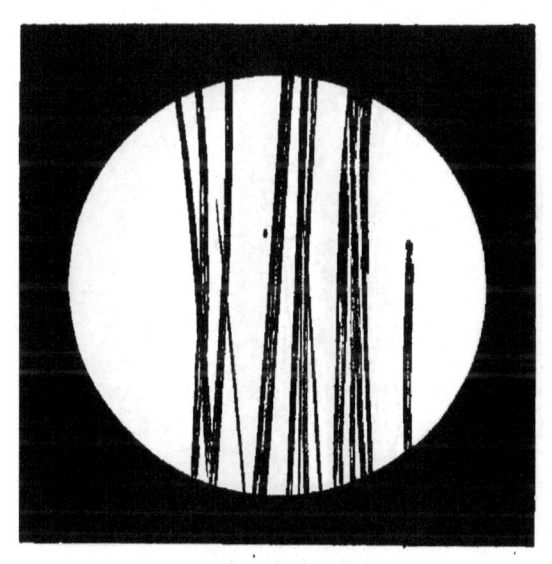

Italian "Flossy."

very beautiful to the eye, and not at all unlike the Italian "Flossy," exhibits a very coarse and irregular appearance under the lens. The ultimate fibres in this also are of extreme tenuity. In the neighbourhood of Queenstown, South Africa, a wild plant grows in profusion, the seed vessels of which are surrounded by a profusion of fibre of extreme delicacy, beautifully soft and silky, and of some tenacity. The name of the plant I am unacquainted with, but it is strange enough and suggestive enough to form another of Africa's "surprises."

Before leaving this interesting subject it may be worth while to note an extreme illustration of the delicacy to which mineral fibres can be drawn out, which was shown by Mr. C. V. Boys, in the paper referred to. Making mention of some quartz fibres which he had drawn out to the millionth part of an inch in diameter, he says, these were of course invisible to the naked eye, but he had in actual use for some time a fibre of the ten thousandth part of an inch in diameter, and in this he found the torsion to be 10,000 times less than that of

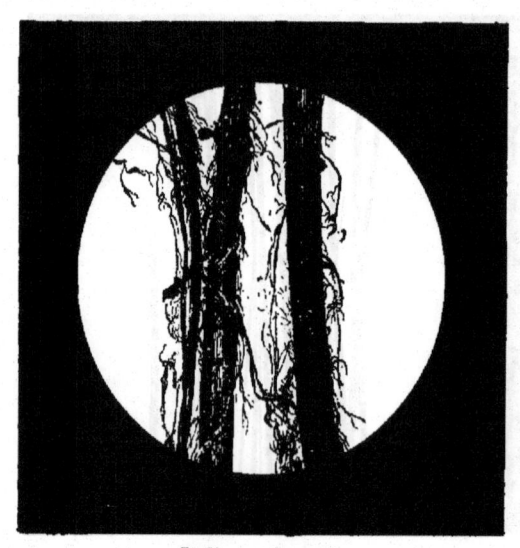

Italian "Grey."

spun glass. These fibres, moreover, were wonderfully uniform in diameter, so uniform, indeed, that the spectrum from end to end consisted of parallel bands, whilst a spider line is so irregular that these bands are hardly observable.

And in regard to strength it appears that as the fibres become finer their relative strength proportionately increases, and actually surpasses that of bar steel, reaching in engineering language as high a figure as 80 tons to the inch, fibres of ordinary size having this strength.

And as the figures of length given can only be realized with difficulty, Mr. Boys illustrates his meaning by saying that a piece of quartz an inch long and an inch in diameter, if drawn out to the degree of fineness alluded to above would be sufficient to go all round the world 658 times, while a grain of sand just visible—say the hundredth part of an inch long and

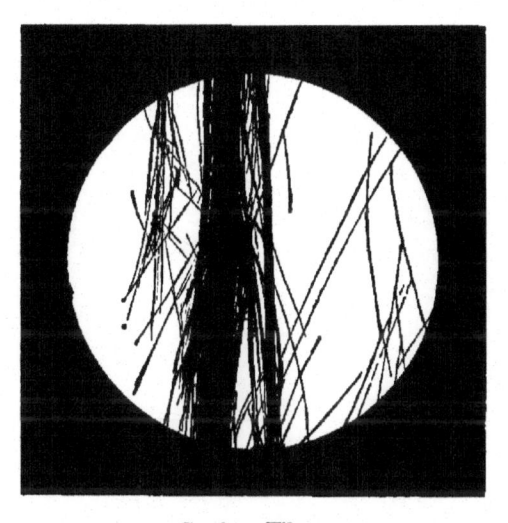

Corsican Fibre.

an hundredth in diameter—would make a thousand miles of such a thread.*

* * * * * *

Having now drawn to a close the description of the very curious and valuable mineral with which the foregoing pages have been concerned, while scientists will have found but little in these pages which is new to them, the writer may say that his own experience has been that, generally speaking, but

* *Jour. Soc. Arts*, June, 1889.

very little is known on the subject of asbestos outside the domains of Science. He trusts, therefore, that his endeavour in this little work to give a clear and popular explanation of the mineral, and the uses to which it is applied, will tend to make it better known, and its many useful qualities more widely appreciated in accordance with its merits.

INDEX.

ABSORPTION of water by slag wool, 196, 198
Accident from contact with electric light, 159
Accident from contact with foot-lights, 159
Actinolite, 19, 21
———— radiated, 19, 76
Adamas, signification of, 10
Adams & Co.'s sewage filtration, 168
Aeronautics, military, 146
African asbestos, 16, 36, 40
Agricola quoted, 3, 4, 70
Air cells, 14, 190, 194
Alaska, asbestos in, 38
Aldini's experiments, 11, 31, 159
Alum, efflorescent, 40
Aluminous asbestos, 40
American asbestos, 33
———————— Company's mine, 99
American Engineer, 192
———— Institute Mining Engineers' visit to Canada, 93
American Journal of Science, 127
Amianthus, 6, 9, 10, 13, 60
Amphibole, 35, 130
Analyses, 47, 48, 59, 61, 73, 92, 103, 185, 186, 203
Anderson & Co.'s slag wool, 188
Anecdotes, 3, 36, 124

Anglo-Canadian Asbestos Co., 96
Ansted, Prof., quoted, 10
Anti-thermal huts, 202
Apatite, 62, 130
Appareil Aldini, Capt. Shaw's account of, 160
Aprons for stokers and firemen, 174
Aqueous origin of asbestos, 95
Arkansas Soapstone Company, 204
Armour plates, protection of, 146
Asbestallicon, 134
Asbestine, 13
Asbestonit, 209
Asbesto-sponge, 143
Asbestos, African, 16, 30, 39, 46
———— American, 33
———— Australian, 38
———— blue, 16
———— British Columbian, 43
———— Broughton, 22, 28, 77, 103
———— Californian, 35
———— Canadian, 43, 58
———— Cape Breton, 76
———— carding of, 25, 30
———— cement, 140, 141
———— Chinese, 39
———— cigarette papers, 177
———— cloth, 3, 6, 55
———— Corsican, 10, 33
———— difficulty in weaving, 4, 211

INDEX.

Asbestos, essentialities of, 30
——— etymology, 13, 59, 70, 212
——— fibres, 218
——— fire-felt, 137, 141
——— general use of, 12, 31
——— immature, 90
——— Italian, 45
——— moulds, 180
——— Newfoundland, 126
——— New South Wales, 38
——— non-fibrous, 19
——— Norwegian, 32, 33, 129
——— packing, varieties of, 133
——— paint, 171
——— paper, 55, 173, 177
——— roofing, 20, 150
——— rope, 175
——— rugs, 183
——— seeds, 52
——— Scandinavian, 33
——— Servian, 33, 41
——— shields, 152
——— Siberian, 33, 37, 52
——— tapestry, 182
——— tobacco, 178
——— true, 14
——— vegetable origin of, 3
Australian foliage, 33
——— asbestos, 38

BÂCHES for military wagons, 149
Baltimorite, 60, 61
Baquet Theatre, fire at, 154
Barberton, rock formation at, 42
Barff, Prof., analyses, 47
Barnum's Exhibition, 162
Barry's "Ivan at Home," 66, 79
Bastard asbestos, 19, 82, 90
Bauer, Prof., quoted, 18
Beetroot sugar refineries, 164
Bell's Asbestos Company, 86
Belmina, 113
Belt, great volcanic, 71

Berlin Opera House, accident at, 159
Big guns, breeches of, 144
— Ham mountain, 72
— Island, 110
Bischoff's experiments, 70
Black Lake mines, 93
Bloxam on slag wool, 198
Blue asbestos, 16
Boiler coverings, 136, 138, 194
Booth & Fisher's asbestos curtains, 151
Bonanza mine, 98
Bonnet on spider webs, 215
Boots, lining for, 179
Borings, trial, 77, 87
Boston Packing Company's mine, 86
Bowman's lectures on wool fibres, 79, 211
Boyd, James, quoted, 5, 163
——————— paper on Italian asbestos, 28, 46, 49, 51
——————— experiments with powder, 148
Boys, C. V., on quartz and other fibres, 215, 216, 224
Boyle quoted, 7
Breeches of big guns, 144
Breyer, Mr., process, 165
Breislakite, 18
"Bridgewater Treatise," 5
British Columbia, 43
Brompton Lake mine, 76
Broughton asbestos, 22, 28, 77, 103
Bruckmann, Prof.'s book, 11, 177
Brumell's Report, 1889, 116, 117
Building laws of America, 150
Byssolite, 18

CALAMINE, 5
Californian asbestos, 35
Canada, cold in, 66
Canadian goldfields, 111
——— maple, 33

anadian Mining Review, 63, 160, 193
────── *Record of Science*, 79
Cape Breton, 76
Captain Shaw on "Fires in Theatres," 155
────── "Fire Protection," 160
Cardboard, 179
Carding, 25, 30
Cariboo Lake, 100
Caron's experiments with magnesia, 8
Carpasian linen, 8
Carriage of explosives, 148
Carystian stone, 8
Cat's eye, 43
Cement, 140, 141
Cerecloth, 7
Chalmers-Spence Company, 137, 177, 180, 182
Chapman, Prof., quoted, 68
Charlemagne's tablecloth, 3
Cheavin's filter, 167
Chinese asbestos, 39
────── medical practice, 39
Cholera belts of slag wool, 197
Chrome iron, 81, 90, 92
Chrysotile, 16, 58, 59
────── Tasmanian, 38
────── British Columbian, 43
────── called amianthus, 23, 60
Cigarette papers, 177
Closing down for winter, 91
Cloth, asbestos, 3, 6, 55
Clothing for firemen, 11, 31, 160
Coating for ironclads, 146
Cobbing, cost of, 122, 123
Cobbold quoted, 39
Cold in Canada, 65, 170
────── Russia, 66
── storage, 163
Coleman's, J. J., paper on non-conductors, 190

Cole's "Micro. Studies," 69
Colour of ore, 82, 105
Coleraine mines, 93
────── mountains, 80, 94
Colonial and Indian Exhibition, 12
Colorado mountains, 68
Commissioner of Crown Lands' Report, 63, 89, 111, 116, 118
Communal Theatre, Amsterdam, burnt, 155
Comparative analyses, 46, 103
────── non-conducting powers, 191
Composition mouldings, 174
Copper, 72
────── and asbestos, 174
Cork, mountain, 14, 15
Corona, Giuseppe della, 11
Corsica, 10, 33
Cottage protected, 201
Cotton fibres, 212
Cost of extraction of ore, 93, 102, 105, 122
Cow Flat copper mines, 18
Cremation cloth, 4
Cremorne Gardens, fire-kings at, 158
Cresswell's filters, 167
────── special marine packing, 135
Crocidolite, 16, 40, 43, 131
Crystal, rock, 7
────── sphere of, 7
Crystals, growth of, 2
Curtains, theatrical: 151
    Booth & Fisher's, 157
    Capt. Heath's, 154
    Chalmers-Spence Company's, 152
    Henry Irving's, 153
    Jodrell Theatre, 154
    Marius' patent, 151
    Terry's Theatre, 152
    United Asbestos Company's, 151

DANA, Prof., quoted, 10, 14, 17, 19, 21, 24, 26, 59, 60, 110, 112, 185, 186
Danville mine, 106
Davies on "Earthy Minerals," 28
Deck cabins of steamers, 164
Decomposed serpentine, 70, 101
Deep borings, 77, 87
Dehydration, 96
De Lapparent quoted, 16, 21, 59, 60, 69, 205
Destruction of theatres by fire, 156
Des Cloizeau quoted, 18
Devonshire everlasting candle, 176
Dewrance steam cocks, 136
Diamond Fields Advertiser, 43
Dick's self-lubricating packing, 135
Difference in fibre, 92
Difficulty in weaving, 5, 211
Diorite, 62, 72, 129
Discolouration, 94, 75, 101
Distinguishing characteristics of ore, 81
Dolomieu, 10
Donald, Prof., quoted, 19, 48, 60, 79, 92, 95, 103
Drink, 124
Drying ore, 95
Dumping, 87, 92
Durable joint, 136
Duriflex packing, 135
Durst, Prof., analyses, 48
Dyeing clothes, cords for, 175
Dykes, effect of, 72, 95, 96
Dynamite shells, 146

EADY, Mr., vi., 195, 218
  Early experiments, 132
Eastern Townships of Quebec, 62, 64, 71
East Broughton, 22, 28, 77, 103
Eastman's asbestallicon packing, 134
Ehrenberg, 208

Electric wires, non-conducting tubes for, 174
Ells, Dr., quoted, 23, 63, 66, 71, 95, 96, 101, 104, 105, 109, 112, 121
Emperors' napkins, 6
Emilie mine, 96
Engineer quoted, 149, 192
Engineering quoted, 31, 52
Engineering uses of asbestos, 132
Erichsen's protective composition, 172
Errors in opening up mines, 87, 92
Eureka mine, 96
Exclusion of heat, 163
Explosives, carriage of, 148

FAILURE, causes of, in mining, 126
Fault, course of the great, 67
Fecteau's discovery of chrysotile, 84
Fibre for stoves, 50, 171
———— spinning, 211
Fibres, asbestos, 218
———— cotton, 212
———— difference in, 92, 94
———— quartz, 218
———— silk, 214
———— slag, 194
———— spider's web, 215
———— spun glass, 209, 217
———— wool, 211
Fiberizing machines, 106, 122, 123
Fibrous actinolite, 20, 26
———— hornblende, 21, 26, 76
———— serpentine, 24
———— tremolite, 20
Filters, construction of, 165
Filters :
      Cheavin's, 167
      Cresswell's, 167
      Judson's, 166
      Lipscombe's, 167
      Maignen's, 166

INDEX.

Filter papers, 164
Filtration purposes, 165
——— of acids, 165
——— sewage, 167
Filtre rapide, 166
Firemen, clothing for, 11, 31, 160
Firemen's and stokers' aprons, 174
Fire at a gas-well, 157
— felt, 139, 140
— fountains of Hawaii, 184
— kings, 158
Fireproof curtains, 150
"Fire Protection," Captain Shaw, 160
Fireside rugs, 183
"Fires in Theatres," Captain Shaw, 155
——— list of, 156
Flax, mountain, 16
Fletcher's gas stoves, 170
Flossy asbestos, 50
Forest fires, 80, 94
Fossil flax, 16
—— meal, 207
Frazer mine, 103
Frechette-Douville mine, 98
French chalk, 203
——— Canadian labour, 124
Furnace linings, 169
Fuses and incandescent circuits, 174
——, time, 145
Fusibility, 2, 9, 22

GAGES' artificial serpentine, 69
Gas shades, 176
Gas stoves, 10, 169
Gaspé, peninsula of, 65, 67, 127
Gas-well on fire, 157
Geikie's "Geology," 21, 23, 69, 184
Geneste, Herscher & Co.'s experiments, 191
Gesner's "Nova Scotia," 76
Gibbon quoted, 8
Gloves, 173

Gold in Eastern Townships, 63
——— Newfoundland, 128
Goldfields of Canada, 111
Goodall, Mr., on soapstone, 205
Gordon Cumming, Miss, 184
Gosselet, M., quoted, 26
Grades of ore, 89
Grading, 121, 123
Granite, effect of, on asbestos, 77
Grant, Baron, 93
Granular structure of rocks, 24
Granulite at Dartmoor, 73
——— effect of, on asbestos, 72, 74, 81, 94, 95
Great volcanic belt, 71
Green garnets, 52
Grey asbestos, 50
Griqualand, 40
Gypsum, 9, 26

HÆCKEL'S "Evolution of Man," 2
Hampden mine, 88
Hanging rods in dye-houses, 175
Harsh fibre, 94
Haussmann, Prof., 17
Heat, conducting powers, 191
——— retaining and excluding, 163
Heath, Captain, curtain, 154
Heddle, Prof., on mountain cork, 15
Helgeland, 131
Herodotus quoted, 4
High prices of asbestos, 34
Hill of silk (Russia), 37
Hippocrates, 11, 39
Hitchins' fireproof plasterings, 198
Hornblende, 14, 21, 60
Housing workmen, 124
Hunt, Dr. J. Sterry, quoted, 60, 65, 127
Hyatt's experiments, 172

ILFRACOMBE (Tasmania) asbestos, 38

Imperfect asbestos, 75, 82, 90
Impresa Mineraria Italiana, 45, 49
Incandescent circuits, 174
Indestructible wicks, 176
Indian dresses of asbestos, 10
Industry, asbestos, in France, 56
Infusibility, 2, 9, 22
Infusorial earth, 207
"Ingwadi Yami," 42
Insulation purposes, 173
Intermediate varieties of ore, 33
Ironclads, coating for, 146
Iron and steel manufacture, 174
Irving's new safety theatre, 153
Isolating dwellings, 201
Italian asbestos, 45, 47, 48, 49
"Ivan at Home," 66, 79

JAGNAUX quoted, 4, 8, 21, 35, 38, 54, 61, 176, 179
James, Mr., actinolite works, 20
Jaspers, 83
Jewellers' blocks, 180
Jodrell Theatre, 154
Johnson Asbestos Company, 12, 85, 219
Joints for hot-air pipes, 143
Jones, Fred., & Co.'s slag wool, 188
Judson's filter, 166

KENNEDY'S discovery, Megantic Mine, 101
Kermesite, 112
Kings, burial dress of, 4
King's mine, 88, 102
Kieselguhr mines, 208

LADDERS, asbestos, 175
Ladewig's process, 179, 209
Lambley & Co.'s mine, 101
Lamps, 8, 10
Lamp wicks, 10, 176

"Lapidarium" quoted, ii, 8
Lapis ollaris, 203
Lapp shoe-grass, 179
La Société Française des Amiantes, 31, 56
"La Vie Souterraine," 28
Leather, mountain, 14, 15
Leeds gas stove, 171
Leuwenhock quoted, 215
Levy quoted, 23
Lightfoot, T. B., experiments, 193
Linings of furnaces, 169
Lint, 149
Lipscombe's filter, 167
Liversedge's "Mineralogy of New South Wales," 18, 38
Locke's "Elementary Natural History" quoted, 1
Logan, Sir W., quoted, 61
Loss of life by fires in theatres, 156
Lucke & Mitchell's mine, 89
Lyell quoted, 23

MACHINE, fiberizing, 106, 102, 123
MacMahon, Major-Gen., quoted, 70
Magnesia, 8, 23, 48
Magnesite, 83
Magnetite, 81, 90
Maignen's filtre rapide, 166
Mail-bags, 149
Manhattan packing, 136
Manufacturers buying mines, 115
Marbles, ornamental, 83
Marco Polo, 6, 10
Mark Twain, 185
Marmolite, 21, 60, 61
Martin mine, 97
Matthews, Dr., in Africa, 42
Meckel quoted, 215
Megantic Mine, 92, 101, 102
Mercier, Hon. W., quoted, 64
Metamorphism, 23
Mica, 10

INDEX. 233

Mica, black, 71
Microscopic studies, Cole's, 69
Millboard, 55
Military balloons, 146
Mineral fibres, delicacy of, 224
——— wool, 187
Minerals of Eastern Townships, 64
——————— New South Wales, 38
——————— Ontario and Quebec, 62
Miners' lamps, 144
Minns & Co.'s packing, 143
Mistakes in opening up mines, 87
Mitchell, Prof., 216
Mode of extraction of ore, 121
Montreal Asbestos Company, 119
Moore's "Ancient Mineralogy," 9
Moseley, Mr., 27
Moulds for type, 180
——————— jewellers, 180
Mountain cork, 14, 15
——————— flax, 16
——————— leather, 14, 15
——————— paper, 14, 15
——————— wood, 14, 82
Mountford's paints, 173
Mummy cloths, 213
Murphy's mine, 89
Murray, Mr. Alexander, 127

NAPKINS of the emperors, 6
Natal asbestos, 40, 169
Native antimony, 112
——— Asbestos Company, 39
New Asbestos Company, 56
Newfoundland, 127
New South Wales asbestos, 38
Nicolet estate, 199
Non-conductors, 191
Non-conducting tubes for electric wires, 174
Non-fibrous asbestos, 19
Norway, 17, 19, 129
"Notes by a Naturalist" (*Challenger*), 27

OBALSKI quoted, 75, 100, 105, 123
Olivine, 70
Ollite, 10, 41, 203
Open fires, 169
Opera Comique, fire at, 152
Ophite and ophiolite, 60, 70
Origin of asbestos, 23
Ottawa valley, 76
Outlook for the trade, 43
Output, cost, &c., 114, 117, 119

PACKINGS, 133
Packings for steam cocks, 136
Packings, Eastwood's asbestalicon, 134
——— Witty & Wyatt's, 134
Paint, 171, 205
Paper, 55, 173, 177
——— wall and ornamental, 176
Paris Exhibition, tests at, 191
Pasty ore, 50, 101
Patent Asbestos Manufacturing Company, 52
——— fire and sound proof plastering, 198
——— ring block, 182
Pausanias quoted, 8
Peculiar properties of asbestos, 2
Pele's hair, 184
Penrose on "Apatite," 62
Percy, Prof., quoted, 186, 198
Peridote, 69
Perpenti, Madame, 11
Petrified wood, 82
Pickett's "Useful Metals" quoted, 40, 187
Picrolite, 18, 38, 60, 61, 75, 82, 129, 130
Pigments, 201
Pikrite, 69
Pilolite, 15
Pipe coverings, 136, 194
——— joints, 136, 143, 168

R

INDEX.

Plaited yarns, 133
Plastic stove-lining, 171
Pliny quoted, 3, 4, 5, 6, 7, 8, 9, 10
Plutarch quoted, 8
Points for consideration before purchasing, 125
Popular Science Monthly, 213, 217
Potstone, 10, 41, 203
Pouchet, M., quoted, 158
Powdery asbestos, 50
Prestwich, Prof., quoted, 23
Price lists printed on asbestos paper, 177
Prices, high, 120
Printing type, 179
Procopius quoted, 159
Profitable nature of asbestos mining, 110, 113, 124
Protection shields, 152
Pseudo-chrysotile in Norway, 130
Pulp, 178
Pyrophyllite, 38
Pyroxene, 14, 21

QUARTZ, 28
 Quartz fibres, 215, 217
" Quartz Fibres," C. V. Boys' paper on, 215
Quebec Central Railway, 91
—— province of, 62
—— river, 91
Quenstedt quoted, 4, 15

RADIANT heat, 170
 " Rambles in Search of Minerals" (Ansted's), 10
Randalite, 143
Rand & Macnally's Atlas, 12
Rannócchia, 70
Ransome's experiments, 172
Redgrave's, Mr. Gilbert, paper on " Slag Wool," 187, 189
Reed, Dr., mine at Coleraine, 100
—————————— Thetford, 90

Reed & Hayden properties, 87
Refuse rock, 123
Removable boiler and pipe coverings, 138
Returns for 1888, 116
—————— 1889, 116
Report of Geological Congress, 26
—— on Yukon District, 43
—————— Mineral Resources of Ontario, 43, 121, 131
Retaining and excluding heat, 163
Ring Strasse Theatre, fire at, 151
Rock crystal, 7
—— wool, 198
Rods in dye-houses, 175
Rogers' experiments, 70
Roll fire-felt, 137
Roman theatres, curtains for, 151
Rope, 175
Roofing slate, 63, 64
Rugs, 183
Russian asbestos, 36, 37
—————— peaches, 79
Rusting, cause of, in ships, 203
Rutile in Norway, 130

SACRED fires, 7
 Safes, 148
Safety lamps, 144
St. Lawrence River, 63, 65, 68
Salting mines in Italy, 51
Scandinavia, physical features of, 129
Schenk's, Dr., Report, 42
Scolecite, 95
Scoria, volcanic, 186
Scott Act, 124
Scottish Canadian Asbestos Company, 97, 104, 119
Selwyn, Dr., quoted, 63, 112
Semenze dell' Amianto, 52
Senarmontite, 112
Seneca quoted, 7
Serpentine, 29, 60, 69, 70, 83

INDEX.

Serpentine, belt, 71
——— decomposed, 70
——— impure, 75
——— marbles, 82
——— Newfoundland, 129
——— Norwegian, 129
——— ornamental, 82
——— soft or pasty, 24, 28, 92, 102, 130
Shaw, Captain, on "Fires in Theatres," 155
——————— "Fire Protection," 160
Shefford, asbestos at, 75
Sheet fire-felt, 141
——— with superator jacket, 141
Sheridan, Mr. Thomas, 77, 86, 87
Shickshock Mountains, 64, 67, 74
Shield curtains, 152
Shoe-grass in Lapland, 179
Siberian asbestos, 36, 37, 87, 52
——— cold, 66
Silicate cotton, 188
Silk fibres, 214
Silky asbestos, 50
Silver at Lake Nicolet, 111
——— in Eastern Townships, 63
Silversmiths' blocks, 180
Simmonds on "Waste Products," 2, 5, 25, 36
Simonin, M., quoted, 28
Singular fact as to Italian asbestos, 51
Slag wool, 187, 193
Slate formation at Broughton, 104
Soapstone, 72, 101, 104, 106, 112, 199, 203
Société Francaise des Amiantes, 56, 149
Soft serpentine, 1, 24, 92, 102
Sources of supply, 32
South Ham mines, 109
Southwark mine, 99
Specimens, fraudulent use of, 81

Speckstein, 199
Spencer, Mr., the aeronaut, 147
Spider's web, 215
Spinning, difficulty of, 30, 211
Spun glass, 209, 217
Steatite, 106, 111, 112, 199, 200
——— from China, 201
Steam pressure, 52
Sterry Hunt, Dr., quoted, 18, 60, 65, 127
Stewart River, 43
Stibnite, 112
Stokers' and firemen's aprons, 174
Stove piping, 174
Strabo quoted, 8
Substitutes and similarities, 184
Sub-varieties, 14
Successful mining, 80
Sudarium, 6
Sugar refineries, 160
Superator, 140, 164
Surface influences, 75, 94

TABLES published by Western Mineral Wool Company, 190
Talc, 34
Tapestry, asbestos, 182
Temagami Lake, 43
Templeton, asbestos at, 76
Terry's Theatre, 153
Theatrical curtains, 150
Theophrastus, 9
Theories of formation, 27
Thetford mines, 84
——— river, 91
Thompson on "Mummy Cloths," 213
Tiger-eye crocidolite, 43
Time fuses, 145
Tobacco paper, 178
Torpedoes, 145
Trade of the province of Quebec, 64
Transport question, 41
Tremolite, 20, 21, 60

Trial borings, 77, 87
True asbestos, 14
Tschermak quoted, 69
Tubes for electric wires, 174
"Twenty-five Years in a Wagon," 41
Tunnelling, 81
Tyndall, Prof., quoted, 19, 25, 181
Type founding, 179

UNITED Asbestos Company, 53, 134, 151, 168
United States asbestos, 33, 35
—— —— Geological Exploring Expedition, 185
Ural, the, 36
Uses of asbestos, 12, 144
Utilization of waste, 106

VALENTINITE, 112
Varieties of asbestos, 13
Varro, 5
Vatican Museum, 5
Vegetable origin, 1, 3
Veins, irregular, 80
—— largest not the best, 79
Vestal virgins' lamps, 8
Victor Hugo, 130
—— metallic packings, 134
—— woven sheeting and tape, 168
Ville, M., 57
Volcanic belt, course of, 71
—— rocks 23, 65, 74

WAGES, 121
Wallace, Prof., 221
Wall and ornamental papers, 176
Ward and Ross mine, 88
Warfare, uses of asbestos in, 144
Warm air stoves, 170
"Waste Products," 2, 5, 25, 36
Waste, utilization of, 106
Watch-case blocks, 180
Weaving, difficulty of, 4, 211
Weight of slag, 190
Wertheim's mine, 99, 160
Western Mineral Wool Company, 188
Whaleite, 210
White's Asbestos Company, 102, 119
Whitehead's torpedoes, 145
Wicks, lamp, 176
Willimott's Report, 111, 131
Wilson's "Science Jottings," 216
Winter work, 91
Witty & Wyatt's packing, 134
Wolfestown, 112
Woodite, 209
Wood, Mr. Charles, 187, 189
Wood wool, 210
Woodwork in buildings, 171
Wool fibres, 79, 211
Writing paper, 177
Wyoming asbestos, 35

YARN, how made, 55
Yarn, a Yankee, 157

7, STATIONERS' HALL COURT, LONDON, E.C.
October, 1889.

A CATALOGUE OF BOOKS

INCLUDING MANY NEW AND STANDARD WORKS IN
ENGINEERING, MECHANICS, ARCHITECTURE,
NATURAL AND APPLIED SCIENCE,
INDUSTRIAL ARTS, TRADE AND COMMERCE, AGRICULTURE,
GARDENING, LAND MANAGEMENT, LAW, &c.

PUBLISHED BY
CROSBY LOCKWOOD & SON.

MECHANICS, MECHANICAL ENGINEERING, etc.

New Manual for Practical Engineers.

THE PRACTICAL ENGINEER'S HAND-BOOK. Comprising a Treatise on Modern Engines and Boilers: Marine, Locomotive and Stationary. And containing a large collection of Rules and Practical Data relating to recent Practice in Designing and Constructing all kinds of Engines, Boilers, and other Engineering work. The whole constituting a comprehensive Key to the Board of Trade and other Examinations for Certificates of Competency in Modern Mechanical Engineering. By WALTER S. HUTTON, Civil and Mechanical Engineer, Author of "The Works' Manager's Handbook for Engineers," &c. With upwards of 370 Illustrations. Third Edition, Revised, with Additions. Medium 8vo, nearly 500 pp., price 18s. Strongly bound. [*Just published.*

☞ *This work is designed as a companion to the Author's* "WORKS' MANAGER'S HAND-BOOK." *It possesses many new and original features, and contains, like its predecessor, a quantity of matter not originally intended for publication, but collected by the author for his own use in the construction of a great variety of modern engineering work.*

The information is given in a condensed and concise form, and is illustrated by upwards of 370 Woodcuts; and comprises a quantity of tabulated matter of great value to all engaged in designing, constructing, or estimating for ENGINES, BOILERS *and* OTHER ENGINEERING WORK.

*** OPINIONS OF THE PRESS.

" We have kept it at hand for several weeks, referring to it as occasion arose, and we have not on a single occasion consulted its pages without finding the information of which we were in quest."—*Athenæum*.

" A thoroughly good practical handbook, which no engineer can go through without learning something that will be of service to him."—*Marine Engineer*.

" An excellent book of reference for engineers, and a valuable text-book for students of engineering."—*Scotsman*.

" This valuable manual embodies the results and experience of the leading authorities on mechanical engineering."—*Building News*.

" The author has collected together a surprising quantity of rules and practical data, and has shown much judgment in the selections he has made. . . . There is no doubt that this book is one of the most useful of its kind published, and will be a very popular compendium."—*Engineer*.

" A mass of information, set down in simple language, and in such a form that it can be easily referred to at any time. The matter is uniformly good and well chosen, and is greatly elucidated by the illustrations. The book will find its way on to most engineers' shelves, where it will rank as one of the most useful books of reference."—*Practical Engineer*.

" Full of useful information, and should be found on the office shelf of all practical engineers." —*English Mechanic.*

B

Handbook for Works' Managers.

THE WORKS' MANAGER'S HANDBOOK OF MODERN RULES, TABLES, AND DATA. For Engineers, Millwrights, and Boiler Makers; Tool Makers, Machinists, and Metal Workers; Iron and Brass Founders, &c. By W. S. HUTTON, Civil and Mechanical Engineer, Author of "The Practical Engineer's Handbook." Third Edition, carefully Revised, with Additions. In One handsome Vol., medium 8vo price 15s. strongly bound.

☞ *The Author having compiled Rules and Data for his own use in a great variety of modern engineering work, and having found his notes extremely useful, decided to publish them—revised to date—believing that a practical work, suited to the* DAILY REQUIREMENTS OF MODERN ENGINEERS, *would be favourably received.*

In the Third Edition, the following among other additions have been made, viz.: Rules for the Proportions of Riveted Joints in Soft Steel Plates, the Results of Experiments by PROFESSOR KENNEDY *for the Institution of Mechanical Engineers—Rules for the Proportions of Turbines—Rules for the Strength of Hollow Shafts of Whitworth's Compressed Steel, &c.*

*** OPINIONS OF THE PRESS.

"The author treats every subject from the point of view of one who has collected workshop notes for application in workshop practice, rather than from the theoretical or literary aspect. The volume contains a great deal of that kind of information which is gained only by practical experience, and is seldom written in books."—*Engineer.*

"The volume is an exceedingly useful one, brimful with engineers' notes, memoranda, and rules, and well worthy of being on every mechanical engineer's bookshelf."—*Mechanical World.*

"A formidable mass of facts and figures, readily accessible through an elaborate index . . . . Such a volume will be found absolutely necessary as a book of reference in all sorts of 'works' connected with the metal trades."—*Ryland's Iron Trades Circular.*

"Brimful of useful information, stated in a concise form, Mr. Hutton's books have met a pressing want among engineers. The book must prove extremely useful to every practical man possessing a copy."—*Practical Engineer.*

"The Modernised Templeton."

THE PRACTICAL MECHANIC'S WORKSHOP COMPANION. Comprising a great variety of the most useful Rules and Formulæ in Mechanical Science, with numerous Tables of Practical Data and Calculated Results for Facilitating Mechanical Operations. By WILLIAM TEMPLETON, Author of "The Engineer's Practical Assistant," &c. &c. Fifteenth Edition, Revised, Modernised, and considerably Enlarged by WALTER S. HUTTON, C.E., Author of "The Works' Manager's Handbook," "The Practical Engineer's Handbook," &c. Fcap. 8vo, nearly 500 pp., with Eight Plates and upwards of 250 Illustrative Diagrams, 6s., strongly bound for workshop or pocket wear and tear.

☞ TEMPLETON'S " MECHANIC'S WORKSHOP COMPANION" *has been for more than a quarter of a century deservedly popular, and, as the well-worn and thumb-marked* vade mecum *of several generations of intelligent and aspiring workmen, it has had the reputation of having been the means of raising many of them in their position in life.*

In consequence of the lapse of time since the Author's death, and the great advances in Mechanical Science, the Publishers have thought it advisable to have it entirely Reconstructed and Modernised; and in its present greatly Enlarged and Improved form, they are sure that it will commend itself to the English workmen of the present day all the world over, and become, like its predecessors, their indispensable friend and referee.

A smaller type having been adopted, and the page increased in size, while the number of pages has advanced from about 330 to nearly 500, the book practically contains double the amount of matter that was comprised in the original work.

*** OPINIONS OF THE PRESS.

"In its modernised form Hutton's 'Templeton' should have a wide sale, for it contains much valuable information which the mechanic will often find of use, and not a few tables and notes which he might look for in vain in other works. This modernised edition will be appreciated by all who have learned to value the original editions of 'Templeton.'"—*English Mechanic.*

"It has met with great success in the engineering workshop, as we can testify; and there are a great many men who, in a great measure, owe their rise in life to this little book."—*Building News.*

"This familiar text-book—well known to all mechanics and engineers—is of essential service to the every-day requirements of engineers, millwrights, and the various trades connected with engineering and building. The new modernised edition is worth its weight in gold."—*Building News.* (Second Notice.)

"The publishers wisely entrusted the task of revision of this popular, valuable and useful book to Mr. Hutton, than whom a more competent man they could not have found."—*Iron.*

MECHANICS, MECHANICAL ENGINEERING, etc.

Stone-working Machinery.
STONE-WORKING MACHINERY, and the Rapid and Economical Conversion of Stone. With Hints on the Arrangement and Management of Stone Works. By M. POWIS BALE, M.I.M.E. Crown 8vo, 9s.

"Should be in the hands of every mason or student of stone-work."—*Colliery Guardian.*
"It is in every sense of the word a standard work upon a subject which the author is fully competent to deal exhaustively with."—*Builder's Weekly Reporter.*
"A capital handbook for all who manipulate stone for building or ornamental purposes."—*Machinery Market.*

Pump Construction and Management.
PUMPS AND PUMPING: A Handbook for Pump Users. Being Notes on Selection, Construction and Management. By M. POWIS BALE, M.I.M.E., Author of "Woodworking Machinery," "Saw Mills," &c. Crown 8vo, 2s. 6d. cloth. [*Just published.*

"The matter is set forth as concisely as possible. In fact, condensation rather than diffuseness has been the author's aim throughout; yet he does not seem to have omitted anything likely to be of use."—*Journal of Gas Lighting.*
"Thoroughly practical and simply and clearly written."—*Glasgow Herald.*

Turning.
LATHE-WORK: A Practical Treatise on the Tools, Appliances, and Processes employed in the Art of Turning. By PAUL N. HASLUCK. Third Edition, Revised and Enlarged. Crown 8vo, 5s. cloth.

"Written by a man who knows, not only how work ought to be done, but who also knows how to do it, and how to convey his knowledge to others. To all turners this book would be valuable."—*Engineering.*
"We can safely recommend the work to young engineers. To the amateur it will simply be invaluable. To the student it will convey a great deal of useful information."—*Engineer.*
"A compact, succinct, and handy guide to lathe-work did not exist in our language until Mr. Hasluck, by the publication of this treatise, gave the turner a true *vade-mecum.*"—*House Decorator.*

Screw-Cutting.
SCREW THREADS: And Methods of Producing Them. With Numerous Tables, and complete directions for using Screw-Cutting Lathes. By PAUL N. HASLUCK, Author of "Lathe-Work," &c. With Fifty Illustrations. Second Edition. Waistcoat-pocket size, price 1s. cloth.

"Full of useful information, hints and practical criticism. Taps, dies and screwing-tools generally are illustrated and their action described."—*Mechanical World.*

Smith's Tables for Mechanics, etc.
TABLES, MEMORANDA, AND CALCULATED RESULTS, FOR MECHANICS, ENGINEERS, ARCHITECTS, BUILDERS, etc. Selected and Arranged by FRANCIS SMITH. Fourth Edition, Revised and Enlarged, 250 pp., waistcoat-pocket size, 1s. 6d. limp leather.

"It would, perhaps, be as difficult to make a small pocket-book selection of notes and formulæ to suit ALL engineers as it would be to make a universal medicine; but Mr. Smith's waistcoat-pocket collection may be looked upon as a successful attempt."—*Engineer.*
"The best example we have ever seen of 250 pages of useful matter packed into the dimensions of a card-case."—*Building News.* "A veritable pocket treasury of knowledge."—*Iron.*

Engineer's and Machinist's Assistant.
THE ENGINEER'S, MILLWRIGHT'S, and MACHINIST'S PRACTICAL ASSISTANT. A collection of Useful Tables, Rules and Data. By WILLIAM TEMPLETON. 7th Edition, with Additions. 18mo, 2s. 6d. cloth.

"Occupies a foremost place among books of this kind. A more suitable present to an apprentice to any of the mechanical trades could not possibly be made."—*Building News.*
"A deservedly popular work, it should be in the 'drawer' of every mechanic."—*English Mechanic.*

Iron and Steel.
"IRON AND STEEL": A Work for the Forge, Foundry, Factory, and Office. Containing ready, useful, and trustworthy Information for Iron-masters and their Stock-takers; Managers of Bar, Rail, Plate, and Sheet Rolling Mills; Iron and Metal Founders; Iron Ship and Bridge Builders; Mecnanical, Mining, and Consulting Engineers; Architects, Builders, and Draughtsmen. By CHARLES HOARE, Author of "The Slide Rule," &c. Eighth Edition, Revised and considerably Enlarged. 32mo, 6s. leather.

"One of the best of the pocket books."—*English Mechanic.*
"We cordially recommend this book to those engaged in considering the details of all kinds of iron and steel works."—*Naval Science.*

Engineering Construction.

PATTERN-MAKING: *A Practical Treatise*, embracing the Main Types of Engineering Construction, and including Gearing, both Hand and Machine made, Engine Work, Sheaves and Pulleys, Pipes and Columns, Screws, Machine Parts, Pumps and Cocks, the Moulding of Patterns in Loam and Greensand, &c., together with the methods of Estimating the weight of Castings; to which is added an Appendix of Tables for Workshop Reference. By a FOREMAN PATTERN MAKER. With upwards of Three Hundred and Seventy Illustrations. Crown 8vo, 7s. 6d. cloth.

"A well-written technical guide, evidently written by a man who understands and has practised what he has written about. We cordially recommend it to engineering students, young journeymen, and others desirous of being initiated into the mysteries of pattern-making."—*Builder*.

"Likely to prove a welcome guide to many workmen, especially to draughtsmen who have lacked a training in the shops, pupils pursuing their practical studies in our factories, and to employers and managers in engineering works."—*Hardware Trade Journal*.

"More than 370 illustrations help to explain the text, which is, however, always clear and explicit, thus rendering the work an excellent *vade mecum* for the apprentice who desires to become master of his trade."—*English Mechanic*.

Dictionary of Mechanical Engineering Terms.

LOCKWOOD'S DICTIONARY OF TERMS USED IN THE PRACTICE OF MECHANICAL ENGINEERING, embracing those current in the Drawing Office, Pattern Shop, Foundry, Fitting, Turning, Smith's and Boiler Shops, &c. &c. Comprising upwards of 6,000 Definitions. Edited by A FOREMAN PATTERN-MAKER, Author of "Pattern Making." Crown 8vo, 7s. 6d. cloth.

"Just the sort of handy dictionary required by the various trades engaged in mechanical engineering. The practical engineering pupil will find the book of great value in his studies, and every foreman engineer and mechanic should have a copy."—*Building News*.

"After a careful examination of the book, and trying all manner of words, we think that the engineer will here find all he is likely to require. It will be largely used."—*Practical Engineer*.

"This admirable dictionary, although primarily intended for the use of draughtsmen and other technical craftsmen, is of much larger value as a book of reference, and will find a ready welcome in many libraries."—*Glasgow Herald*.

"One of the most useful books which can be presented to a mechanic or student."—*English Mechanic*.

"Not merely a dictionary, but, to a certain extent, also a most valuable guide. It strikes us as a happy idea to combine with a definition of the phrase useful information on the subject of which it treats."—*Machinery Market*.

"This carefully-compiled volume forms a kind of pocket cyclopædia of the extensive subject to which it is devoted. No word having connection with any branch of constructive engineering seems to be omitted. No more comprehensive work has been, so far, issued."—*Knowledge*.

"We strongly commend this useful and reliable adviser to our friends in the workshop, and to students everywhere."—*Colliery Guardian*.

Steam Boilers.

A TREATISE ON STEAM BOILERS: *Their Strength, Construction, and Economical Working*. By ROBERT WILSON, C.E. Fifth Edition. 12mo, 6s. cloth.

"The best treatise that has ever been published on steam boilers."—*Engineer*.

"The author shows himself perfect master of his subject, and we heartily recommend all employing steam power to possess themselves of the work."—*Ryland's Iron Trade Circular*.

Boiler Chimneys.

BOILER AND FACTORY CHIMNEYS; *Their Draught-Power and Stability*. With a Chapter on *Lightning Conductors*. By ROBERT WILSON, C.E., Author of "A Treatise on Steam Boilers," &c. Second Edition. Crown 8vo, 3s. 6d. cloth.

"Full of useful information, definite in statement, and thoroughly practical in treatment."—*The Local Government Chronicle*.

"A valuable contribution to the literature of scientific building. . . . The whole subject is a very interesting and important one, and it is gratifying to know that it has fallen into such competent hands."—*The Builder*.

Boiler Making.

THE BOILER-MAKER'S READY RECKONER. With Examples of Practical Geometry and Templating, for the Use of Platers, Smiths and Riveters. By JOHN COURTNEY, Edited by D. K. CLARK, M.I.C.E. Second Edition, Revised, with Additions, 12mo, 5s. half-bound.

"No workman or apprentice should be without this book."—*Iron Trade Circular*.

"A reliable guide to the working boiler-maker."—*Iron*.

"Boiler-makers will readily recognise the value of this volume. . . . The tables are clearly printed, and so arranged that they can be referred to with the greatest facility, so that it cannot be doubted that they will be generally appreciated and much used."—*Mining Journal*.

Steam Engine.

TEXT-BOOK ON THE STEAM ENGINE. With a Supplement on Gas Engines. By T. M. GOODEVE, M.A., Barrister-at-Law, Author of "The Elements of Mechanism," &c. Tenth Edition, En'arged. With numerous Illustrations. Crown 8vo, 6s. cloth. [*Just published.*

"Professor Goodeve has given us a treatise on the steam engine which will bear comparison with anything written by Huxley or Maxwell, and we can award it no higher praise."—*Engineer.*

"Professor Goodeve's book is ably and clearly written. It is a sound work."—*Athenæum.*

"Mr. Goodeve's text-book is a work of which every young engineer should possess himself."—*Mining Journal.*

"Essentially practical in ts aim. The manner of exposition leaves nothing to be desired."—*Scotsman.*

Gas Engines.

ON GAS-ENGINES. Being a Reprint, with some Additions, of the Supplement to the *Text-book on the Steam Engine*, by T. M. GOODEVE, M.A. Crown 8vo, 2s. 6d. cloth. [*Just published.*

"Like all Mr. Goodeve's writings, the present s no exception in point of general excellence. It is a valuable little volume."—*Mechanical World.*

"This little book will be useful to those who desire to understand how the gas-engine works.'—*English Mechanic.*

Steam.

THE SAFE USE OF STEAM. Containing Rules for Unprofessional Steam-users. By an ENGINEER. Sixth Edition. Sewed, 6d.

"If steam-users would but learn this little book by heart boiler explosions would become sensations by their rarity."—*English Mechanic.*

Coal and Speed Tables.

A POCKET BOOK OF COAL AND SPEED TABLES, for Engineers and Steam-users. By NELSON FOLEY, Author of "Boiler Construction." Pocket-size, 3s. 6d. cloth; 4s. leather.

"This is a very useful book, containing very useful tables. The results given are well chosen, and the volume contains evidence that the author really understands his subject. We can recommend the work with pleasure."—*Mechanical World.*

"These tables are designed to meet the requirements of every-day use; they are of sufficient scope for most practical purposes, and may be commended to engineers and users of steam."—*Iron.*

"This pocket-book well merits the attention of the practical engineer. Mr. Foley has compiled a very useful set of tables, the information contained in which is frequently required by engineers, coal consumers and users of steam."—*Iron and Coal Trades Review.*

Fire Engineering.

FIRES, FIRE-ENGINES, AND FIRE-BRIGADES. With a History of Fire-Engines, their Construction, Use, and Management; Remarks on Fire-Proof Buildings, and the Preservation of Life from Fire; Statistics of the Fire Appliances in English Towns; Foreign Fire Systems; Hints on Fire Brigades, &c. &c. By CHARLES F. T. YOUNG, C.E. With numerous Illustrations, 544 pp., demy 8vo, £1 4s. cloth.

"To such of our readers as are interested in the subject of fires and fire apparatus, we can most heartily commend this book. It is really the only English work we now have upon the subject."—*Engineering.*

"It displays much evidence of careful research; and Mr. Young has put his facts neatly together. It is evident enough that his acquaintance with the practical details of the construction of steam fire engines, old and new, and the conditions with which it is necessary they should comply, is accurate and full."—*Engineer.*

Gas Lighting.

COMMON SENSE FOR GAS-USERS: A Catechism of Gas-Lighting for Householders, Gasfitters, Millowners, Architects, Engineers, etc. By ROBERT WILSON, C.E., Author of "A Treatise on Steam Boilers." Second Edition, with Folding Plates and Wood Engravings. Crown 8vo, price 1s. in wrapper.

"All gas-users will decidedly benefit, both in pocket and comfort, if they will avail themselves of Mr. Wilson's counsels."—*Engineering.*

Dynamo Construction.

HOW TO MAKE A DYNAMO: A Practical Treatise for Amateurs. Containing numerous Illustrations and Detailed Instructions for Constructing a Small Dynamo, to Produce the Electric Light. By ALFRED CROFTS. Second Edition, Revised and Enlarged. Crown 8vo, 2s. cloth. [*Just published.*

"The instructions given in this unpretentious little book are suffi iently clear and explicit to enable any amateur mechanic possessed of average skill and the usual tools to be found in an amateur's workshop, to build a practical dynamo machine."—*Electrician.*

THE POPULAR WORKS OF MICHAEL REYNOLDS
("The Engine Driver's Friend").

Locomotive-Engine Driving.
LOCOMOTIVE-ENGINE DRIVING: A Practical Manual for Engineers in charge of Locomotive Engines. By MICHAEL REYNOLDS, Member of the Society of Engineers, formerly Locomotive Inspector L. B. and S. C. R. Eighth Edition. Including a KEY TO THE LOCOMOTIVE ENGINE. With Illustrations and Portrait of Author. Crown 8vo, 4s. 6d. cloth.

"Mr. Reynolds has supplied a want, and has supplied it well. We can confidently recommend the book, not only to the practical driver, but to everyone who takes an interest in the performance of locomotive engines."—*The Engineer*.

"Mr. Reynolds has opened a new chapter in the literature of the day. This admirable practical treatise, of the practical utility of which we have to speak in terms of warm commendation."—*Athenæum*.

"Evidently the work of one who knows his subject thoroughly."—*Railway Service Gazette*.

"Were the cautions and rules given in the book to become part of the every-day working of our engine-drivers, we might have fewer distressing accidents to deplore."—*Scotsman*.

Stationary Engine Driving.
STATIONARY ENGINE DRIVING: A Practical Manual for Engineers in charge of Stationary Engines. By MICHAEL REYNOLDS. Third Edition, Enlarged. With Plates and Woodcuts. Crown 8vo, 4s. 6d. cloth.

"The author is thoroughly acquainted with his subjects, and his advice on the various points treated is clear and practical. . . . He has produced a manual which is an exceedingly useful one for the class for whom it is specially intended."—*Engineering*.

"Our author leaves no stone unturned. He is determined that his readers shall not only know something about the stationary engine, but all about it."—*Engineer*.

"An engineman who has mastered the contents of Mr. Reynolds's book will require but little actual experience with boilers and engines before he can be trusted to look after them."—*English Mechanic*.

The Engineer, Fireman, and Engine-Boy.
THE MODEL LOCOMOTIVE ENGINEER, FIREMAN, and ENGINE-BOY. Comprising a Historical Notice of the Pioneer Locomotive Engines and their Inventors. By MICHAEL REYNOLDS. With numerous Illustrations and a fine Portrait of George Stephenson. Crown 8vo, 4s. 6d. cloth.

"From the technical knowledge of the author it will appeal to the railway man of to-day more forcibly than anything written by Dr. Smiles. . . . The volume contains information of a technical kind, and facts that every driver should be familiar with."—*English Mechanic*.

"We should be glad to see this book in the possession of everyone in the kingdom who has ever laid, or is to lay, hands on a locomotive engine."—*Iron*.

Continuous Railway Brakes.
CONTINUOUS RAILWAY BRAKES: A Practical Treatise on the several Systems in Use in the United Kingdom; their Construction and Performance. With copious Illustrations and numerous Tables. By MICHAEL REYNOLDS. Large crown 8vo, 9s. cloth.

"A popular explanation of the different brakes. It will be of great assistance in forming public opinion, and will be studied with benefit by those who take an interest in the brake."—*English Mechanic*.

"Written with sufficient technical detail to enable the principle and relative connection of the various parts of each particular brake to be readily grasped."—*Mechanical World*.

Engine-Driving Life.
ENGINE-DRIVING LIFE: Stirring Adventures and Incidents in the Lives of Locomotive-Engine Drivers. By MICHAEL REYNOLDS. Second Edition, with Additional Chapters. Crown 8vo, 2s. cloth. [*Just published*.

"From first to last perfectly fascinating. Wilkie Collins's most thrilling conceptions are thrown into the shade by true incidents, endless in their variety, related in every page."—*North British Mail*.

"Anyone who wishes to get a real insight into railway life cannot do better than read 'Engine-Driving Life' for himself; and if he once take it up he will find that the author's enthusiasm and real love of the engine-driving profession will carry him on till he has read every page."—*Saturday Review*.

Pocket Companion for Enginemen.
THE ENGINEMAN'S POCKET COMPANION AND PRACTICAL EDUCATOR FOR ENGINEMEN, BOILER ATTENDANTS, AND MECHANICS. By MICHAEL REYNOLDS. With Forty-five Illustrations and numerous Diagrams. Second Edition, Revised. Royal 18mo, 3s. 6d., strongly bound for pocket wear.

"This admirable work is well suited to accomplish its object, being the honest workmanship of a competent engineer."—*Glasgow Herald*.

"A most meritorious work, giving in a succinct and practical form all the information an engineminder desirous of mastering the scientific principles of his daily calling would require."—*Miller*.

"A boon to those who are striving to become efficient mechanics."—*Daily Chronicle*.

French-English Glossary for Engineers, etc.

A POCKET GLOSSARY of TECHNICAL TERMS: ENGLISH-FRENCH, FRENCH-ENGLISH; with Tables suitable for the Architectural, Engineering, Manufacturing and Nautical Professions. By JOHN JAMES FLETCHER, Engineer and Surveyor; 200 pp. Waistcoat-pocket size, 1s. 6d., limp leather.

"It ought certainly to be in the waistcoat-pocket of every professional man. — *Iron.*
"It is a very great advantage for readers and correspondents in France and England to have so large a number of the words relating to engineering and manufacturers collected in a liliputian volume. The little book will be useful both to students and travellers."—*Architect.*
"The glossary of terms is very complete, and many of the tables are new and well arranged. We cordially commend the book."—*Mechanical World.*

Portable Engines.

THE PORTABLE ENGINE; ITS CONSTRUCTION AND MANAGEMENT. A Practical Manual for Owners and Users of Steam Engines generally. By WILLIAM DYSON WANSBROUGH. With 90 Illustrations. Crown 8vo, 3s. 6d. cloth.

"This is a work of value to those who use steam machinery. . . . Should be read by everyone who has a steam engine, on a farm or elsewhere."—*Mark Lane Express.*
"We cordially commend this work to buyers and owners of steam engines, and to those who have to do with their construction or use."—*Timber Trades Journal.*
"Such a general knowledge of the steam engine as Mr. Wansbrough furnishes to the reader should be acquired by all intelligent owners and others who use the steam engine."—*Building News.*

CIVIL ENGINEERING, SURVEYING, etc.

MR. HUMBER'S IMPORTANT ENGINEERING BOOKS.

The Water Supply of Cities and Towns.

A COMPREHENSIVE TREATISE on the WATER-SUPPLY OF CITIES AND TOWNS. By WILLIAM HUMBER, A-M.Inst.C.E., and M. Inst. M.E., Author of "Cast and Wrought Iron Bridge Construction," &c. &c. Illustrated with 50 Double Plates, 1 Single Plate, Coloured Frontispiece, and upwards of 250 Woodcuts, and containing 400 pages of Text. Imp. 4to, £6 6s. elegantly and substantially half-bound in morocco.

List of Contents.

I. Historical Sketch of some of the means that have been adopted for the Supply of Water to Cities and Towns.—II. Water and the Foreign Matter usually associated with it.—III. Rainfall and Evaporation.—IV. Springs and the water-bearing formations of various districts.—V. Measurement and Estimation of the flow of Water—VI. On the Selection of the Source of Supply.—VII. Wells.—VIII. Reservoirs.—IX. The Purification of Water.—X. Pumps. — XI. Pumping Machinery.— XII. Conduits.—XIII. Distribution of Water.—XIV. Meters, Service Pipes, and House Fittings.—XV. The Law and Economy of Water Works.—XVI. Constant and Intermittent Supply.—XVII. Description of Plates. — Appendices, giving Tables of Rates of Supply, Velocities, &c. &c., together with Specifications of several Works illustrated, among which will be found: Aberdeen, Bideford, Canterbury, Dundee, Halifax, Lambeth, Rotherham, Dublin, and others.

"The most systematic and valuable work upon water supply hitherto produced in English, or in any other language. . . . Mr. Humber's work is characterised almost throughout by an exhaustiveness much more distinctive of French and German than of English technical treatises."—*Engineer.*
"We can congratulate Mr. Humber on having been able to give so large an amount of information on a subject so important as the water supply of cities and towns. The plates, fifty in number, are mostly drawings of executed works, and alone would have commanded the attention of every engineer whose practice may lie in this branch of the profession."—*Builder.*

Cast and Wrought Iron Bridge Construction.

A COMPLETE AND PRACTICAL TREATISE ON CAST AND WROUGHT IRON BRIDGE CONSTRUCTION, including Iron Foundations. In Three Parts—Theoretical, Practical, and Descriptive. By WILLIAM HUMBER, A.M.Inst.C.E., and M.Inst.M.E. Third Edition, Revised and much improved, with 115 Double Plates (20 of which now first appear in this edition), and numerous Additions to the Text. In Two Vols., imp. 4to, £6 16s. 6d. half-bound in morocco.

"A very valuable contribution to the standard literature of civil engineering. In addition to elevations, plans and sections, large scale details are given which very much enhance the instructive worth of those illustrations."—*Civil Engineer and Architect's Journal.*
"Mr. Humber's stately volumes, lately issued—in which the most important bridges erected during the last five years, under the direction of the late Mr. Brunel, Sir W. Cubitt, Mr. Hawkshaw, Mr. Page, Mr. Fowler, Mr. Hemans, and others among our most eminent engineers, are drawn and specified in great detail."—*Engineer*

MR. HUMBER'S GREAT WORK ON MODERN ENGINEERING.

Complete in Four Volumes, imperial 4to, price £12 12s., half-morocco. Each Volume sold separately as follows:—

A RECORD OF THE PROGRESS OF MODERN ENGINEERING.
FIRST SERIES. Comprising Civil, Mechanical, Marine, Hydraulic, Railway, Bridge, and other Engineering Works, &c. By WILLIAM HUMBER, A-M.Inst.C.E., &c. Imp. 4to, with 36 Double Plates, drawn to a large scale, Photographic Portrait of John Hawkshaw, C.E., F.R.S., &c., and copious descriptive Letterpress, Specifications, &c., £3 3s. half-morocco.

List of the Plates and Diagrams.

Victoria Station and Roof, L. B. & S. C. R. (8 plates); Southport Pier (2 plates); Victoria Station and Roof, L. C. & D. and G. W. R. (6 plates); Roof of Cremorne Music Hall; Bridge over G. N. Railway; Roof of Station, Dutch Rhenish Rail (2 plates); Bridge over the Thames, West London Extension Railway (5 plates); Armour Plates: Suspension Bridge, Thames (4 plates); The Allen Engine; Suspension Bridge, Avon (3 plates); Underground Railway (3 plates).

"Handsomely lithographed and printed. It will find favour with many who desire to preserve in a permanent form copies of the plans and specifications prepared for the guidance of the contractors for many important engineering works."—*Engineer.*

HUMBER'S RECORD OF MODERN ENGINEERING. SECOND
SERIES. Imp. 4to, with 36 Double Plates, Photographic Portrait of Robert Stephenson, C.E., M.P., F.R.S., &c., and copious descriptive Letterpress, Specifications, &c., £3 3s. half-morocco.

List of the Plates and Diagrams.

Birkenhead Docks, Low Water Basin (15 plates); Charing Cross Station Roof, C. C. Railway (3 plates); Digswell Viaduct, Great Northern Railway; Robbery Wood Viaduct, Great Northern Railway; Iron Permanent Way; Clydach Viaduct, Merthyr, Tredegar, and Abergavenny Railway; Ebbw Viaduct, Merthyr, Tredegar, and Abergavenny Railway; College Wood Viaduct, Cornwall Railway; Dublin Winter Palace Roof (3 plates); Bridge over the Thames, L. C. & D. Railway (6 plates); Albert Harbour, Greenock (4 plates).

"Mr. Humber has done the profession good and true service, by the fine collection of examples he has here brought before the profession and the public."—*Practical Mechanic's Journal.*

HUMBER'S RECORD OF MODERN ENGINEERING. THIRD
SERIES. Imp. 4to, with 40 Double Plates, Photographic Portrait of J. R. M'Clean, late Pres. Inst. C.E., and copious descriptive Letterpress, Specifications, &c., £3 3s. half-morocco.

List of the Plates and Diagrams.

MAIN DRAINAGE, METROPOLIS.—*North Side.*—Map showing Interception of Sewers; Middle Level Sewer (2 plates); Outfall Sewer, Bridge over River Lea (3 plates); Outfall Sewer, Bridge over Marsh Lane, North Woolwich Railway, and Bow and Barking Railway Junction; Outfall Sewer, Bridge over Bow and Barking Railway (3 plates); Outfall Sewer, Bridge over East London Waterworks' Feeder (2 plates); Outfall Sewer, Reservoir (2 plates); Outfall Sewer, Tumbling Bay and Outlet; Outfall Sewer, Penstocks. *South Side.*—Outfall Sewer, Bermondsey Branch (2 plates); Outfall Sewer, Reservoir and Outlet (4 plates); Outfall Sewer, Filth Hoist; Sections of Sewers (North and South Sides).
THAMES EMBANKMENT.—Section of River Wall; Steamboat Pier, Westminster (2 plates); Landing Stairs between Charing Cross and Waterloo Bridges; York Gate (2 plates); Overflow and Outlet at Savoy Street Sewer (3 plates); Steamboat Pier, Waterloo Bridge (3 plates); Junction of Sewers, Plans and Sections; Gullies, Plans and Sections; Rolling Stock; Granite and Iron Forts.

"The drawings have a constantly increasing value, and whoever desires to possess clear representations of the two great works carried out by our Metropolitan Board will obtain Mr. Humber's volume."—*Engineer.*

HUMBER'S RECORD OF MODERN ENGINEERING. FOURTH
SERIES. Imp. 4to, with 36 Double Plates, Photographic Portrait of John Fowler, late Pres. Inst. C.E., and copious descriptive Letterpress, Specifications, &c., £3 3s. half-morocco.

List of the Plates and Diagrams.

Abbey Mills Pumping Station, Main Drainage, Metropolis (4 plates); Barrow Docks (5 plates); Manquis Viaduct, Santiago and Valparaiso Railway (2 plates); Adam's Locomotive, St. Helen's Canal Railway (2 plates); Cannon Street Station Roof, Charing Cross Railway (3 plates); Road Bridge over the River Moka (2 plates); Telegraphic Apparatus for Mesopotamia; Viaduct over the River Wye, Midland Railway (3 plates); St. Germans Viaduct, Cornwall Railway (2 plates); Wrought-Iron Cylinder for Diving Bell; Millwall Docks (6 plates); Milroy's Patent Excavator; Metropolitan District Railway (6 plates); Harbours, Ports, and Breakwaters (3 plates).

"We gladly welcome another year's issue of this valuable publication from the able pen of Mr. Humber. The accuracy and general excellence of this work are well known, while its usefulness in giving the measurements and details of some of the latest examples of engineering, as carried out by the most eminent men in the profession, cannot be too highly prized."—*Artisan.*

CIVIL ENGINEERING, SURVEYING, etc.

MR. HUMBER'S ENGINEERING BOOKS—continued.

Strains, Calculation of.

A HANDY BOOK FOR THE CALCULATION OF STRAINS IN GIRDERS AND SIMILAR STRUCTURES, AND THEIR STRENGTH. Consisting of Formulæ and Corresponding Diagrams, with numerous details for Practical Application, &c. By WILLIAM HUMBER, A-M.Inst.C.E., &c. Fourth Edition. Crown 8vo, nearly 100 Woodcuts and 3 Plates, 7s. 6d. cloth.

"The formulæ are neatly expressed, and the diagrams good."—*Athenæum.*
"We heartily commend this really *handy* book to our engineer and architect readers."—*English Mechanic.*

Barlow's Strength of Materials, enlarged by Humber

A TREATISE ON THE STRENGTH OF MATERIALS; with Rules for Application in Architecture, the Construction of Suspension Bridges, Railways, &c. By PETER BARLOW, F.R.S. A New Edition, revised by his Sons, P. W. BARLOW, F.R.S., and W. H. BARLOW, F.R.S.; to which are added, Experiments by HODGKINSON, FAIRBAIRN, and KIRKALDY; and Formulæ for Calculating Girders, &c. Arranged and Edited by W. HUMBER, A-M.Inst.C.E. Demy 8vo, 400 pp., with 19 large Plates and numerous Woodcuts, 18s. cloth.

"Valuable alike to the student, tyro, and the experienced practitioner, it will always rank in future, as it has hitherto done, as the standard treatise on that particular subject."—*Engineer.*
"There is no greater authority than Barlow."—*Building News.*
"As a scientific work of the first class. it deserves a foremost place on the bookshelves of every civil engineer and practical mechanic."—*English Mechanic.*

Trigonometrical Surveying.

AN OUTLINE OF THE METHOD OF CONDUCTING A TRIGONOMETRICAL SURVEY, for the Formation of Geographical and Topographical Maps and Plans, Military Reconnaissance, Levelling, &c., with Useful Problems, Formulæ, and Tables. By Lieut.-General FROME, R.E. Fourth Edition, Revised and partly Re-written by Major General Sir CHARLES WARREN, G.C.M.G., R.E. With 19 Plates and 115 Woodcuts, royal 8vo, 16s. cloth.

"The simple fact that a fourth edition has been called for is the best testimony to its merits. No words of praise from us can strengthen the position so well and so steadily maintained by this work. Sir Charles Warren has revised the entire work, and made such additions as were necessary to bring every portion of the contents up to the present date."—*Broad Arrow.*

Oblique Bridges.

A PRACTICAL AND THEORETICAL ESSAY ON OBLIQUE BRIDGES. With 13 large Plates. By the late GEORGE WATSON BUCK, M.I.C.E. Third Edition, revised by his Son, J. H. WATSON BUCK, M.I.C.E.; and with the addition of Description to Diagrams for Facilitating the Construction of Oblique Bridges, by W. H. BARLOW, M.I.C.E. Royal 8vo, 12s. cloth.

"The standard text-book for all engineers regarding skew arches is Mr. Buck's treatise, and it would be impossible to consult a better."—*Engineer.*
"Mr. Buck's treatise is recognised as a standard text-book, and his treatment has divested the subject of many of the intricacies supposed to belong to it. As a guide to the engineer and architect, on a confessedly difficult subject, Mr. Buck's work is unsurpassed."—*Building News.*

Water Storage, Conveyance and Utilisation.

WATER ENGINEERING: A Practical Treatise on the Measurement, Storage, Conveyance and Utilisation of Water for the Supply of Towns, for Mill Power, and for other Purposes. By CHARLES SLAGG, Water and Drainage Engineer, A.M.Inst.C.E., Author of "Sanitary Work in the Smaller Towns, and in Villages," &c. With numerous Illustrations. Crown 8vo, 7s. 6d. cloth. [*Just published.*

"As a small practical treatise on the water supply of towns, and on some applications of water-power, the work is in many respects exellent."—*Engineering.*
"The author has collated the results deduced from the experiments of the most eminent authorities, and has presented them in a compact and practical form, accompanied by very clear and detailed explanations. . . . The application of water as a motive power is treated very carefully and exhaustively"—*Builder.*
"For anyone who desires to begin the study of hydraulics with a consideration of the practical applications of the science there is no better guide.'—*Architect.*

Statics, Graphic and Analytic.

GRAPHIC AND ANALYTIC STATICS, in their Practical Application to the Treatment of Stresses in Roofs, Solid Girders, Lattice, Bowstring and Suspension Bridges, Braced Iron Arches and Piers, and other Frameworks. By R. HUDSON GRAHAM, C.E. Containing Diagrams and Plates to Scale. With numerous Examples, many taken from existing Structures. Specially arranged for Class-work in Colleges and Universities. Second Edition, Revised and Enlarged. 8vo, 16s. cloth.

"Mr. Graham's book will find a place wherever graphic and analytic statics are used or studied."—*Engineer*.

"The work is excellent from a practical point of view, and has evidently been prepared with much care. The directions for working are ample, and are illustrated by an abundance of well-selected examples. It is an excellent text-book for the practical draughtsman."—*Athenæum*.

Student's Text-Book on Surveying.

PRACTICAL SURVEYING: A Text-Book for Students preparing for Examination or for Survey-work in the Colonies. By GEORGE W. USILL, A.M.I.C.E., Author of "The Statistics of the Water Supply of Great Britain." With Four Lithographic Plates and upwards of 330 Illustrations. Crown 8vo, 7s. 6d. cloth. [*Just published*.

"The best forms of instruments are described as to their construction, uses and modes of employment, and there are innumerable hints on work and equipment such as the author, in his experience as surveyor, draughtsman and teacher, has found necessary, and which the student in his inexperience will find most serviceable."—*Engineer*.

"We have no hesitation in saying that the student will find this treatise a better guide than any of its predecessors. . . . It deserves to be recognised as the first book which should be put in the hands of a pupil of Civil Engineering, and every gentleman of education who sets out for the Colonies would find it well to have a copy."—*Architect*.

"A very useful, practical handbook on field practice. Clear, accurate and not too condensed."—*Journal of Education*.

Survey Practice.

AID TO SURVEY PRACTICE, for Reference in Surveying, Levelling, Setting-out and in Route Surveys of Travellers by Land and Sea. With Tables, Illustrations, and Records. By LOWIS D'A. JACKSON, A.M.I.C.E., Author of "Hydraulic Manual," "Modern Metrology," &c. Second Edition, Enlarged. Large crown 8vo, 12s. 6d. cloth.

"Mr. Jackson has produced a valuable *vade-mecum* for the surveyor. We can recommend this book as containing an admirable supplement to the teaching of the accomplished surveyor."—*Athenæum*.

"As a text-book we should advise all surveyors to place it in their libraries, and study well the matured instructions afforded in its pages."—*Colliery Guardian*.

"The author brings to his work a fortunate union of theory and practical experience which, aided by a clear and lucid style of writing, renders the book a very useful one."—*Builder*.

Surveying, Land and Marine.

LAND AND MARINE SURVEYING, in Reference to the Preparation of Plans for Roads and Railways; Canals, Rivers, Towns' Water Supplies; Docks and Harbours. With Description and Use of Surveying Instruments. By W. D. HASKOLL, C.E., Author of "Bridge and Viaduct Construction," &c. Second Edition, with Additions. Large crown 8vo, 9s. cloth.

"This book must prove of great value to the student. We have no hesitation in recommending it, feeling assured that it will more than repay a careful study."—*Mechanical World*.

"We can strongly recommend it as a carefully-written and valuable text-book. It enjoys a well-deserved repute among surveyors."—*Builder*.

"This volume cannot fail to prove of the utmost practical utility. It may be safely recommended to all students who aspire to become clean and expert surveyors."—*Mining Journal*.

Tunnelling.

PRACTICAL TUNNELLING. Explaining in detail the Setting-out of the works, Shaft-sinking and Heading-driving, Ranging the Lines and Levelling underground, Sub-Excavating, Timbering, and the Construction of the Brickwork of Tunnels, with the amount of Labour required for, and the Cost of, the various portions of the work. By FREDERICK W. SIMMS, F.G.S., M.Inst.C.E. Third Edition, Revised and Extended by D. KINNEAR CLARK, M.Inst.C.E.; Imperial 8vo, with 21 Folding Plates and numerous Wood Engravings, 30s. cloth.

"The estimation in which Mr. Simms's book on tunnelling has been held for over thirty years cannot be more truly expressed than in the words of the late Prof. Rankine:—'The best source of information on the subject of tunnels is Mr. F. W. Simms's work on Practical Tunnelling.'"—*Architect*.

"It has been regarded from the first as a text book of the subject. . . . Mr. Clarke has added immensely to the value of the book."—*Engineer*.

CIVIL ENGINEERING, SURVEYING, etc.

Levelling.

A TREATISE ON THE PRINCIPLES AND PRACTICE OF LEVELLING. Showing its Application to purposes of Railway and Civil Engineering, in the Construction of Roads; with Mr. TELFORD's Rules for the same. By FREDERICK W. SIMMS, F.G.S., M.Inst.C.E. Seventh Edition, with the addition of LAW's Practical Examples for Setting-out Railway Curves, and TRAUTWINE's Field Practice of Laying-out Circular Curves. With 7 Plates and numerous Woodcuts, 8vo, 8s. 6d. cloth. *⁎* TRAUTWINE on Curves may be had separate, 5s.

"The text-book on levelling in most of our engineering schools and colleges."—*Engineer.*
"The publishers have rendered a substantial service to the profession, especially to the younger members, by bringing out the present edition of Mr. Simms's useful work."—*Engineering.*

Heat, Expansion by.

EXPANSION OF STRUCTURES BY HEAT. By JOHN KEILY, C.E., late of the Indian Public Works and Victorian Railway Departments. Crown 8vo, 3s. 6d. cloth.

SUMMARY OF CONTENTS.

Section I. FORMULAS AND DATA.
Section II. METAL BARS.
Section III. SIMPLE FRAMES.
Section IV. COMPLEX FRAMES AND PLATES.
Section V. THERMAL CONDUCTIVITY.
Section VI. MECHANICAL FORCE OF HEAT.
Section VII. WORK OF EXPANSION AND CONTRACTION.
Section VIII. SUSPENSION BRIDGES.
Section IX. MASONRY STRUCTURES.

"The aim the author has set before him, viz., to show the effects of heat upon metallic and other structures, is a laudable one, for this is a branch of physics upon which the engineer or architect can find but little reliable and comprehensive data in books."—*Builder.*
"Whoever is concerned to know the effect of changes of temperature on such structures as suspension bridges and the like, could not do better than consult Mr. Keily's valuable and handy exposition of the geometrical principles involved in these changes."—*Scotsman.*

Practical Mathematics.

MATHEMATICS FOR PRACTICAL MEN: Being a Commonplace Book of Pure and Mixed Mathematics. Designed chiefly for the use of Civil Engineers, Architects and Surveyors. By OLINTHUS GREGORY, LL.D., F.R.A.S., Enlarged by HENRY LAW, C.E. 4th Edition, carefully Revised by J. R. YOUNG, formerly Professor of Mathematics, Belfast College. With 13 Plates, 8vo, £1 1s. cloth.

"The engineer or architect will here find ready to his hand rules for solving nearly every mathematical difficulty that may arise in his practice The rules are in all cases explained by means of examples, in which every step of the process is clearly worked out."—*Builder.*
"It is an instructive book for the student, and a text-book for him who, having once mastered the subjects it treats of, needs occasionally to refresh his memory upon them."—*Building News.*

Hydraulic Tables.

HYDRAULIC TABLES, CO-EFFICIENTS, and FORMULÆ for finding the Discharge of Water from Orifices, Notches, Weirs, Pipes, and Rivers. With New Formulæ, Tables, and General Information on Rainfall, Catchment-Basins, Drainage, Sewerage, Water Supply for Towns and Mill Power. By JOHN NEVILLE, Civil Engineer, M.R.I.A. Third Edition, carefully Revised, with Additions. Numerous Illustrations. Cr. 8vo, 14s. cloth.

"Alike valuable to students and engineers in practice; its study will prevent the annoyance of avoidable failures, and assist them to select the readiest means of successfully carrying out any given work connected with hydraulic engineering."—*Mining Journal.*
"It is, of all English books on the subject, the one nearest to completeness. . . . From the good arrangement of the matter, the clear explanations, and abundance of formulæ, the carefully calculated tables, and, above all, the thorough acquaintance with both theory and construction, which is displayed from first to last, the book will be found to be an acquisition."—*Architect.*

Hydraulics.

HYDRAULIC MANUAL. Consisting of Working Tables and Explanatory Text. Intended as a Guide in Hydraulic Calculations and Field Operations. By LOWIS D'A. JACKSON, Author of "Aid to Survey Practice," "Modern Metrology," &c. Fourth Edition, Enlarged. Large cr. 8vo, 16s. cl.

"The author has had a wide experience in hydraulic engineering and has been a careful observer of the facts which have come under his notice, and from the great mass of material at his command he has constructed a manual which may be accepted as a trustworthy guide to this branch of the engineer's profession. We can heartily recommend this volume to all who desire to be acquainted with the latest development of this important subject."—*Engineering.*
"The most useful feature of this work is its freedom from what is superannuated, and its thorough adoption of recent experiments; the text is, in fact, in great part a short account of the great modern experiments."—*Nature.*

Drainage.

ON THE DRAINAGE OF LANDS, TOWNS AND BUILDINGS. By G. D. DEMPSEY, C.E., Author of "The Practical Railway Engineer," &c. Revised, with large Additions on RECENT PRACTICE IN DRAINAGE ENGINEERING, by D. KINNEAR CLARK, M.Inst.C.E. Author of "Tramways; Their Construction and Working," "A Manual of Rules, Tables, and Data for Mechanical Engineers," &c. &c. Crown 8vo, 7s. 6d. cloth.

"The new matter added to Mr. Dempsey's excellent work is characterised by the comprehensive grasp and accuracy of detail for which the name of Mr. D. K. Clark is a sufficient voucher."—*Athenæum.*

"As a work on recent practice in drainage engineering, the book is to be commended to all who are making that branch of engineering science their special study."—*Iron.*

"A comprehensive manual on drainage engineering, and a useful introduction to the student."—*Building News.*

Tramways and their Working.

TRAMWAYS: THEIR CONSTRUCTION AND WORKING. Embracing a Comprehensive History of the System; with an exhaustive Analysis of the various Modes of Traction, including Horse-Power, Steam, Heated Water, and Compressed Air; a Description of the Varieties of Rolling Stock; and ample Details of Cost and Working Expenses: the Progress recently made in Tramway Construction, &c. &c. By D. KINNEAR CLARK, M.Inst.C.E. With over 200 Wood Engravings, and 13 Folding Plates. Two Vols., large crown 8vo, 30s. cloth.

"All interested in tramways must refer to it, as all railway engineers have turned to the author's work 'Railway Machinery.'"—*Engineer.*

"An exhaustive and practical work on tramways, in which the history of this kind of locomotion, and a description and cost of the various modes of laying tramways, are to be found."—*Building News.*

"The best form of rails, the best mode of construction, and the best mechanical appliances are so fairly indicated in the work under review, that any engineer about to construct a tramway will be enabled at once to obtain the practical information which will be of most service to him."—*Athenæum.*

Oblique Arches.

A PRACTICAL TREATISE ON THE CONSTRUCTION OF OBLIQUE ARCHES. By JOHN HART. Third Edition, with Plates. Imperial 8vo, 8s. cloth.

Curves, Tables for Setting-out.

TABLES OF TANGENTIAL ANGLES AND MULTIPLES *for Setting-out Curves from 5 to 200 Radius.* By ALEXANDER BEAZELEY, M.Inst.C.E. Third Edition. Printed on 48 Cards, and sold in a cloth box, waistcoat-pocket size, 3s. 6d.

"Each table is printed on a small card, which, being placed on the theodolite, leaves the hands free to manipulate the instrument—no small advantage as regards the rapidity of work."—*Engineer.*

"Very handy; a man may know that all his day's work must fall on two of these cards, which he puts into his own card-case, and leaves the rest behind."—*Athenæum.*

Earthwork.

EARTHWORK TABLES. Showing the Contents in Cubic Yards of Embankments, Cuttings, &c., of Heights or Depths up to an average of 80 feet. By JOSEPH BROADBENT, C.E., and FRANCIS CAMPIN, C.E. Crown 8vo, 5s. cloth.

"The way in which accuracy is attained, by a simple division of each cross section into three elements, two in which are constant and one variable, is ingenious."—*Athenæum.*

Tunnel Shafts.

THE CONSTRUCTION OF LARGE TUNNEL SHAFTS: A Practical and Theoretical Essay. By J. H. WATSON BUCK, M.Inst.C.E., Resident Engineer, London and North-Western Railway. Illustrated with Folding Plates, royal 8vo, 12s. cloth.

"Many of the methods given are of extreme practical value to the mason; and the observations on the form of arch, the rules for ordering the stone, and the construction of the templates will be found of considerable use. We commend the book to the engineering profession."—*Building News.*

"Will be regarded by civil engineers as of the utmost value, and calculated to save much time and obviate many mistakes."—*Colliery Guardian.*

Girders, Strength of.

GRAPHIC TABLE FOR FACILITATING THE COMPUTATION OF THE WEIGHTS OF WROUGHT IRON AND STEEL GIRDERS, etc., for Parliamentary and other Estimates. By J. H. WATSON BUCK, M.Inst.C.E. On a Sheet, 2s.6d.

River Engineering.

RIVER BARS: *The Causes of their Formation, and their Treatment by " Induced Tidal Scour;"* with a Description of the Successful Reduction by this Method of the Bar at Dublin. By A. J. MANN, Assist. Eng. to the Dublin Port and Docks Board. Royal 8vo, 7s. 6d. cloth.

"We recommend all interested in harbour works—and, indeed, those concerned in the improvements of rivers generally—to read Mr. Mann's interesting work on the treatment of river bars."—*Engineer.*

Trusses.

TRUSSES OF WOOD AND IRON. *Practical Applications of Science in Determining the Stresses, Breaking Weights, Safe Loads, Scantlings, and Details of Construction,* with Complete Working Drawings. By WILLIAM GRIFFITHS, Surveyor, Assistant Master, Tranmere School of Science and Art. Oblong 8vo, 4s. 6d. cloth.

"This handy little book enters so minutely into every detail connected with the construction of roof trusses, that no student need be ignorant of these matters."—*Practical Engineer.*

Railway Working.

SAFE RAILWAY WORKING. *A Treatise on Railway Accidents: Their Cause and Prevention;* with a Description of Modern Appliances and Systems. By CLEMENT E. STRETTON, C.E., Vice-President and Consulting Engineer, Amalgamated Society of Railway Servants. With Illustrations and Coloured Plates, crown 8vo, 4s. 6d. strongly bound.

"A book for the engineer, the directors, the managers; and, in short, all who wish for information on railway matters will find a perfect encyclopædia in 'Safe Railway Working.'"—*Railway Review.*

"We commend the remarks on railway signalling to all railway managers, especially where a uniform code and practice is advocated."—*Herepath's Railway Journal.*

"The author may be congratulated on having collected, in a very convenient form, much valuable information on the principal questions affecting the safe working of railways."—*Railway Engineer.*

Field-Book for Engineers.

THE ENGINEER'S, MINING SURVEYOR'S, AND CONTRACTOR'S FIELD-BOOK. Consisting of a Series of Tables, with Rules, Explanations of Systems, and use of Theodolite for Traverse Surveying and Plotting the Work with minute accuracy by means of Straight Edge and Set Square only; Levelling with the Theodolite, Casting-out and Reducing Levels to Datum, and Plotting Sections in the ordinary manner; setting-out Curves with the Theodolite by Tangential Angles and Multiples, with Right and Left-hand Readings of the Instrument: Setting-out Curves without Theodolite, on the System of Tangential Angles by sets of Tangents and Offsets: and Earthwork Tables to 80 feet deep, calculated for every 6 inches in depth. By W. DAVIS HASKOLL, C.E. With numerous Woodcuts. Fourth Edition, Enlarged. Crown 8vo, 12s. cloth.

"The book is very handy; the separate tables of sines and tangents to every minute will make it useful for many other purposes, the genuine traverse tables existing all the same."—*Athenæum.*

"Every person engaged in engineering field operations will estimate the importance of such a work and the amount of valuable time which will be saved by reference to a set of reliable tables prepared with the accuracy and fulness of those given in this volume."—*Railway News.*

Earthwork, Measurement of.

A MANUAL ON EARTHWORK. By ALEX. J. S. GRAHAM, C.E. With numerous Diagrams. 18mo, 2s. 6d. cloth.

"A great amount of practical information, very admirably arranged, and available for rough estimates, as well as for the more exact calculations required in the engineer's and contractor's offices."—*Artisan.*

Strains in Ironwork.

THE STRAINS ON STRUCTURES OF IRONWORK; with Practical Remarks on Iron Construction. By F. W. SHEILDS, M.Inst.C.E. Second Edition, with 5 Plates. Royal 8vo, 5s. cloth.

"The student cannot find a better little book on this subject."—*Engineer.*

Cast Iron and other Metals, Strength of.

A PRACTICAL ESSAY ON THE STRENGTH OF CAST IRON AND OTHER METALS. By THOMAS TREDGOLD, C.E. Fifth Edition, including HODGKINSON'S Experimental Researches. 8vo, 12s. cloth.

ARCHITECTURE, BUILDING, etc.

Construction.
THE SCIENCE OF BUILDING: An Elementary Treatise on the Principles of Construction. By E. WYNDHAM TARN, M.A., Architect. Second Edition, Revised, with 58 Engravings. Crown 8vo, 7s. 6d. cloth.

"A very valuable book, which we strongly recommend to all students."—*Builder.*

"No architectural student should be without this handbook of constructional knowledge."—*Architect.*

Villa Architecture.
A HANDY BOOK OF VILLA ARCHITECTURE: Being a Series of Designs for Villa Residences in various Styles. With Outline Specifications and Estimates. By C. WICKES, Architect, Author of "The Spires and Towers of England," &c. 61 Plates, 4to, £1 11s. 6d. half-morocco, gilt edges.

"The whole of the designs bear evidence of their being the work of an artistic architect, and they will prove very valuable and suggestive."—*Building News.*

Text-Book for Architects.
THE ARCHITECT'S GUIDE: Being a Text-Book of Useful Information for Architects, Engineers, Surveyors, Contractors, Clerks of Works, &c. &c. By FREDERICK ROGERS, Architect, Author of "Specifications for Practical Architecture," &c. Second Edition, Revised and Enlarged. With numerous Illustrations. Crown 8vo, 6s. cloth.

"As a text-book of useful information for architects, engineers, surveyors, &c., it would be hard to find a handier or more complete little volume."—*Standard.*

"A young architect could hardly have a better guide-book."—*Timber Trades Journal.*

Taylor and Cresy's Rome.
THE ARCHITECTURAL ANTIQUITIES OF ROME. By the late G. L. TAYLOR, Esq., F.R.I.B.A., and EDWARD CRESY, Esq. New Edition, thoroughly Revised by the Rev. ALEXANDER TAYLOR, M.A. (son of the late G. L. Taylor, Esq.), Fellow of Queen's College, Oxford, and Chaplain of Gray's Inn. Large folio, with 130 Plates, half-bound, £3 3s.

N.B.—*This is the only book which gives on a large scale, and with the precision of architectural measurement, the principal Monuments of Ancient Rome in plan, elevation, and detail.*

"Taylor and Cresy's work has from its first publication been ranked among those professional books which cannot be bettered. . . . It would be difficult to find examples of drawings, even among those of the most painstaking students of Gothic, more thoroughly worked out than are the one hundred and thirty plates in this volume."—*Architect.*

Architectural Drawing.
PRACTICAL RULES ON DRAWING, for the Operative Builder and Young Student in Architecture. By GEORGE PYNE. With 14 Plates, 4to, 7s. 6d. boards.

Civil Architecture.
THE DECORATIVE PART OF CIVIL ARCHITECTURE. By Sir WILLIAM CHAMBERS, F.R.S. With Illustrations, Notes, and an Examination of Grecian Architecture, by JOSEPH GWILT, F.S.A. Edited by W. H. LEEDS. 66 Plates, 4to, 21s. cloth.

House Building and Repairing.
THE HOUSE-OWNER'S ESTIMATOR; or, What will it Cost to Build, Alter, or Repair? A Price Book adapted to the Use of Unprofessional People, as well as for the Architectural Surveyor and Builder. By JAMES D. SIMON, A.R.I.B.A. Edited and Revised by FRANCIS T. W. MILLER, A.R.I.B.A. With numerous Illustrations. Fourth Edition, Revised. Crown 8vo, 3s. 6d. cloth. [*Just published.*

"In two years it will repay its cost a hundred times over"—*Field.*

"A very handy book."—*English Mechanic.*

Designing, Measuring, and Valuing.

THE STUDENT'S GUIDE to the PRACTICE of MEASURING AND VALUING ARTIFICERS' WORKS. Containing Directions for taking Dimensions, Abstracting the same, and bringing the Quantities into Bill, with Tables of Constants for Valuation of Labour, and for the Calculation of Areas and Solidities. Originally edited by EDWARD DOBSON, Architect. Revised, with considerable Additions on Mensuration and Construction, and a New Chapter on Dilapidations, Repairs, and Contracts, by E. WYNDHAM TARN, M.A. Sixth Edition, including a Complete Form of a Bill of Quantities. With 8 Plates and 63 Woodcuts. Crown 8vo, 7s. 6d. clo [*Just published.*

"Well fulfils the promise of its title-page, and we can thoroughly recommend it to the class for whose use it has been compiled. Mr. Tarn's additions and revisions have much increased the usefulness of the work, and have especially augmented its value to students."—*Engineering.*

"This edition will be found the most complete treatise on the principles of measuring and valuing artificers' work that has yet been published."—*Building News.*

Pocket Estimator and Technical Guide.

THE POCKET TECHNICAL GUIDE, MEASURER AND ESTIMATOR FOR BUILDERS AND SURVEYORS. Containing Technical Directions for Measuring Work in all the Building Trades, with a Treatise on the Measurement of Timber and Complete Specifications for Houses, Roads, and Drains, and an easy Method of Estimating the various parts of a Building collectively. By A. C. BEATON, Author of "Quantities and Measurements," &c. Fifth Edition, carefully Revised and Priced according to the Present Value of Materials and Labour, with 53 Woodcuts, leather, waistcoat-pocket size, 1s. 6d. gilt edges. [*Just published.*

"No builder, architect, surveyor, or valuer should be without his 'Beaton.'"—*Building News.*

"Contains an extraordinary amount of information in daily requisition in measuring and estimating. Its presence in the pocket will save valuable time and trouble."—*Building World.*

Donaldson on Specifications.

THE HANDBOOK OF SPECIFICATIONS; or, Practical Guide to the Architect, Engineer, Surveyor, and Builder, in drawing up Specifications and Contracts for Works and Constructions. Illustrated by Precedents of Buildings actually executed by eminent Architects and Engineers. By Professor T. L. DONALDSON, P.R.I.B.A., &c. New Edition, in One large Vol., 8vo, with upwards of 1,000 pages of Text, and 33 Plates, £1 11s. 6d. cloth

"In this work forty-four specifications of executed works are given, including the specifications for parts of the new Houses of Parliament, by Sir Charles Barry, and for the new Royal Exchange, by Mr. Tite, M.P. The latter, in particular, is a very complete and remarkable document. It embodies, to a great extent, as Mr. Donaldson mentions, 'the bill of quantities with the description of the works.' . . . It is valuable as a record, and more valuable still as a book of precedents. . . . Suffice it to say that Donaldson's 'Handbook of Specifications' must be bought by all architects."—*Builder.*

Bartholomew and Rogers' Specifications.

SPECIFICATIONS FOR PRACTICAL ARCHITECTURE. A Guide to the Architect, Engineer, Surveyor, and Builder. With an Essay on the Structure and Science of Modern Buildings. Upon the Basis of the Work by ALFRED BARTHOLOMEW, thoroughly Revised, Corrected, and greatly added to by FREDERICK ROGERS, Architect. Second Edition, Revised, with Additions. With numerous Illustrations, medium 8vo, 15s. cloth.

"The collection of specifications prepared by Mr. Rogers on the basis of Bartholomew's work is too well known to need any recommendation from us. It is one of the books with which every young architect must be equipped ; for time has shown that the specifications cannot be set aside through any defect in them."—*Architect.*

"Good forms for specifications are of considerable value, and it was an excellent idea to compile a work on the subject upon the basis of the late Alfred Bartholomew's valuable work. The second edition of Mr. Rogers's book is evidence of the want of a book dealing with modern requirements and materials."—*Building News.*

Building; Civil and Ecclesiastical.

A BOOK ON BUILDING, Civil and Ecclesiastical, including Church Restoration; with the Theory of Domes and the Great Pyramid, &c. By Sir EDMUND BECKETT, Bart., LL.D., F.R.A.S., Author of "Clocks and Watches, and Bells," &c. Second Edition, Enlarged. Fcap. 8vo, 5s. cloth.

"A book which is always amusing and nearly always instructive. The style throughout is in the highest degree condensed and epigrammatic."—*Times.*

Geometry for the Architect, Engineer, etc.

PRACTICAL GEOMETRY, for the Architect, Engineer and Mechanic. Giving Rules for the Delineation and Application of various Geometrical Lines, Figures and Curves. By E. W. TARN, M.A., Architect, Author of "The Science of Building," &c. Second Edition. With Appendices on Diagrams of Strains and Isometrical Projection. With 172 Illustrations, demy 8vo, 9s. cloth.

"No book with the same objects in view has ever been published in which the clearness of the rules laid down and the illustrative diagrams have been so satisfactory."—*Scotsman.*

"This is a manual for the practical man, whether architect, engineer, or mechanic. . . . The object of the author being to avoid all abstruse formulæ or complicated methods, and to enable persons with but a moderate knowledge of geometry to work out the problems required."—*English Mechanic.*

The Science of Geometry.

THE GEOMETRY OF COMPASSES; or, Problems Resolved by the mere Description of Circles, and the use of Coloured Diagrams and Symbols. By OLIVER BYRNE. Coloured Plates. Crown 8vo, 3s. 6d. cloth.

"The treatise is a good one, and remarkable—like all Mr. Byrne's contributions to the science of geometry—for the lucid character of its teaching."—*Building News.*

DECORATIVE ARTS, etc.

Woods and Marbles (Imitation of).

SCHOOL OF PAINTING FOR THE IMITATION OF WOODS AND MARBLES, as Taught and Practised by A. R. VAN DER BURG and P. VAN DER BURG, Directors of the Rotterdam Painting Institution. Royal folio, 18¾ by 12¼ in., Illustrated with 24 full-size Coloured Plates: also 12 plain Plates, comprising 154 Figures. Second and Cheaper Edition. Price £1 11s. 6d.

List of Plates.

1. Various Tools required for Wood Painting—2, 3. Walnut: Preliminary Stages of Graining and Finished Specimen—4. Tools used for Marble Painting and Method of Manipulation—5, 6. St. Remi Marble: Earlier Operations and Finished Specimen—7. Methods of Sketching different Grains, Knots, &c.—8, 9. Ash: Preliminary Stages and Finished Specimen—10. Methods of Sketching Marble Grains—11, 12. Breche Marble: Preliminary Stages of Working and Finished Specimen—13. Maple: Methods of Producing the different Grains—14, 15. Bird's-eye Maple: Preliminary Stages and Finished Specimen—16. Methods of Sketching the different Species of White Marble—17, 18. White Marble: Preliminary Stages of Process and Finished Specimen—19. Mahogany: Specimens of various Grains and Methods of Manipulation—20, 21. Mahogany: Earlier Stages and Finished Specimen—22, 23, 24. Sienna Marble: Varieties of Grain, Preliminary Stages and Finished Specimen—25, 26, 27. Juniper Wood: Methods of producing Grain, &c.: Preliminary Stages and Finished Specimen—28, 29, 30. Vert de Mer Marble: Varieties of Grain and Methods of Working Unfinished and Finished Specimens—31, 32, 33. Oak: Varieties of Grain, Tools Employed, and Methods of Manipulation, Preliminary Stages and Finished Specimen—34, 35, 36. Waulsort Marble: Varieties of Grain, Unfinished and Finished Specimens.

*** OPINIONS OF THE PRESS.

"Those who desire to attain skill in the art of painting woods and marbles will find advantage in consulting this book. . . . Some of the Working Men's Clubs should give their young men the opportunity to study it."—*Builder.*

"A comprehensive guide to the art. The explanations of the processes, the manipulation and management of the colours, and the beautifully executed plates will not be the least valuable to the student who aims at making his work a faithful transcript of nature."—*Building News.*

"Students and novices are fortunate who are able to become the possessors of so noble a work."—*Architect.*

House Decoration.

ELEMENTARY DECORATION. A Guide to the Simpler Forms of Everyday Art, as applied to the Interior and Exterior Decoration of Dwelling Houses, &c. By JAMES W. FACEY, Jun. With 68 Cuts. 12mo, 2s. cloth limp.

"As a technical guide-book to the decorative painter it will be found reliable."—*Building News.*

PRACTICAL HOUSE DECORATION: A Guide to the Art of Ornamental Painting, the Arrangement of Colours in Apartments, and the principles of Decorative Design. With some Remarks upon the Nature and Properties of Pigments. By JAMES WILLIAM FACEY, Author of "Elementary Decoration," &c. With numerous Illustrations. 12mo, 2s. 6d. cloth limp.

N.B.—*The above Two Works together in One Vol., strongly half-bound, 5s.*

Colour.

A GRAMMAR OF COLOURING. Applied to Decorative Painting and the Arts. By GEORGE FIELD. New Edition, Revised, Enlarged, and adapted to the use of the Ornamental Painter and Designer. By ELLIS A. DAVIDSON. With New Coloured Diagrams and Engravings. 12mo, 3s. 6d. cloth boards.

"The book is a most useful *resume* of the properties of pigments."—*Builder.*

House Painting, Graining, etc.

HOUSE PAINTING, GRAINING, MARBLING, AND SIGN WRITING, A Practical Manual of. By ELLIS A. DAVIDSON. Fifth Edition. With Coloured Plates and Wood Engravings. 12mo, 6s. cloth boards.

"A mass of information, of use to the amateur and of value to the practical man."—*English Mechanic.*

"Simply invaluable to the youngster entering upon this particular calling, and highly serviceable to the man who is practising it."—*Furniture Gazette.*

Decorators, Receipts for.

THE DECORATOR'S ASSISTANT: A Modern Guide to Decorative Artists and Amateurs, Painters, Writers, Gilders, &c. Containing upwards of 600 Receipts, Rules and Instructions; with a variety of Information for General Work connected with every Class of Interior and Exterior Decorations, &c. Third Edition, Revised. 152 pp., crown 8vo, 1s. in wrapper.

"Full of receipts of value to decorators, painters, gilders, &c. The book contains the gist of larger treatises on colour and technical processes. It would be difficult to meet with a work so full of varied information on the painter's art."—*Building News.*

"We recommend the work to all who, whether for pleasure or profit, require a guide to decoration."—*Plumber and Decorator.*

Moyr Smith on Interior Decoration.

ORNAMENTAL INTERIORS, ANCIENT AND MODERN. By J. MOYR SMITH. Super-royal 8vo, with 32 full-page Plates and numerous smaller Illustrations, handsomely bound in cloth, gilt top, price 18s.

☞ In "ORNAMENTAL INTERIORS" *the designs of more than thirty artist-decorators and architects of high standing have been illustrated. The book may therefore fairly claim to give a good general view of the works of the modern school of decoration, besides giving characteristic examples of earlier decorative arrangements.*

"ORNAMENTAL INTERIORS" *gives a short account of the styles of Interior Decoration as practised by the Ancients in Egypt, Greece, Assyria, Rome and Byzantium. This part is illustrated by characteristic designs.*

*** OPINIONS OF THE PRESS.

"The book is well illustrated and handsomely got up, and contains some true criticism and a good many good examples of decorative treatment."—*The Builder.*

"Well fitted for the dilettante, amateur, and professional designer."—*Decoration.*

"This is the most elaborate, and beautiful work on the artistic decoration of interiors that we have seen.... The scrolls, panels and other designs from the author's own pen are very beautiful and chaste; but he takes care that the designs of other men shall figure even more than his own."—*Liverpool Albion.*

"To all who take an interest in elaborate domestic ornament this handsome volume will be welcome."—*Graphic.*

"Mr. Moyr Smith deserves the thanks of art workers for having placed within their reach a book that seems eminently adapted to afford, by example and precept, that guidance of which most craftsmen stand in need."—*Furniture Gazette.*

British and Foreign Marbles.

MARBLE DECORATION and the Terminology of British and Foreign Marbles. A Handbook for Students. By GEORGE H. BLAGROVE, Author of "Shoring and its Application," &c. With 28 Illustrations. Crown 8vo, 3s. 6d. cloth.

"This most useful and much wanted handbook should be in the hands of every architect and builder."—*Building World.*

"It is an excellent manual for students, and interesting to artistic readers generally."—*Saturday Review.*

"A carefully and usefully written eatise; the work is essentially practical."—*Scotsman.*

Marble Working, etc.

MARBLE AND MARBLE WORKERS: A Handbook for Architects, Artists, Masons and Students. By ARTHUR LEE, Author of "A Visit to Carrara," "The Working of Marble," &c. Small crown 8vo, 2s. cloth.

"A really valuable addition to the technical literature of architects and masons."—*Building News.*

DELAMOTTE'S WORKS ON ILLUMINATION AND ALPHABETS.

A PRIMER OF THE ART OF ILLUMINATION, *for the Use of Beginners*: with a Rudimentary Treatise on the Art, Practical Directions for its exercise, and Examples taken from Illuminated MSS., printed in Gold and Colours. By F. DELAMOTTE. New and Cheaper Edition. Small 4to, 6s. ornamental boards.

"The examples of ancient MSS. recommended to the student, which, with much good sense, the author chooses from collections accessible to all, are selected with judgment and knowledge, as well as taste."—*Athenæum*.

ORNAMENTAL ALPHABETS, Ancient and Mediæval, from the Eighth Century, with Numerals; including Gothic, Church-Text, large and small, German, Italian, Arabesque, Initials for Illumination, Monograms, Crosses, &c. &c., for the use of Architectural and Engineering Draughtsmen, Missal Painters, Masons, Decorative Painters, Lithographers, Engravers, Carvers, &c. &c. Collected and Engraved by F. DELAMOTTE, and printed in Colours. New and Cheaper Edition. Royal 8vo, oblong, 2s. 6d. ornamental boards.

"For those who insert enamelled sentences round gilded chalices, who blazon shop legends over shop-doors, who letter church walls with pithy sentences from the Decalogue, this book will be useful."—*Athenæum*.

EXAMPLES OF MODERN ALPHABETS, Plain and Ornamental; including German, Old English, Saxon, Italic, Perspective, Greek, Hebrew, Court Hand, Engrossing, Tuscan, Riband, Gothic, Rustic, and Arabesque; with several Original Designs, and an Analysis of the Roman and Old English Alphabets, large and small, and Numerals, for the use of Draughtsmen, Surveyors, Masons, Decorative Painters, Lithographers, Engravers, Carvers, &c. Collected and Engraved by F. DELAMOTTE, and printed in Colours. New and Cheaper Edition. Royal 8vo, oblong, 2s. 6d. ornamental boards.

"There is comprised in it every possible shape into which the letters of the alphabet and numerals can be formed, and the talent which has been expended in the conception of the various plain and ornamental letters is wonderful."—*Standard*.

MEDIÆVAL ALPHABETS AND INITIALS FOR ILLUMINATORS. By G. DELAMOTTE. Containing 21 Plates and Illuminated Title, printed in Gold and Colours. With an Introduction by J. WILLIS BROOKS. Fourth and Cheaper Edition. Small 4to, 4s. ornamental boards.

"A volume in which the letters of the alphabet come forth glorified in gilding and all the colours of the prism interwoven and intertwined and intermingled."—*Sun*.

THE EMBROIDERER'S BOOK OF DESIGN. Containing Initials, Emblems, Cyphers, Monograms, Ornamental Borders, Ecclesiastical Devices, Mediæval and Modern Alphabets, and National Emblems. Collected by F. DELAMOTTE, and printed in Colours. Oblong royal 8vo, 1s. 6d. ornamental wrapper.

"The book will be of great assistance to ladies and young children who are endowed with the art of plying the needle in this most ornamental and useful pretty work."—*East Anglian Times*.

Wood Carving.

INSTRUCTIONS IN WOOD-CARVING, for Amateurs; with Hints on Design. By A LADY. With Ten large Plates, 2s. 6d. in emblematic wrapper.

"The handicraft of the wood-carver, so well as a book can impart it, may be learnt from 'A Lady's' publication."—*Athenæum*.
"The directions given are plain and easily understood."—*English Mechanic*.

Glass Painting.

GLASS STAINING AND THE ART OF PAINTING ON GLASS. From the German of Dr. GESSERT and EMANUEL OTTO FROMBERG. With an Appendix on THE ART OF ENAMELLING. 12mo, 2s. 6d. cloth limp.

Letter Painting.

THE ART OF LETTER PAINTING MADE EASY. By JAMES GREIG BADENOCH. With 12 full-page Engravings of Examples, 1s. 6d. cloth limp.

"The system is a simple one, but quite original, and well worth the careful attention of letter painters. It can be easily mastered and remembered."—*Building News*.

CARPENTRY, TIMBER, etc.

Tredgold's Carpentry, Enlarged by Tarn.
THE ELEMENTARY PRINCIPLES OF CARPENTRY. A Treatise on the Pressure and Equilibrium of Timber Framing, the Resistance of Timber, and the Construction of Floors, Arches, Bridges, Roofs, Uniting Iron and Stone with Timber, &c. To which is added an Essay on the Nature and Properties of Timber, &c., with Descriptions of the kinds of Wood used in Building; also numerous Tables of the Scantlings of Timber for different purposes, the Specific Gravities of Materials, &c. By THOMAS TREDGOLD, C.E. With an Appendix of Specimens of Various Roofs of Iron and Stone, Illustrated. Seventh Edition, thoroughly revised and considerably enlarged by E. WYNDHAM TARN, M.A., Author of "The Science of Building," &c. With 61 Plates, Portrait of the Author, and several Woodcuts. In one large vol., 4to, price £1 5s. cloth.

"Ought to be in every architect's and every builder's library."—*Builder.*

"A work whose monumental excellence must commend it wherever skilful carpentry is concerned. The author's principles are rather confirmed than impaired by time. The additional plates are of great intrinsic value."—*Building News.*

Woodworking Machinery.
WOODWORKING MACHINERY: Its Rise, Progress, and Construction. With Hints on the Management of Saw Mills and the Economical Conversion of Timber. Illustrated with Examples of Recent Designs by leading English, French, and American Engineers. By M. POWIS BALE, A.M.Inst.C.E., M.I.M.E. Large crown 8vo, 12s. 6d. cloth.

"Mr. Bale is evidently an expert on the subject and he has collected so much information that his book is all-sufficient for builders and others engaged in the conversion of timber."—*Architect.*

"The most comprehensive compendium of wood-working machinery we have seen. The author is a thorough master of his subject."—*Building News.*

"The appearance of this book at the present time will, we should think, give a considerable impetus to the onward march of the machinist engaged in the designing and manufacture of wood-working machines. It should be in the office of every wood-working factory."—*English Mechanic.*

Saw Mills.
SAW MILLS: Their Arrangement and Management, and the Economical Conversion of Timber. (A Companion Volume to "Woodworking Machinery.") By M. POWIS BALE. With numerous Illustrations. Crown 8vo, 10s. 6d. cloth.

"The *administration* of a large sawing establishment is discussed, and the subject examined from a financial standpoint. Hence the size, shape, order, and disposition of saw mills and the like are gone into in detail, and the course of the timber is traced from its reception to its delivery in its converted state. We could not desire a more complete or practical treatise."—*Builder.*

"We highly recommend Mr. Bale's work to the attention and perusal of all those who are engaged in the art of wood conversion, or who are about building or remodelling saw-mills on improved principles."—*Building News.*

Carpentering.
THE CARPENTER'S NEW GUIDE; or, Book of Lines for Carpenters; comprising all the Elementary Principles essential for acquiring a knowledge of Carpentry. Founded on the late PETER NICHOLSON'S Standard Work. A New Edition, Revised by ARTHUR ASHPITEL, F.S.A. Together with Practical Rules on Drawing, by GEORGE PYNE. With 74 Plates, 4to, £1 1s. cloth.

Handrailing.
A PRACTICAL TREATISE ON HANDRAILING: Showing New and Simple Methods for Finding the Pitch of the Plank, Drawing the Moulds, Bevelling, Jointing-up, and Squaring the Wreath. By GEORGE COLLINGS. Illustrated with Plates and Diagrams. 12mo, 1s. 6d. cloth limp.

"Will be found of practical utility in the execution of this difficult branch of joinery."—*Builder.*

"Almost every difficult phase of this somewhat intricate branch of joinery is elucidated by the aid of plates and explanatory letterpress."—*Furniture Gazette.*

Circular Work.
CIRCULAR WORK IN CARPENTRY AND JOINERY: A Practical Treatise on Circular Work of Single and Double Curvature. By GEORGE COLLINGS, Author of "A Practical Treatise on Handrailing." Illustrated with numerous Diagrams. 12mo, 2s. 6d. cloth limp.

"An excellent example of what a book of this kind should be. Cheap in price, clear in definition and practical in the examples selected."—*Builder.*

Timber Merchant's Companion.

THE TIMBER MERCHANT'S AND BUILDER'S COMPANION. Containing New and Copious Tables of the Reduced Weight and Measurement of Deals and Battens, of all sizes, from One to a Thousand Pieces, and the relative Price that each size bears per Lineal Foot to any given Price per Petersburg Standard Hundred; the Price per Cube Foot of Square Timber to any given Price per Load of 50 Feet; the proportionate Value of Deals and Battens by the Standard, to Square Timber by the Load of 50 Feet; the readiest mode of ascertaining the Price of Scantling per Lineal Foot of any size, to any given Figure per Cube Foot, &c. &c. By WILLIAM DOWSING. Fourth Edition, Revised and Corrected. Cr. 8vo, 3s. cl.

"Everything is as concise and clear as it can possibly be made. There can be no doubt that every timber merchant and builder ought to possess it."—*Hull Advertiser.*
"We are glad to see a fourth edition of these admirable tables, which for correctness and simplicity of arrangement leave nothing to be desired."—*Timber Trades Journal.*
"An exceedingly well-arranged, clear, and concise manual of tables for the use of all who buy or sell timber."—*Journal of Forestry.*

Practical Timber Merchant.

THE PRACTICAL TIMBER MERCHANT. Being a Guide for the use of Building Contractors, Surveyors, Builders, &c., comprising useful Tables for all purposes connected with the Timber Trade, Marks of Wood, Essay on the Strength of Timber, Remarks on the Growth of Timber, &c. By W. RICHARDSON. Fcap. 8vo, 3s. 6d. cloth.

"Contains much valuable information for the use of timber merchants, builders, foresters, and all others connected with the growth, sale, and manufacture of timber."—*Journal of Forestry.*

Timber Freight Book.

THE TIMBER MERCHANT'S, SAW MILLER'S, AND IMPORTER'S FREIGHT BOOK AND ASSISTANT. Comprising Rules, Tables, and Memoranda relating to the Timber Trade. By WILLIAM RICHARDSON, Timber Broker; together with a Chapter on "SPEEDS OF SAW MILL MACHINERY," by M. POWIS BALE, M.I.M.E., &c. 12mo, 3s. 6d. cl. boards.

"A very useful manual of rules, tables, and memoranda relating to the timber trade. We recommend it as a compendium of calculation to all timber measurers and merchants, and as supplying a real want in the trade."—*Building News.*

Packing-Case Makers, Tables for.

PACKING-CASE TABLES; showing the number of Superficial Feet in Boxes or Packing-Cases, from six inches square and upwards. By W. RICHARDSON, Timber Broker. Second Edition. Oblong 4to, 3s. 6d. cl.

"Invaluable labour-saving tables."—*Ironmonger.*
"Will save much labour and calculation."—*Grocer.*

Superficial Measurement.

THE TRADESMAN'S GUIDE TO SUPERFICIAL MEASUREMENT. Tables calculated from 1 to 200 inches in length, by 1 to 108 inches in breadth. For the use of Architects, Surveyors, Engineers, Timber Merchants, Builders, &c. By JAMES HAWKINGS. Third Edition. Fcap., 3s. 6d. cloth.

"A useful collection of tables to facilitate rapid calculation of surfaces. The exact area of any surface of which the limits have been ascertained can be instantly determined. The book will be found of the greatest utility to all engaged in building operations."—*Scotsman.*
"These tables will be found of great assistance to all who require to make calculations in superficial measurement."—*English Mechanic.*

Forestry.

THE ELEMENTS OF FORESTRY. Designed to afford Information concerning the Planting and Care of Forest Trees for Ornament or Profit, with Suggestions upon the Creation and Care of Woodlands. By F. B. HOUGH. Large crown 8vo, 10s. cloth.

Timber Importer's Guide.

THE TIMBER IMPORTER'S, TIMBER MERCHANT'S AND BUILDER'S STANDARD GUIDE. By RICHARD E. GRANDY. Comprising an Analysis of Deal Standards, Home and Foreign with Comparative Values and Tabular Arrangements for fixing Nett Landed Cost on Baltic and North American Deals, including all intermediate Expenses, Freight, Insurance, &c. &c. Together with copious Information for the Retailer and Builder. Third Edition, Revised. 12mo, 2s. cloth limp.

"Everything it pretends to be: built up gradually, it leads one from a forest to a treenail, and throws in, as a makeweight, a host of material concerning bricks, columns, cisterns, &c."—*English Mechanic.*

MARINE ENGINEERING, NAVIGATION, etc.

Chain Cables.

CHAIN CABLES AND CHAINS. Comprising Sizes and Curves of Links, Studs, &c., Iron for Cables and Chains, Chain Cable and Chain Making, Forming and Welding Links, Strength of Cables and Chains, Certificates for Cables, Marking Cables, Prices of Chain Cables and Chains, Historical Notes, Acts of Parliament, Statutory Tests, Charges for Testing, List of Manufacturers of Cables, &c. &c. By THOMAS W. TRAILL, F.E.R.N., M. Inst. C.E., Engineer Surveyor in Chief, Board of Trade, Inspector of Chain Cable and Anchor Proving Establishments, and General Superintendent, Lloyd's Committee on Proving Establishments. With numerous Tables, Illustrations and Lithographic Drawings. Folio, £2 2s. cloth.

"It contains a vast amount of valuable information. Nothing seems to be wanting to make it a complete and standard work of reference on the subject."—*Nautical Magazine.*

Marine Engineering.

MARINE ENGINES AND STEAM VESSELS (A Treatise on). By ROBERT MURRAY, C.E. Eighth Edition, thoroughly Revised, with considerable Additions by the Author and by GEORGE CARLISLE, C.E., Senior Surveyor to the Board of Trade at Liverpool. 12mo, 5s. cloth boards.

"Well adapted to give the young steamship engineer or marine engine and boiler maker a general introduction into his practical work."—*Mechanical World.*

"We feel sure that this thoroughly revised edition will continue to be as popular in the future as it has been in the past, as for its size, it contains more useful information than any similar treatise."—*Industries.*

"The information given is both sound and sensible, and well qualified to direct young sea-going hands on the straight road to the extra chief's certificate."—*Glasgow Herald.*

"An indispensable manual for the student of marine engineering."—*Liverpool Mercury.*

Pocket-Book for Naval Architects and Shipbuilders.

THE NAVAL ARCHITECT'S AND SHIPBUILDER'S POCKET-BOOK of Formulæ, Rules, and Tables, and MARINE ENGINEER'S AND SURVEYOR'S Handy Book of Reference. By CLEMENT MACKROW, Member of the Institution of Naval Architects, Naval Draughtsman. Third Edition, Revised. With numerous Diagrams, &c. Fcap., 12s. 6d. leather.

"Should be used by all who are engaged in the construction or design of vessels. . . . Will be found to contain the most useful tables and formulæ required by shipbuilders, carefully collected from the best authorities, and put together in a popular and simple form."—*Engineer.*

"The professional shipbuilder has now, in a convenient and accessible form, reliable data for solving many of the numerous problems that present themselves in the course of his work."—*Iron.*

"There is scarcely a subject on which a naval architect or shipbuilder can require to refresh his memory which will not be found within the covers of Mr. Mackrow's book."—*English Mechanic.*

Pocket-Book for Marine Engineers.

A POCKET-BOOK OF USEFUL TABLES AND FORMULÆ FOR MARINE ENGINEERS. By FRANK PROCTOR, A.I.N.A. Third Edition. Royal 32mo, leather, gilt edges, with strap, 4s.

"We recommend it to our readers as going far to supply a long-felt want."—*Naval Science.*

"A most useful companion to all marine engineers."—*United Service Gazette.*

Introduction to Marine Engineering.

ELEMENTARY ENGINEERING: A Manual for Young Marine Engineers and Apprentices. In the Form of Questions and Answers on Metals, Alloys, Strength of Materials, Construction and Management of Marine Engines, &c. &c. With an Appendix of Useful Tables. By J. S. BREWER, Government Marine Surveyor, Hongkong. Small crown 8vo, 2s. 6d. cloth. [*Just published.*

"Contains much valuable information for the class for whom it is intended, especially in the chapters on the management of boilers and engines."—*Nautical Magazine.*

"A useful introduction to the more elaborate text books."—*Scotsman.*

"To a student who has the requisite desire and resolve to attain a thorough knowledge, Mr. Brewer offers decidedly useful help."—*Athenæum.*

Navigation.

PRACTICAL NAVIGATION. Consisting of THE SAILOR'S SEA-BOOK, by JAMES GREENWOOD and W. H ROSSER; together with the requisite Mathematical and Nautical Tables for the Working of the Problems. By HENRY LAW, C.E., and Professor J. R. YOUNG. Illustrated. 12mo, 7s. strongly half-bound.

MINING AND MINING INDUSTRIES.

Metalliferous Mining.

BRITISH MINING: A Treatise on the History, Discovery, Practical Development, and Future Prospects of Metalliferous Mines in the United Kingdom. By ROBERT HUNT, F.R.S., Keeper of Mining Records; Editor of "Ure's Dictionary of Arts, Manufactures, and Mines," &c. Upwards of 950 pp., with 230 Illustrations. Second Edition, Revised. Super-royal 8vo, £2 2s. cloth.

"One of the most valuable works of reference of modern times. Mr. Hunt, as keeper of mining records of the United Kingdom, has had opportunities for such a task not enjoyed by anyone else, and has evidently made the most of them. . . . The language and style adopted are good, and the treatment of the various subjects laborious, conscientious, and scientific."—*Engineering*.

"The book is, in fact, a treasure-house of statistical information on mining subjects, and we know of no other work embodying so great a mass of matter of this kind. Were this the only merit of Mr. Hunt's volume, it would be sufficient to render it indispensable in the library of everyone interested in the development of the mining and metallurgical industries of the country."—*Athenæum*.

"A mass of information not elsewhere available, and of the greatest value to those who may be interested in our great mineral industries."—*Engineer*.

"A sound, business-like collection of interesting facts. . . . The amount of information Mr. Hunt has brought together is enormous. . . . The volume appears likely to convey more instruction upon the subject than any work hitherto published."—*Mining Journal*.

"The work will be for the mining industry what Dr. Percy's celebrated treatise has been for the metallurgical—a book that cannot with advantage be omitted from the library."—*Iron and Coal Trades Review*.

"The volume is massive and exhaustive, and the high intellectual powers and patient, persistent application which characterise the author have evidently been brought into play in its production. Its contents are invaluable."—*Colliery Guardian*.

Coal and Iron.

THE COAL AND IRON INDUSTRIES OF THE UNITED KINGDOM. Comprising a Description of the Coal Fields, with Returns of their Produce and its Distribution, and Analyses of Special Varieties. Also an Account of the occurrence of Iron Ores in Veins or Seams; Analyses of each Variety; and a History of the Rise and Progress of Pig Iron Manufacture since the year 1740. By RICHARD MEADE, Assistant Keeper of Mining Records. With Maps of the Coal Fields and Ironstone Deposits of the United Kingdom. 8vo, £1 8s. cloth.

"The book is one which must find a place on the shelves of all interested in coal and iron production, and in the iron, steel, and other metallurgical industries."—*Engineer*.

"Of this book we may unreservedly say that it is the best of its class which we have ever met. . . . A book of reference which no one engaged in the iron or coal trades should omit from his library."—*Iron and Coal Trades Review*.

"An exhaustive treatise and a valuable work of reference."—*Mining Journal*.

Prospecting for Gold and other Metals.

THE PROSPECTOR'S HANDBOOK: A Guide for the Prospector and Traveller in Search of Metal-Bearing or other Valuable Minerals. By J. W. ANDERSON, M.A. (Camb.), F.R.G.S., Author of "Fiji and New Caledonia." Fourth Edition, thoroughly Revised and Enlarged. Small crown 8vo, 3s. 6d. cloth. [*Just published*.

"Will supply a much felt want, especially among Colonists, in whose way are so often thrown many mineralogical specimens the value of which it is difficult for anyone, not a specialist, to determine. The author has placed his instructions before his readers in the plainest possible terms, and his book is the best of its kind."—*Engineer*.

"How to find commercial minerals, and how to identify them when they are found, are the leading points to which attention is directed. The author has managed to pack as much practical detail into his pages as would supply material for a book three times its size."—*Mining Journal*.

"Those toilers who explore the trodden or untrodden tracks on the face of the globe will find much that is useful to them in this book."—*Athenæum*.

Mining Notes and Formulæ.

NOTES AND FORMULÆ FOR MINING STUDENTS. By JOHN HERMAN MERIVALE, M.A., Certificated Colliery Manager, Professor of Mining in the Durham College of Science, Newcastle-upon-Tyne. Second Edition, carefully Revised. Small crown 8vo, cloth, price 2s. 6d.

"Invaluable to anyone who is working up for an examination on mining subjects."—*Coal and Iron Trades Review*.

"The author has done his work in an exceedingly creditable manner, and has produced a book that will be of service to students, and those who are practically engaged in mining operations."—*Engineer*

"A vast amount of technical matter of the utmost value to mining engineers, and of considerable interest to students."—*Schoolmaster*.

Gold, Metallurgy of.

THE METALLURGY OF GOLD: A Practical Treatise on the Metallurgical Treatment of Gold-bearing Ores. Including the Processes of Concentration and Chlorination, and the Assaying, Melting and Refining of Gold. By M. EISSLER, Mining Engineer and Metallurgical Chemist, formerly Assistant Assayer of the U. S. Mint, San Francisco. Second Edition, Revised and much Enlarged. With 132 Illustrations. Crown 8vo, 9s. cloth.
[*Just published.*

"This book thoroughly deserves its title of a 'Practical Treatise.' The whole process of gold milling, from the breaking of the quartz to the assay of the bullion, is described in clear and orderly narrative and with much, but not too much, fulness of detail."—*Saturday Review.*
"The work is a storehouse of information and valuable data, and we strongly recommend it o all professional men engaged in the gold-mining industry."—*Mining Journal.*
"Anyone who wishes to have an intelligent acquaintance with the characteristics of gold and gold ores, the methods of extracting the metal, concentrating and chlorinating it, and further on of refining and assaying it, will find all he wants in Mr. Eissler's book."—*Financial News.*

Silver, Metallurgy of.

THE METALLURGY OF SILVER: A Practical Treatise on the Amalgamation, Roasting and Lixiviation of Silver Ores. Including the Assaying, Melting and Refining of Silver Bullion. By M. EISSLER, Author of "The Metallurgy of Gold." With 124 Illustrations. Crown 8vo, 10s. 6d. cloth.
[*Just published.*

"A practical treatise, and a technical work which we are convinced will supply a long-felt want amongst practical men, and at the same time be of value to students and others indirectly connected with the industries."—*Mining Journal.*
"From first to last the book is thoroughly sound and reliable."—*Colliery Guardian.*
"For chemists, practical miners, assayers and investors alike, we do not know of any work on the subject so handy and yet so comprehensive."—*Glasgow Herald.*

Mineral Surveying and Valuing.

THE MINERAL SURVEYOR AND VALUER'S COMPLETE GUIDE, comprising a Treatise on Improved Mining Surveying and the Valuation of Mining Properties, with New Traverse Tables. By WM. LINTERN, Mining and Civil Engineer. Third Edition, with an Appendix on "Magnetic and Angular Surveying," With Four Plates. 12mo, 4s. cloth.

"An enormous fund of information of great value."—*Mining Journal.*
"Mr. Lintern's book forms a valuable and thoroughly trustworthy guide."—*Iron and Coal Trades Review.*
"This new edition must be of the highest value to colliery surveyors, proprietors and managers."—*Colliery Guardian.*

Metalliferous Minerals and Mining.

TREATISE ON METALLIFEROUS MINERALS AND MINING. By D. C. DAVIES, F.G.S., Mining Engineer, &c., Author of "A Treatise on Slate and Slate Quarrying." Illustrated with numerous Wood Engravings. Fourth Edition, carefully Revised. Crown 8vo, 12s. 6d. cloth.

"Neither the practical miner nor the general reader interested in mines can have a better book or his companion and his guide."—*Mining Journal.*
"The volume is one which no student of mineralogy should be without."—*Colliery Guardian.*
"A book that will not only be useful to the geologist, the practical miner, and the metallurgist, but also very interesting to the general public."—*Iron.*
"As a history of the present state of mining throughout the world this book has a real value, and it supplies an actual want, for no such information has hitherto been brought together within such limited space."—*Athenæum.*

Earthy Minerals and Mining.

TREATISE ON EARTHY AND OTHER MINERALS AND MINING. By D. C. DAVIES, F.G.S. Uniform with, and forming a Companion Volume to, the same Author's "Metalliferous Minerals and Mining." With 76 Wood Engravings. Second Edition. Crown 8vo, 12s. 6d. cloth.

"It is essentially a practical work, intended primarily for the use of practical men. . . . We do not remember to have met with any English work on mining matters that contains the same amount of information packed in equally convenient form."—*Academy.*
"The book is clearly the result of many years' careful work and thought, and we should be inclined to rank it as among the very best of the handy technical and trades manuals which have recently appeared."—*British Quarterly Review.*
"The volume contains a great mass of practical information carefully methodised and presented in a very intelligible shape."—*Scotsman.*
"The subject matter of the volume will be found of high value by all—and they are a numerous class—who trade in earthy minerals."—*Athenæum.*

Underground Pumping Machinery.

MINE DRAINAGE. Being a Complete and Practical Treatise on Direct-Acting Underground Steam Pumping Machinery, with a Description of a large number of the best known Engines, their General Utility and the Special Sphere of their Action, the Mode of their Application, and their merits compared with other forms of Pumping Machinery. By STEPHEN MICHELL. 8vo, 15s. cloth.

"Will be highly esteemed by colliery owners and lessees, mining engineers, and students generally who require to be acquainted with the best means of securing the drainage of mines. It is a most valuable work, and stands almost alone in the literature of steam pumping machinery."—*Colliery Guardian.*

"Much valuable information is given, so that the book is thoroughly worthy of an extensive circulation amongst practical men and purchasers of machinery."—*Mining Journal.*

Mining Tools.

A MANUAL OF MINING TOOLS. For the Use of Mine Managers, Agents, Students, &c. By WILLIAM MORGANS, Lecturer on Practical Mining at the Bristol School of Mines. 12mo, 2s. 6d. cloth limp.

ATLAS OF ENGRAVINGS to Illustrate the above, containing 235 Illustrations of Mining Tools, drawn to scale. 4to, 4s. 6d. cloth.

"Students in the science of mining, and overmen, captains, managers, and viewers may gain practical knowledge and useful hints by the study of Mr. Morgans' manual."—*Colliery Guardian.*

"A valuable work, which will tend materially to improve our mining literature."—*Mining Journal.*

Coal Mining.

COAL AND COAL MINING: A Rudimentary Treatise on. By Sir WARINGTON W. SMYTH, M.A., F.R.S., &c., Chief Inspector of the Mines of the Crown. New Edition, Revised and Corrected. With numerous Illustrations. 12mo, 4s. cloth boards.

"As an outline is given of every known coal-field in this and other countries, as well as of the principal methods of working, the book will doubtless interest a very large number of readers."—*Mining Journal.*

Granite Quarrying.

GRANITES AND OUR GRANITE INDUSTRIES. By GEORGE F. HARRIS, F.G.S., Membre de la Société Belge de Géologie, Lecturer on Economic Geology at the Birkbeck Institution, &c. With Illustrations. Crown 8vo, 2s. 6d. cloth.

"A clearly and well-written manual for persons engaged or interested in the granite industry."—*Scotsman.*

"An interesting work, which will be deservedly esteemed. We advise the author to write again."—*Colliery Guardian.*

"An exceedingly interesting and valuable monograph, on a subject which has hitherto received unaccountably little attention in the shape of systematic literary treatment."—*Scottish Leader.*

NATURAL AND APPLIED SCIENCE.

Text Book of Electricity.

THE STUDENT'S TEXT-BOOK OF ELECTRICITY. By HENRY M. NOAD, Ph.D., F.R.S., F.C.S. New Edition, carefully Revised. With an Introduction and Additional Chapters, by W. H. PREECE, M.I.C.E., Vice-President of the Society of Telegraph Engineers, &c. With 470 Illustrations. Crown 8vo, 12s. 6d. cloth.

"The original plan of this book has been carefully adhered to so as to make it a reflex of the existing state of electrical science, adapted for students. . . . Discovery seems to have progressed with marvellous strides; nevertheless it has now apparently ceased, and practical applications have commenced their career; and it is to give a faithful account of these that this fresh edition of Dr. Noad's valuable text-book is launched forth."—*Extract from Introduction by W. H. Preece, Esq.*

"We can recommend Dr. Noad's book for clear style, great range of subject, a good index and a plethora of woodcuts. Such collections as the present are indispensable."—*Athenæum.*

"An admirable text book for every student — beginner or advanced — of electricity."—*Engineering.*

Electricity.

A MANUAL OF ELECTRICITY: Including Galvanism, Magnetism, Dia-Magnetism, Electro-Dynamics, Magno-Electricity, and the Electric Telegraph. By HENRY M. NOAD, Ph.D., F.R.S., F.C.S. Fourth Edition. With 500 Woodcuts. 8vo, £1 4s. cloth.

"It is worthy of a place in the library of every public institution."—*Mining Journal.*

NATURAL AND APPLIED SCIENCE.

Electric Light.
ELECTRIC LIGHT: Its Production and Use. Embodying Plain Directions for the Treatment of Voltaic Batteries, Electric Lamps, and Dynamo-Electric Machines. By J. W. URQUHART, C.E., Author of "Electroplating: A Practical Handbook." Edited by F. C. WEBB, M.I.C.E., M.S.T.E. Second Edition, Revised, with large Additions and 128 Illusts. 7s. 6d. cloth.

"The book is by far the best that we have yet met with on the subject."—*Athenæum.*

"It is the only work at present available which gives, in language intelligible for the most part to the ordinary reader, a general but concise history of the means which have been adopted up to the present time in producing the electric light."—*Metropolitan.*

"The book contains a general account of the means adopted in producing the electric light, not only as obtained from voltaic or galvanic batteries, but treats at length of the dynamo-electric machine in several of its forms."—*Colliery Guardian.*

Electric Lighting.
THE ELEMENTARY PRINCIPLES OF ELECTRIC LIGHTING. By ALAN A. CAMPBELL SWINTON, Associate I.E.E. Second Edition, Enlarged and Revised. With 16 Illustrations. Crown 8vo, 1s. 6d. cloth.

"Anyone who desires a short and thoroughly clear exposition of the elementary principles of electric-lighting cannot do better than read this little work."—*Bradford Observer.*

Dr. Lardner's School Handbooks.
NATURAL PHILOSOPHY FOR SCHOOLS. By Dr. LARDNER. 328 Illustrations. Sixth Edition. One Vol., 3s. 6d. cloth.

"A very convenient class-book for junior students in private schools. It is intended to convey, in clear and precise terms, general notions of all the principal divisions of Physical Science."—*British Quarterly Review.*

ANIMAL PHYSIOLOGY FOR SCHOOLS. By Dr. LARDNER. With 190 Illustrations. Second Edition. One Vol., 3s. 6d. cloth.

"Clearly written, well arranged, and excellently illustrated."—*Gardener's Chronicle.*

Dr. Lardner's Electric Telegraph.
THE ELECTRIC TELEGRAPH. By Dr. LARDNER. Revised and Re-written by E. B. BRIGHT, F.R.A.S. 140 Illustrations. Small 8vo, 2s. 6d. cloth.

"One of the most readable books extant on the Electric Telegraph."—*English Mechanic.*

Astronomy.
ASTRONOMY. By the late Rev. ROBERT MAIN, M.A., F.R.S., formerly Radcliffe Observer at Oxford. Third Edition, Revised and Corrected to the present time, by WILLIAM THYNNE LYNN, B.A., F.R.A.S., formerly of the Royal Observatory, Greenwich. 12mo, 2s cloth limp.

"A sound and simple treatise, very carefully edited, and a capital book for beginners."—*Knowledge.*

"Accurately brought down to the requirements of the present time by Mr. Lynn."—*Educational Times.*

The Blowpipe.
THE BLOWPIPE IN CHEMISTRY, MINERALOGY, AND GEOLOGY. Containing all known Methods of Anhydrous Analysis, many Working Examples, and Instructions for Making Apparatus. By Lieut.-Colonel W. A. Ross, R.A., F.G.S. With 120 Illustrations. Second Edition, Revised and Enlarged. Crown 8vo, 5s. cloth. [*Just published.*

"The student who goes conscientiously through the course of experimentation here laid down will gain a better insight into inorganic chemistry and mineralogy than if he had 'got up' any of the best text-books of the day, and passed any number of examinations in their contents."—*Chemical News.*

The Military Sciences.
AIDE-MEMOIRE TO THE MILITARY SCIENCES. Framed from Contributions of Officers and others connected with the different Services. Originally edited by a Committee of the Corps of Royal Engineers. Second Edition, most carefully Revised by au Officer of the Corps, with many Additions; containing nearly 350 Engravings and many hundred Woodcuts. Three Vols., royal 8vo, extra cloth boards, and lettered, £4 10s.

"A compendious encyclopædia of military knowledge, to which we are greatly indebted."—*Edinburgh Review.*

"The most comprehensive book of reference to the military and collateral sciences."—*Volunteer Service Gazette.*

Field Fortification.
A TREATISE ON FIELD FORTIFICATION, THE ATTACK OF FORTRESSES, MILITARY MINING, AND RECONNOITRING. By Colonel I. S. MACAULAY, late Professor of Fortification in the R.M.A., Woolwich. Sixth Edition, crown 8vo, cloth, with separate Atlas of 12 Plates, 12s.

Temperaments.

OUR TEMPERAMENTS, THEIR STUDY AND THEIR TEACHING. A Popular Outline. By ALEXANDER STEWART, F.R.C.S. Edin. In one large 8vo volume, with 30 Illustrations, including A Selection from Lodge's "Historical Portraits," showing the Chief Forms of Faces. Price 15s. cloth, gilt top.

"The book is exceedingly interesting, even for those who are not systematic students of anthropology. . . . To those who think the proper study of mankind is man, it will be full of attraction."—*Daily Telegraph.*

"The author's object is to enable a student to read a man's temperament in his aspect. The work is well adapted to its end. It is worthy of the attention of students of human nature."—*Scotsman.*

"The volume is heavy to hold, but light to read. Though the author has treated his subject exhaustively, he writes in a popular and pleasant manner that renders it attractive to the general reader."—*Punch.*

Antiseptic Nursing.

ANTISEPTICS: A Handbook for Nurses. Being an Epitome of Antiseptic Treatment. With Notes on Antiseptic Substances, Disinfection, Monthly Nursing, &c. By Mrs. ANNIE HEWER, late Hospital Sister, Diplomée Obs. Soc. Lond. Crown 8vo, 1s. 6d. cloth. [*Just published.*

"This excellent little work . . . is very readable and contains much information. We can strongly recommend it to those who are undergoing training at the various hospitals and also to those who are engaged in the practice of nursing, as they cannot fail to obtain practical hints from its perusal."—*Lancet.*

"The student or the busy practitioner would do well to look through its pages, offering as they do a suggestive and faithful picture of antiseptic methods."—*Hospital Gazette.*

"A clear, concise, and excellent little handbook."—*The Hospital.*

Pneumatics and Acoustics.

PNEUMATICS: including Acoustics and the Phenomena of Wind Currents, for the Use of Beginners. By CHARLES TOMLINSON, F.R.S., F.C.S., &c. Fourth Edition, Enlarged. With numerous Illustrations. 12mo, 1s. 6d. cloth.

"Beginners in the study of this important application of science could not have a better manual."—*Scotsman.*

"A valuable and suitable text-book for students of Acoustics and the Phenomena of Wind Currents."—*Schoolmaster.*

Conchology.

A MANUAL OF THE MOLLUSCA: Being a Treatise on Recent and Fossil Shells. By S. P. WOODWARD, A.L.S., F.G.S., late Assistant Palæontologist in the British Museum. Fifth Edition. With an Appendix on *Recent and Fossil Conchological Discoveries,* by RALPH TATE, A.L.S., F.G.S. Illustrated by A. N. WATERHOUSE and JOSEPH WILSON LOWRY. With 23 Plates and upwards of 300 Woodcuts. Crown 8vo, 7s. 6d. cloth boards.

"A most valuable storehouse of conchological and geological information."—*Science Gossip.*

Geology.

RUDIMENTARY TREATISE ON GEOLOGY, PHYSICAL AND HISTORICAL. Consisting of "Physical Geology," which sets forth the leading Principles of the Science; and "Historical Geology," which treats of the Mineral and Organic Conditions of the Earth at each successive epoch, especial reference being made to the British Series of Rocks. By RALPH TATE, A.L.S., F.G.S., &c., &c. With 250 Illustrations. 12mo, 5s. cloth boards.

"The fulness of the matter has elevated the book into a manual. Its information is exhaustive and well arranged."—*School Board Chronicle.*

Geology and Genesis.

THE TWIN RECORDS OF CREATION; or, Geology and Genesis: their Perfect Harmony and Wonderful Concord. By GEORGE W. VICTOR LE VAUX. Numerous Illustrations. Fcap. 8vo, 5s. cloth.

"A valuable contribution to the evidences of Revelation, and disposes very conclusively of the arguments of those who would set God's Works against God's Word. No real difficulty is shirked, and no sophistry is left unexposed."—*The Rock.*

"The remarkable peculiarity of this author is that he combines an unbounded admiration of science with an unbounded admiration of the Written record. The two impulses are balanced to a nicety; and the consequence is that difficulties, which to minds less evenly poised would be serious, find immediate solutions of the happiest kinds."—*London Review.*

NATURAL AND APPLIED SCIENCE.

DR. LARDNER'S HANDBOOKS OF NATURAL PHILOSOPHY.

THE HANDBOOK OF MECHANICS. Enlarged and almost rewritten by BENJAMIN LOEWY, F.R.A.S. With 378 Illustrations. Post 8vo, 6s. cloth.

"The perspicuity of the original has been retained, and chapters which had become obsolete have been replaced by others of more modern character. The explanations throughout are studiously popular, and care has been taken to show the application of the various branches of physics to the industrial arts, and to the practical business of life."—*Mining Journal*.

"Mr. Loewy has carefully revised the book, and brought it up to modern requirements."—*Nature*.

"Natural philosophy has had few exponents more able or better skilled in the art of popularising the subject than Dr. Lardner; and Mr. Loewy is doing good service in fitting this treatise, and the others of the series, for use at the present time."—*Scotsman*.

THE HANDBOOK OF HYDROSTATICS AND PNEUMATICS. New Edition, Revised and Enlarged, by BENJAMIN LOEWY, F.R.A.S. With 236 Illustrations. Post 8vo, 5s. cloth.

"For those 'who desire to attain an accurate knowledge of physical science without the profound methods of mathematical investigation,' this work is not merely intended, but well adapted."—*Chemical News*.

"The volume before us has been carefully edited, augmented to nearly twice the bulk of the former edition, and all the most recent matter has been added. . . . It is a valuable text-book."—*Nature*.

"Candidates for pass examinations will find it, we think, specially suited to their requirements."—*English Mechanic*.

THE HANDBOOK OF HEAT. Edited and almost entirely rewritten by BENJAMIN LOEWY, F.R.A.S., &c. 117 Illustrations. Post 8vo, 6s. cloth.

"The style is always clear and precise, and conveys instruction without leaving any cloudiness or lurking doubts behind."—*Engineering*.

"A most exhaustive book on the subject on which it treats, and is so arranged that it can be understood by all who desire to attain an accurate knowledge of physical science. . . . Mr. Loewy has included all the latest discoveries in the varied laws and effects of heat."—*Standard*.

"A complete and handy text-book for the use of students and general readers."—*English Mechanic*.

THE HANDBOOK OF OPTICS. By DIONYSIUS LARDNER, D.C.L., formerly Professor of Natural Philosophy and Astronomy in University College, London. New Edition. Edited by T. OLVER HARDING, B.A. Lond., of University College, London. With 298 Illustrations. Small 8vo, 448 pages, 5s. cloth.

"Written by one of the ablest English scientific writers, beautifully and elaborately illustrated. *Mechanic's Magazine*.

THE HANDBOOK OF ELECTRICITY, MAGNETISM, AND ACOUSTICS. By Dr. LARDNER. Ninth Thousand. Edit. by GEORGE CAREY FOSTER, B.A., F.C S. With 400 Illustrations. Small 8vo, 5s. cloth.

"The book could not have been entrusted to anyone better calculated to preserve the terse and lucid style of Lardner, while correcting his errors and bringing up his work to the present state of scientific knowledge."—*Popular Science Review*.

*** *The above Five Volumes, though each is Complete in itself, form* A COMPLETE COURSE OF NATURAL PHILOSOPHY.

Dr. Lardner's Handbook of Astronomy.

THE HANDBOOK OF ASTRONOMY. Forming a Companion to the "Handbook of Natural Philosophy." By DIONYSIUS LARDNER, D.C.L., formerly Professor of Natural Philosophy and Astronomy in University College, London. Fourth Edition. Revised and Edited by EDWIN DUNKIN, F.R.A.S., Royal Observatory, Greenwich. With 38 Plates and upwards of 100 Woodcuts. In One Vol., small 8vo, 550 pages, 9s. 6d. cloth.

"Probably no other book contains the same amount of information in so compendious and well-arranged a form—certainly none at the price at which this is offered to the public."—*Athenæum*.

"We can do no other than pronounce this work a most valuable manual of astronomy, and we strongly recommend it to all who wish to acquire a general—but at the same time correct—acquaintance with this sublime science."—*Quarterly Journal of Science*.

"One of the most deservedly popular books on the subject . . . We would recommend not only the student of the elementary principles of the science, but he who aims at mastering the higher and mathematical branches of astronomy, not to be without this work beside him."—*Practical Magazine*.

DR. LARDNER'S MUSEUM OF SCIENCE AND ART.

THE MUSEUM OF SCIENCE AND ART. Edited by DIONYSIUS LARDNER, D.C.L., formerly Professor of Natural Philosophy and Astronomy in University College, London. With upwards of 1,200 Engravings on Wood. In 6 Double Volumes, £1 1s., in a new and elegant cloth binding; or handsomely bound in half-morocco, 31s. 6d.

Contents:

The Planets: Are they Inhabited Worlds?—Weather Prognostics—Popular Fallacies in Questions of Physical Science—Latitudes and Longitudes—Lunar Influences—Meteoric Stones and Shooting Stars—Railway Accidents—Light—Common Things: Air—Locomotion in the United States—Cometary Influences—Common Things: Water—The Potter's Art—Common Things: Fire—Locomotion and Transport, their Influence and Progress—The Moon—Common Things: The Earth—The Electric Telegraph—Terrestrial Heat—The Sun—Earthquakes and Volcanoes—Barometer, Safety Lamp, and Whitworth's Micrometric Apparatus—Steam—The Steam Engine—The Eye—The Atmosphere—Time—Common Things: Pumps—Common Things: Spectacles, the Kaleidoscope—Clocks and Watches—Microscopic Drawing and Engraving—Locomotive—Thermometer—New Planets: Leverrier and Adams's Planet—Magnitude and Minuteness—Common Things: The Almanack—Optical Images—How to observe the Heavens—Common Things: The Looking-glass—Stellar Universe—The Tides—Colour—Common Things: Man—Magnifying Glasses—Instinct and Intelligence—The Solar Microscope—The Camera Lucida—The Magic Lantern—The Camera Obscura—The Microscope—The White Ants: Their Manners and Habits—The Surface of the Earth, or First Notions of Geography—Science and Poetry—The Bee—Steam Navigation—Electro-Motive Power—Thunder, Lightning, and the Aurora Borealis—The Printing Press—The Crust of the Earth—Comets—The Stereoscope—The Pre-Adamite Earth—Eclipses—Sound.

*** OPINIONS OF THE PRESS.

"This series, besides affording popular but sound instruction on scientific subjects, with which the humblest man in the country ought to be acquainted, also undertakes that teaching of 'Common Things' which every well-wisher of his kind is anxious to promote. Many thousand copies of this serviceable publication have been printed, in the belief and hope that the desire for instruction and improvement widely prevails; and we have no fear that such enlightened faith will meet with disappointment."—*Times.*

"A cheap and interesting publication, alike informing and attractive. The papers combine subjects of importance and great scientific knowledge, considerable inductive powers, and a popular style of treatment."—*Spectator.*

"The 'Museum of Science and Art' is the most valuable contribution that has ever been made to the Scientific Instruction of every class of society."—Sir DAVID BREWSTER, in the *North British Review.*

"Whether we consider the liberality and beauty of the illustrations, the charm of the writing, or the durable interest of the matter, we must express our belief that there is hardly to be found among the new books one that would be welcomed by people of so many ages and classes as a valuable present."—*Examiner.*

*** *Separate books formed from the above, suitable for Workmen's Libraries, Science Classes, etc.*

Common Things Explained. Containing Air, Earth, Fire, Water, Time, Man, the Eye, Locomotion, Colour, Clocks and Watches, &c. 233 Illustrations, cloth gilt, 5s.

The Microscope. Containing Optical Images, Magnifying Glasses, Origin and Description of the Microscope, Microscopic Objects, the Solar Microscope, Microscopic Drawing and Engraving, &c. 147 Illustrations, cloth gilt, 2s.

Popular Geology. Containing Earthquakes and Volcanoes, the Crust of the Earth, &c. 201 Illustrations, cloth gilt, 2s. 6d.

Popular Physics. Containing Magnitude and Minuteness, the Atmosphere, Meteoric Stones, Popular Fallacies, Weather Prognostics, the Thermometer, the Barometer, Sound, &c. 85 Illustrations, cloth gilt, 2s. 6d.

Steam and its Uses. Including the Steam Engine, the Locomotive, and Steam Navigation. 89 Illustrations, cloth gilt, 2s.

Popular Astronomy. Containing How to observe the Heavens—The Earth, Sun, Moon, Planets, Light, Comets, Eclipses, Astronomical Influences, &c. 182 Illustrations, 4s. 6d.

The Bee and White Ants: Their Manners and Habits. With Illustrations of Animal Instinct and Intelligence. 135 Illustrations, cloth gilt, 2s.

The Electric Telegraph Popularized. To render intelligible to all who can Read, irrespective of any previous Scientific Acquirements, the various forms of Telegraphy in Actual Operation. 100 Illustrations, cloth gilt, 1s. 6d.

COUNTING-HOUSE WORK, TABLES, etc.

Accounts for Manufacturers.
FACTORY ACCOUNTS: Their Principles and Practice. A Handbook for Accountants and Manufacturers, with Appendices on the Nomenclature of Machine Details; the Income Tax Acts; the Rating of Factories; Fire and Boiler Insurance; the Factory and Workshop Acts, &c., including also a Glossary of Terms and a large number of Specimen Rulings. By EMILE GARCKE and J. M. FELLS. Third Edition. Demy 8vo, 250 pages, price 6s strongly bound. [*Just published.*

"A very interesting description of the requirements of Factory Accounts. . . . the principle of assimilating the Factory Accounts to the general commercial books is one which we thoroughly agree with."—*Accountants' Journal.*

"Characterised by extreme thoroughness. There are few owners of Factories who would not derive great benefit from the perusal of this most admirable work."—*Local Government Chronicle.*

Foreign Commercial Correspondence.
THE FOREIGN COMMERCIAL CORRESPONDENT: Being Aids to Commercial Correspondence in Five Languages—English, French, German, Italian and Spanish. By CONRAD E. BAKER. Second Edition, Revised. Crown 8vo, 3s. 6d. cloth. [*Just published.*

"Whoever wishes to correspond in all the languages mentioned by Mr. Baker cannot do better than study this work, the materials of which are excellent and conveniently arranged. They consist not of entire specimen letters, but what are far more useful—short passages, sentences, or phrases expressing the same general idea in various forms."—*Athenæum.*

"A careful examination has convinced us that it is unusually complete, well arranged and reliable. The book is a thoroughly good one."—*Schoolmaster.*

Intuitive Calculations.
THE COMPENDIOUS CALCULATOR; or, Easy and Concise Methods of Performing the various Arithmetical Operations required in Commercial and Business Transactions, together with Useful Tables. By DANIEL O'GORMAN. Corrected and Extended by J. R. YOUNG, formerly Professor of Mathematics at Belfast College. Twenty-seventh Edition, carefully Revised by C. NORRIS. Fcap. 8vo, 3s. 6d. strongly half-bound in leather.

"It would be difficult to exaggerate the usefulness of a book like this to everyone engaged in commerce or manufacturing industry. It is crammed full of rules and formulæ for shortening and employing calculations."—*Knowledge.*

"Supplies special and rapid methods for all kinds of calculations. Of great utility to persons engaged in any kind of commercial transactions."—*Scotsman.*

Modern Metrical Units and Systems.
MODERN METROLOGY: A Manual of the Metrical Units and Systems of the Present Century. With an Appendix containing a proposed English System. By LOWIS D'A. JACKSON, A.M.Inst.C.E., Author of "Aid to Survey Practice," &c. Large crown 8vo, 12s. 6d. cloth.

"The author has brought together much valuable and interesting information. . . . We cannot but recommend the work to the consideration of all interested in the practical reform of our weights and measures."—*Nature.*

"For exhaustive tables of equivalent weights and measures of all sorts, and for clear demonstrations of the effects of the various systems that have been proposed or adopted, Mr. Jackson's treatise is without a rival."—*Academy.*

The Metric System and the British Standards.
A SERIES OF METRIC TABLES, in which the British Standard Measures and Weights are compared with those of the Metric System at present in Use on the Continent. By C. H. DOWLING, C.E. 8vo, 10s. 6d. strongly bound.

"Their accuracy has been certified by Professor Airy, the Astronomer-Royal."—*Builder.*

"Mr. Dowling's Tables are well put together as a ready-reckoner for the conversion of one system into the other."—*Athenæum.*

Iron and Metal Trades' Calculator.
THE IRON AND METAL TRADES' COMPANION. For expeditiously ascertaining the Value of any Goods bought or sold by Weight, from 1s. per cwt. to 112s. per cwt., and from one farthing per pound to one shilling per pound. Each Table extends from one pound to 100 tons. To which are appended Rules on Decimals, Square and Cube Root, Mensuration of Superficies and Solids, &c.; Tables of Weights of Materials, and other Useful Memoranda. By THOS. DOWNIE. 396 pp., 9s. Strongly bound in leather.

"A most useful set of tables, and will supply a want, for nothing like them before existed."—*Building News.*

"Although specially adapted to the iron and metal trades, the tables will be found useful in every other business in which merchandise is bought and sold by weight."—*Railway News.*

Calculator for Numbers and Weights Combined.

THE NUMBER AND WEIGHT CALCULATOR. Containing upwards of 250,000 Separate Calculations, showing at a glance the value at 421 different rates, ranging from 1/32th of a Penny to 20s. each, or per cwt., and £20 per ton, of any number of articles consecutively, from 1 to 470.—Any number of cwts., qrs., and lbs., from 1 cwt. to 470 cwts.—Any number ot tons, cwts., qrs., and lbs., from 1 to 23½ tons. By WILLIAM CHADWICK, Public Accountant. Second Edition, Revised and Improved, and specially adapted for the Apportionment of Mileage Charges for Railway Traffic. 8vo, price 18s., strongly bound for Office wear and tear. [*Just published.*

☞ *This comprehensive and entirely unique and original Calculator is adapted for the use of Accountants and Auditors, Railway Companies, Canal Companies, Shippers, Shipping Agents, General Carriers, etc. Ironfounders, Brassfounders, Metal Merchants, Iron Manufacturers, Ironmongers, Engineers, Machinists, Boiler Makers, Millwrights, Roofing, Bridge and Girder Makers, Colliery Proprietors, etc. Timber Merchants, Builders, Contractors, Architects, Surveyors, Auctioneers, Valuers, Brokers, Mill Owners and Manufacturers, Mill Furnishers, Merchants and General Wholesale Tradesmen.*

*** OPINIONS OF THE PRESS.

The book contains the answers to questions, and not simply a set of ingenious puzzle methods of arriving at results. It is as easy of reference for any answer or any number of answers as a dictionary, and the references are even more quickly made. For making up accounts or estimates, the book must prove invaluable to all who have any considerable quantity of calculations involving price and measure in any combination to do."—*Engineer.*

"The most complete and practical ready reckoner which it has been our fortune yet to see. It is difficult to imagine a trade or occupation in which it could not be of the greatest use, either in saving human labour or in checking work. The Publishers have placed within the reach ot every commercial man an invaluable and unfailing assistant."—*The Miller.*

"The most perfect work of the kind yet prepared."—*Glasgow Herald.*

Comprehensive Weight Calculator.

THE WEIGHT CALCULATOR. Being a Series of Tables upon a New and Comprehensive Plan, exhibiting at One Reference the exact Value of any Weight from 1 lb. to 15 tons, at 300 Progressive Rates, from 1d. to 168s. per cwt., and containing 186,000 Direct Answers, which, with their Combinations, consisting of a single addition (mostly to be performed at sight), will afford an aggregate of 10,266,000 Answers; the whole being calculated and designed to ensure correctness and promote despatch. By HENRY HARBEN, Accountant. Fourth Edition, carefully Corrected. Royal 8vo, strongly half-bound, £1 5s.

"A practical and useful work of reference for men of business generally; it is the best of the kind we have seen."—*Ironmonger.*

"Of priceless value to business men. It is a necessary book in all mercantile offices."—*Sheffield Independent.*

Comprehensive Discount Guide.

THE DISCOUNT GUIDE. Comprising several Series of Tables for the use of Merchants, Manufacturers, Ironmongers, and others, by which may be ascertained the exact Profit arising from any mode of using Discounts, either in the Purchase or Sale of Goods, and the method of either Altering a Rate of Discount or Advancing a Price, so as to produce, by one operation, a sum that will realise any required profit after allowing one or more Discounts: to which are added Tables of Profit or Advance from 1¼ to 90 per cent., Tables of Discount from 1¼ to 98¾ per cent., and Tables of Commission, &c., from ⅛ to 10 per cent. By HENRY HARBEN, Accountant, Author of "The Weight Calculator." New Edition, carefully Revised and Corrected. Demy 8vo, 544 pp. half-bound, £1 5s.

"A book such as this can only be appreciated by business men, to whom the saving of time means saving of money. We have the high authority of Professor J. R. Young that the tables throughout the work are constructed upon strictly accurate principles. The work is a model of typographical clearness, and must prove of great value to merchants, manufacturers, and general traders."—*British Trade Journal.*

Iron Shipbuilders' and Merchants' Weight Tables.

IRON-PLATE WEIGHT TABLES: For *Iron Shipbuilders, Engineers and Iron Merchants.* Containing the Calculated Weights of upwards of 150,000 different sizes of Iron Plates, from 1 foot by 6 in. by ¼ in. to 10 feet by 5 feet by 1 in. Worked out on the basis of 40 lbs. to the square foot of Iron of 1 inch in thickness. Carefully compiled and thoroughly Revised by H. BURLINSON and W. H. SIMPSON. Oblong 4to, 25s. half-bound.

"This work will be found of great utility. The authors have had much practical experience of what is wanting in making estimates; and the use of the book will save much time in making elaborate calculations.—*English Mechanic.*

INDUSTRIAL AND USEFUL ARTS.

Soap-making.

THE ART OF SOAP-MAKING: A Practical Handbook of the Manufacture of Hard and Soft Soaps, Toilet Soaps, etc. Including many New Processes, and a Chapter on the Recovery of Glycerine from Waste Leys. By ALEXANDER WATT, Author of "Electro-Metallurgy Practically Treated," &c. With numerous Illustrations. Third Edition, Revised. Crown 8vo, 7s. 6d. cloth.

"The work will prove very useful, not merely to the technological student, but to the practical soap-boiler who wishes to understand the theory of his art."—*Chemical News.*

"Really an excellent example of a technical manual, entering, as it does, thoroughly and exhaustively both into the theory and practice of soap manufacture. The book is well and honestly done, and deserves the considerable circulation with which it will doubtless meet."—*Knowledge.*

"Mr. Watt's book is a thoroughly practical treatise on an art which has almost no literature in our language. We congratulate the author on the success of his endeavour to fill a void in English technical literature."—*Nature.*

Paper Making.

THE ART OF PAPER MANUFACTURE: A Practical Handbook of the Manufacture of Paper from Rags, Esparto, Wood and other Fibres. By ALEXANDER WATT, Author of "The Art of Soap-Making," "The Art of Leather Manufacture," &c. With numerous Illustrations. Cr. 8vo. [*In the press.*

Leather Manufacture.

THE ART OF LEATHER MANUFACTURE. Being a Practical Handbook, in which the Operations of Tanning, Currying, and Leather Dressing are fully Described, and the Principles of Tanning Explained, and many Recent Processes introduced; as also Methods for the Estimation of Tannin, and a Description of the Arts of Glue Boiling, Gut Dressing, &c. By ALEXANDER WATT, Author of "Soap-Making," "Electro-Metallurgy," &c. With numerous Illustrations. Second Edition. Crown 8vo, 9s. cloth.

"A sound, comprehensive treatise on tanning and its accessories. . . . An eminently valuable production, which redounds to the credit of both author and publishers."—*Chemical Review.*

"This volume is technical without being tedious, comprehensive and complete without being prosy, and it bears on every page the impress of a master hand. We have never come across a better trade treatise, nor one that so thoroughly supplied an absolute want."—*Shoe and Leather Trades' Chronicle.*

Boot and Shoe Making.

THE ART OF BOOT AND SHOE-MAKING. A Practical Handbook, including Measurement, Last-Fitting, Cutting-Out, Closing and Making, with a Description of the most approved Machinery employed. By JOHN B. LENO, late Editor of *St. Crispin*, and *The Boot and Shoe-Maker*. With numerous Illustrations. Third Edition. 12mo, 2s. cloth limp.

"This excellent treatise is by far the best work ever written on the subject. A new work, embracing all modern improvements, was much wanted. This want is now satisfied. The chapter on clicking, which shows how waste may be prevented, will save fifty times the price of the book."—*Scottish Leather Trader.*

"This volume is replete with matter well worthy the perusal of boot and shoe manufacturers and experienced craftsmen, and instructive and valuable in the highest degree to all young beginners and craftsmen in the trade of which it treats."—*Leather Trades' Circular.*

Dentistry.

MECHANICAL DENTISTRY: A Practical Treatise on the Construction of the various kinds of Artificial Dentures. Comprising also Useful Formulæ, Tables and Receipts for Gold Plate, Clasps, Solders, &c. &c. By CHARLES HUNTER. Third Edition, Revised. With upwards of 100 Wood Engravings. Crown 8vo, 3s. 6d. cloth.

"The work is very practical."—*Monthly Review of Dental Surgery.*

"We can strongly recommend Mr. Hunter's treatise to all students preparing for the profession of dentistry, as well as to every mechanical dentist."—*Dublin Journal of Medical Science.*

"A work in a concise form that few could read without gaining information from."—*British Journal of Dental Science.*

Wood Engraving.

A PRACTICAL MANUAL OF WOOD ENGRAVING. With a Brief Account of the History of the Art. By WILLIAM NORMAN BROWN. With numerous Illustrations. Crown 8vo, 2s. cloth.

"The author deals with the subject in a thoroughly practical and easy series of representative lessons."—*Paper and Printing Trades Journal.*

"The book is clear and complete, and will be useful to anyone wanting to understand the first elements of the beautiful art of wood engraving."—*Graphic.*

HANDYBOOKS FOR HANDICRAFTS. By PAUL N. HASLUCK.

☞ *These Handybooks are written to supply Handicraftsmen with information on workshop practice, and are intended to convey, in plain language, technical knowledge of the several crafts. Workshop terms are used, and workshop practice described, the text being freely illustrated with drawings of modern tools, appliances and processes.*

N.B. The following Volumes are already published, and others are in preparation.

Metal Turning.

THE METAL TURNER'S HANDYBOOK. A Practical Manual for Workers at the Foot-Lathe: Embracing Information on the Tools, Appliances and Processes employed in Metal Turning. By PAUL N. HASLUCK, Author of "Lathe-Work." With upwards of One Hundred Illustrations. Second Edition, Revised. Crown 8vo, 2s. cloth.

"Altogether admirably adapted to initiate students into the art of turning."—*Leicester Post.*
"Clearly and concisely written, excellent in every way, we heartily commend it to all interested in metal turning."—*Mechanical World.*

Wood Turning.

THE WOOD TURNER'S HANDYBOOK. A Practical Manual for Workers at the Lathe: Embracing Information on the Tools, Appliances and Processes Employed in Wood Turning. By PAUL N. HASLUCK. With upwards of One Hundred Illustrations. Crown 8vo, 2s. cloth.

"We recommend the book to young turners and amateurs. A multitude of workmen have hitherto sought in vain for a manual of this special industry."—*Mechanical World.*

Watch Repairing.

THE WATCH JOBBER'S HANDYBOOK. A Practical Manual on Cleaning, Repairing and Adjusting. Embracing Information on the Tools, Materials, Appliances and Processes Employed in Watchwork. By PAUL N. HASLUCK. With upwards of One Hundred Illustrations. Cr. 8vo, 2s. cloth.

"All young persons connected with the trade should acquire and study this excellent, and at the same time, inexpensive work."—*Clerkenwell Chronicle.*

Pattern Making.

THE PATTERN MAKER'S HANDYBOOK. A Practical Manual, embracing Information on the Tools, Materials and Appliances employed in Constructing Patterns for Founders. By PAUL N. HASLUCK. With One Hundred Illustrations. Crown 8vo, 2s. cloth.

"We commend it to all who are interested in the counsels it so ably gives."—*Colliery Guardian.*
"This handy volume contains sound information of considerable value to students and artificers."—*Hardware Trades Journal.*

Mechanical Manipulation.

THE MECHANIC'S WORKSHOP HANDYBOOK. A Practical Manual on Mechanical Manipulation. Embracing Information on various Handicraft Processes, with Useful Notes and Miscellaneous Memoranda. By PAUL N. HASLUCK. Crown 8vo, 2s. cloth.

"It is a book which should be found in every workshop, as it is one which will be continually referred to for a very great amount of standard information."—*Saturday Review.*

Model Engineering.

THE MODEL ENGINEER'S HANDYBOOK: A Practical Manual on Model Steam Engines. Embracing Information on the Tools. Materials and Processes Employed in their Construction. By PAUL N. HASLUCK. With upwards of 100 Illustrations. Crown 8vo, 2s. cloth.

"Mr. Hasluck's latest volume is of greater importance than would at first appear; and indeed he has produced a very good little book."—*Builder.*
"By carefully going through the work, amateurs may pick up an excellent notion of the construction of full-sized steam engines."—*Telegraphic Journal.*

Clock Repairing.

THE CLOCK JOBBER'S HANDYBOOK: A Practical Manual on Cleaning, Repairing and Adjusting. Embracing Information on the Tools, Materials, Appliances and Processes Employed in Clockwork. By PAUL N. HASLUCK. With upwards of 100 Illustrations. Cr. 8vo. 2s. cloth. [*Just ready.*

INDUSTRIAL AND USEFUL ARTS. 33

Electrolysis of Gold, Silver, Copper, etc.
ELECTRO-DEPOSITION: A Practical Treatise on the Electrolysis of Gold, Silver, Copper, Nickel, and other Metals and Alloys. With descriptions of Voltaic Batteries, Magneto and Dynamo-Electric Machines, Thermopiles, and of the Materials and Processes used in every Department of the Art, and several Chapters on Electro-Metallurgy. By ALEXANDER WATT, Author of "Electro-Metallurgy," &c. With numerous Illustrations. Third Edition, Revised and Enlarged. Crown 8vo, 9s. cloth.
"Eminently a book for the practical worker in electro-deposition. It contains minute and practical descriptions of methods, processes and materials as actually pursued and used in the workshop. Mr. Watt's book recommends itself to all interested in its subjects."—*Engineer.*

Electro-Metallurgy.
ELECTRO-METALLURGY; Practically Treated. By ALEXANDER WATT, Author of "Electro Deposition," &c. Ninth Edition, including the most recent Processes. 12mo, 4s. cloth boards.
"From this book both amateur and artisan may learn everything necessary for the successful prosecution of electroplating."—*Iron.*

Electroplating.
ELECTROPLATING: A Practical Handbook on the Deposition of Copper, Silver, Nickel, Gold, Aluminium, Brass, Platinum, &c. &c. With Descriptions of the Chemicals, Materials, Batteries and Dynamo Machines used in the Art. By J. W. URQUHART, C.E., Author of "Electric Light," &c. Second Edition, Revised, with Additions. Numerous Illustrations. Crown 8vo, 5s. cloth.
"An excellent practical manual."—*Engineering.*
"This book will show any person how to become an expert in electro-deposition."—*Builder.*
"An excellent work, giving the newest information."—*Horological Journal.*

Electrotyping.
ELECTROTYPING: The Reproduction and Multiplication of Printing Surfaces and Works of Art by the Electro-deposition of Metals. By J. W. URQUHART, C.E. Crown 8vo, 5s. cloth.
"The book is thoroughly practical. The reader is, therefore, conducted through the leading laws of electricity, then through the metals used by electrotypers, the apparatus, and the depositing processes, up to the final preparation of the work."—*Art Journal.*

Goldsmiths' Work.
THE GOLDSMITH'S HANDBOOK. By GEORGE E. GEE, Jeweller, &c. Third Edition, considerably Enlarged. 12mo, 3s. 6d. cloth.
"A good, sound, technical educator, and will be generally accepted as an authority.."—*Horological Journal.*
"A standard book which few will care to be without."—*Jeweller and Metalworker.*

Silversmiths' Work.
THE SILVERSMITH'S HANDBOOK. By GEORGE E. GEE, Jeweller, &c. Second Edition, Revised, with Illustrations. 12mo, 3s. 6d. cloth.
"The chief merit of the work is its practical character. . . . The workers in the trade will speedily discover its merits when they sit down to study it."—*English Mechanic.*
*** The above two works together, strongly half-bound, price 7s.

Bread and Biscuit Baking.
THE BREAD AND BISCUIT BAKER'S AND SUGAR-BOILER'S ASSISTANT. Including a large variety of Modern Recipes. With Remarks on the Art of Bread-making. By ROBERT WELLS, Practical Baker. Crown 8vo, 2s. cloth. [*Just published.*
"A large number of wrinkles for the ordinary cook, as well as the baker."—*Saturday Review.*
"A book of instruction for learners and for daily reference in the bakehouse.'—*Baker's Times.*

Confectionery.
THE PASTRYCOOK AND CONFECTIONER'S GUIDE. For Hotels, Restaurants and the Trade in general, adapted also for Family Use. By ROBERT WELLS, Author of "The Bread and Biscuit Baker's and Sugar Boiler's Assistant." Crown 8vo, 2s. cloth. [*Just published.*
"We cannot speak too highly of this really excellent work. In these days of keen competition our readers cannot do better than purchase this book."—*Baker's Times.*
"Will be found as serviceable by private families as by restaurant *chefs* and victuallers in general."—*Miller.*

Laundry Work.
A HANDBOOK OF LAUNDRY MANAGEMENT. For Use in Steam and Hand-Power Laundries and Private Houses. By the Editor of THE LAUNDRY JOURNAL. Crown 8vo, 2s. 6d. cloth. [*Just published.*

Horology.

***A TREATISE ON MODERN HOROLOGY**, in Theory and Practice.* Translated from the French of CLAUDIUS SAUNIER, ex-Director of the School of Horology at Macon, by JULIEN TRIPPLIN, F.R.A.S., Besancon, Watch Manufacturer, and EDWARD RIGG, M.A., Assayer in the Royal Mint. With Seventy-eight Woodcuts and Twenty-two Coloured Copper Plates. Second Edition. Super-royal 8vo £2 2s cloth; £2 10s. half-calf.

"There is no horological work in the English language at all to be compared to this production of M. Saunier's for clearness and completeness. It is alike good as a guide for the student and as a reference for the experienced horologist and skilled workman."—*Horological Journal.*

"The latest, the most complete, and the most reliable of those literary productions to which continental watchmakers are indebted for the mechanical superiority over their English brethren—in fact, the Book of Books, is M. Saunier's 'Treatise.'"—*Watchmaker, Jeweller and Silversmith.*

Watchmaking.

THE WATCHMAKER'S HANDBOOK. Translated from the French of CLAUDIUS SAUNIER, and considerably Enlarged by JULIEN TRIPPLIN, F.R.A.S., Vice-President of the Horological Institute, and EDWARD RIGG, M.A., Assayer in the Royal Mint. With Numerous Woodcuts and Fourteen Copper Plates. Second Edition, Revised. With Appendix. Cr. 8vo, 9s. cloth.

"Each part is truly a treatise in itself. The arrangement is good and the language is clear and concise. It is an admirable guide for the young watchmaker."—*Engineering.*

"It is impossible to speak too highly of its excellence. It fulfils every requirement in a handbook intended for the use of a workman. Should be found in every workshop."—*Watch and Clockmaker.*

CHEMICAL MANUFACTURES & COMMERCE.

Alkali Trade, Manufacture of Sulphuric Acid, etc.

A MANUAL OF THE ALKALI TRADE, including the Manufacture of Sulphuric Acid, Sulphate of Soda, and Bleaching Powder. By JOHN LOMAS, Alkali Manufacturer, Newcastle-upon-Tyne and London. With 232 Illustrations and Working Drawings, and containing 390 pages of Text. Second Edition, with Additions. Super-royal 8vo, £1 10s. cloth.

"This book is written by a manufacturer for manufacturers. The working details of the most approved forms of apparatus are given, and these are accompanied by no less than 232 wood engravings, all of which may be used for the purposes of construction. Every step in the manufacture is very fully described in this manual, and each improvement explained.'—*Athenæum.*

"We find here not merely a sound and luminous explanation of the chemical principles of the trade, but a notice of numerous matters which have a most important bearing on the successful conduct of alkali works, but which are generally overlooked by even experienced technological authors."—*Chemical Review.*

Brewing.

A HANDBOOK FOR YOUNG BREWERS. By HERBERT EDWARDS WRIGHT, B.A. Crown 8vo, 3s. 6d. cloth.

"This little volume, containing such a large amount of good sense in so small a compass, ough to recommend itself to every brewery pupil, and many who have passed that stage."—*Brewers Guardian.*

"The book is very clearly written, and the author has successfully brought his scientific knowledge to bear upon the various processes and details of brewing."—*Brewer.*

Commercial Chemical Analysis.

THE COMMERCIAL HANDBOOK OF CHEMICAL ANALYSIS; or, Practical Instructions for the determination of the Intrinsic or Commercial Value of Substances used in Manufactures, in Trades, and in the Arts. By A. NORMANDY, Editor of Rose's "Treatise on Chemical Analysis." New Edition, to a great extent Re-written by HENRY M. NOAD, Ph.D., F.R.S. With numerous Illustrations. Crown 8vo, 12s. 6d. cloth

"We strongly recommend this book to our readers as a guide, alike indispensable to the housewife as to the pharmaceutical practitioner."—*Medical Times.*

"Essential to the analysts appointed under the new Act. The most recent results are given, and the work is well edited and carefully written."—*Nature.*

Explosives.

A HANDBOOK OF MODERN EXPLOSIVES. Being a Practical Treatise on the Manufacture and Application of Dynamite, Gun-Cotton, Nitro-Glycerine, and other Explosive Compounds. By M. EISSLER, Mining Engineer, Author of "The Metallurgy of Gold," "The Metallurgy of Silver," &c. With about 100 Illustrations. Crown 8vo. [*In the press.*

Dye-Wares and Colours.

THE MANUAL OF COLOURS AND DYE-WARES: Their Properties, Applications, Valuation, Impurities, and Sophistications. For the use of Dyers, Printers, Drysalters, Brokers, &c. By J. W. SLATER. Second Edition, Revised and greatly Enlarged. Crown 8vo, 7s. 6d. cloth.

"A complete encyclopædia of the *materia tinctoria*. The information given respecting each article is full and precise, and the methods of determining the value of articles such as these, so liable to sophistication, are given with clearness, and are practical as well as valuable."—*Chemist and Druggist.*

"There is no other work which covers precisely the same ground. To students preparing for examinations in dyeing and printing it will prove exceedingly useful."—*Chemical News.*

Pigments.

THE ARTIST'S MANUAL OF PIGMENTS. Showing their Composition, Conditions of Permanency, Non-Permanency, and Adulterations; Effects in Combination with Each Other and with Vehicles, and the most Reliable Tests of Purity. Together with the Science and Arts Department's Examination Questions on Painting. By H. C. STANDAGE. Second Edition, Revised Small crown 8vo, 2s 6d. cloth.

"This work is indeed *multum-in-parvo*, and we can with good conscience, recommend it to all who come in contact with pigments, whether as makers, dealers or users."—*Chemica Review.*

"This manual cannot fail to be a very valuable aid to all painters who wish their work to endure and be of a sound character; it is complete and comprehensive."—*Spectator.*

"The author supplies a great deal of very valuable information and memoranda as to the chemical qualities and artistic effect of the principal pigments used by painters."—*Builder.*

Gauging. Tables and Rules for Revenue Officers, Brewers, etc.

A POCKET BOOK OF MENSURATION AND GAUGING: Containing Tables, Rules and Memoranda for Revenue Officers, Brewers, Spirit Merchants, &c. By J. B. MANT (Inland Revenue). Oblong 18mo, 4s. leather, with elastic band.

"This handy and useful book is adapted to the requirements of the Inland Revenue Department, and will be a favourite book of reference. The range of subjects is comprehensive, and the arrangement simple and clear."—*Civilian.*

"A most useful book. It should be in the hands of every practical brewer."—*Brewers' Journal.*

AGRICULTURE, FARMING, GARDENING, etc.

Agricultural Facts and Figures.

NOTE-BOOK OF AGRICULTURAL FACTS AND FIGURES FOR FARMERS AND FARM STUDENTS. By PRIMROSE MCCONNELL, Fellow of the Highland and Agricultural Society; late Professor of Agriculture, Glasgow Veterinary College. Third Edition. Royal 32mo, full roan, gilt edges, with elastic band, 4s.

"The most complete and comprehensive Note-book for Farmers and Farm Students that we have seen. It literally teems with information, and we can cordially recommend it to all connected with agriculture."—*North British Agriculturist.*

Youatt and Burn's Complete Grazier.

THE COMPLETE GRAZIER, and FARMER'S and CATTLE-BREEDER'S ASSISTANT. A Compendium of Husbandry; especially in the departments connected with the Breeding, Rearing, Feeding, and General Management of Stock; the Management of the Dairy, &c. With Directions for the Culture and Management of Grass Land, of Grain and Root Crops, the Arrangement of Farm Offices, the use of Implements and Machines, and on Draining, Irrigation, Warping, &c.; and the Application and Relative Value of Manures. By WILLIAM YOUATT, Esq., V.S. Twelfth Edition, Enlarged by ROBERT SCOTT BURN, Author of "Outlines of Modern Farming," "Systematic Small Farming," &c. One large 8vo volume, 860 pp., with 244 Illustrations. £1 1s. half-bound.

"The standard and text-book with the farmer and grazier."—*Farmer's Magazine.*

"A treatise which will remain a standard work on the subject as long as British agriculture endures."—*Mark Lane Express* (First Notice).

"The book deals with all departments of agriculture, and contains an immense amount of valuable information. It is, in fact, an encyclopædia of agriculture put into readable form, and it is the only work equally comprehensive brought down to present date. It is excellently printed on thick paper, and strongly bound, and deserves a place in the library of every agriculturist."—*Mark Lane Express* (Second Notice).

"This esteemed work is well worthy of a place in the libraries of agriculturists."—*North British Agriculturist.*

Flour Manufacture, Milling, etc.

FLOUR MANUFACTURE: A Treatise on Milling Science and Practice. By FRIEDRICH KICK, Imperial Regierungsrath, Professor of Mechanical Technology in the Imperial German Polytechnic Institute, Prague. Translated from the Second Enlarged and Revised Edition with Supplement. By H. H. P. POWLES, A.M.I.C.E. Nearly 400 pp. Illustrated with 28 Folding Plates, and 167 Woodcuts. Royal 8vo, 25s. cloth.

"This valuable work is, and will remain, the standard authority on the science of milling... The miller who has read and digested this work will have laid the foundation, so to speak, of a successful career: he will have acquired a number of general principles which he can proceed to apply... It is permissible to hope that at last we have the accepted text-book of modern milling in good sound English without leaving, if any, trace of the German idiom."—*The Miller.*

"The appearance of his celebrated work in English is very opportune, and British millers will, we are sure, not be slow in availing themselves of its pages."—*Millers' Gazette.*

Small Farming.

SYSTEMATIC SMALL FARMING; *or, The Lessons of my Farm.* Being an Introduction to Modern Farm Practice for Small Farmers. By ROBERT SCOTT BURN, Author of "Outlines of Modern Farming." With numerous Illustrations, crown 8vo, 6s. cloth.

"This is the completest book of its class we have seen, and one which every amateur farmer will read with pleasure and accept as a guide."—*Field.*

"The volume contains a vast amount of useful information. No branch of farming is left untouched, from the labour to be done to the results achieved. It may be safely recommended to all who think they will be in paradise when they buy or rent a three-acre farm."—*Glasgow Herald.*

Modern Farming.

OUTLINES OF MODERN FARMING. By R. SCOTT BURN. Soils, Manures, and Crops—Farming and Farming Economy—Cattle, Sheep, and Horses—Management of Dairy, Pigs and Poultry—Utilisation of Town-Sewage, Irrigation, &c. Sixth Edition. In One Vol., 1,250 pp., half-bound, profusely Illustrated, 12s.

"The aim of the author has been to make his work at once comprehensive and trustworthy, and in this aim he has succeeded to a degree which entitles him to much credit."—*Morning Advertiser.* "No farmer should be without this book."—*Banbury Guardian.*

Agricultural Engineering.

FARM ENGINEERING, THE COMPLETE TEXT-BOOK OF. Comprising Draining and Embanking; Irrigation and Water Supply; Farm Roads, Fences, and Gates; Farm Buildings, their Arrangement and Construction, with Plans and Estimates; Barn Implements and Machines; Field Implements and Machines; Agricultural Surveying, Levelling, &c. By Prof. JOHN SCOTT, Professor of Agriculture at the Royal Agricultural College, Cirencester, &c. In One Vol., 1,150 pages, half-bound, 600 Illustrations, 12s.

"Written with great care, as well as with knowledge and ability. The author has done his work well; we have found him a very trustworthy guide wherever we have tested his statements. The volume will be of great value to agricultural students."—*Mark Lane Express.*

"For a young agriculturist we know of no handy volume so likely to be more usefully studied."—*Bell's Weekly Messenger.*

English Agriculture.

THE FIELDS OF GREAT BRITAIN: A Text-Book of Agriculture, adapted to the Syllabus of the Science and Art Department. For Elementary and Advanced Students. By HUGH CLEMENTS (Board of Trade). Second Edition, Revised and Enlarged. 18mo, 2s. 6d. cloth.

"A most comprehensive volume, giving a mass of information."—*Agricultural Economist.*

"It is a long time since we have seen a book which has pleased us more, or which contains such a vast and useful fund of knowledge."—*Educational Times.*

New Pocket Book for Farmers.

TABLES, MEMORANDA, AND CALCULATED RESULTS for Farmers, Graziers, Agricultural Students, Surveyors, Land Agents Auctioneers, etc. With a New System of Farm Book-keeping. Selected and Arranged by SIDNEY FRANCIS. Second Edition, Revised. 272 pp., waistcoat-pocket size, 1s. 6d., limp leather. [*Just published.*

"Weighing less than 1 oz., and occupying no more space than a match box, it contains a mass of facts and calculations which has never before, in such handy form, been obtainable. Every operation on the farm is dealt with. The work may be taken as thoroughly accurate, having been revised by Dr. Fream. We cordially recommend it."—*Bell's Weekly Messenger.*

"A marvellous little book... The agriculturist who possesses himself of it will not be disappointed with his investment."—*The Farm.*

AGRICULTURE, FARMING, GARDENING, etc.

Farm and Estate Book-keeping.
BOOK-KEEPING FOR FARMERS & ESTATE OWNERS. A Practical Treatise, presenting, in Three Plans, a System adapted to all Classes of Farms. By JOHNSON M. WOODMAN, Chartered Accountant. Second Edition, Revised. Crown 8vo, 3s. 6d. cloth boards; or 2s. 6d. cloth limp.
"The volume is a capital study of a most important subject."—*Agricultural Gazette.*
"Will be found of great assistance by those who intend to commence a system of book-keeping, the author's examples being clear and explicit, and his explanations, while full and accurate, being to a large extent free from technicalities."—*Live Stock Journal.*

Farm Account Book.
WOODMAN'S YEARLY FARM ACCOUNT BOOK. Giving a Weekly Labour Account and Diary, and showing the Income and Expenditure under each Department of Crops, Live Stock, Dairy, &c. &c. With Valuation, Profit and Loss Account, and Balance Sheet at the end of the Year, and an Appendix of Forms. Ruled and Headed for Entering a Complete Record of the Farming Operations. By JOHNSON M. WOODMAN, Chartered Accountant, Author of "Book-keeping for Farmers." Folio, 7s. 6d. half bound. [*culture.*
"Contains every requisite orm for keeping farm accounts readily and accurately."—*Agri-*

Early Fruits, Flowers and Vegetables.
THE FORCING GARDEN; or, How to Grow Early Fruits, Flowers, and Vegetables. With Plans and Estimates for Building Glasshouses, Pits and Frames. Containing also Original Plans for Double Glazing, a New Method of Growing the Gooseberry under Glass, &c. &c., and on Ventilation, &c. With Illustrations. By SAMUEL WOOD. Crown 8vo, 3s. 6d. cloth.
"A good book, and fairly fills a place that was in some degree vacant. The book is written with great care, and contains a great deal of valuable teaching."—*Gardeners' Magazine.*
"Mr. Wood's book is an original and exhaustive answer to the question 'How to Grow Early Fruits, Flowers and Vegetables?'"—*Land and Water.*

Good Gardening.
A PLAIN GUIDE TO GOOD GARDENING; or, How to Grow Vegetables, Fruits, and Flowers. With Practical Notes on Soils, Manures, Seeds, Planting, Laying-out of Gardens and Grounds, &c. By S. WOOD. Third Edition, with considerable Additions, &c., and numerous Illustrations. Crown 8vo, 5s. cloth.
"A very good book, and one to be highly recommended as a practical guide. The practical directions are excellent."—*Athenæum.*
"May be recommended to young gardeners, cottagers and amateurs, for the plain and trustworthy information it gives on common matters too often neglected."—*Gardeners' Chronicle.*

Gainful Gardening.
MULTUM-IN-PARVO GARDENING; or, How to make One Acre of Land produce £620 a-year by the Cultivation of Fruits and Vegetables; also, How to Grow Flowers in Three Glass Houses, so as to realise £176 per annum clear Profit. By SAMUEL WOOD, Author of "Good Gardening," &c. Fourth and cheaper Edition, Revised, with Additions. Crown 8vo, 1s. sewed.
"We are bound to recommend it as not only suited to the case of the amateur and gentleman's gardener, but to the market grower."—*Gardeners' Magazine.*

Gardening for Ladies.
THE LADIES' MULTUM-IN-PARVO FLOWER GARDEN, and Amateurs' Complete Guide. By S. WOOD. Crown 8vo, 3s. 6d. cloth.
"This volume contains a good deal of sound, common sense instruction."—*Florist.*
"Full of shrewd hints and useful instructions, based on a lifetime of experience."—*Scotsman.*

Receipts for Gardeners.
GARDEN RECEIPTS. Edited by CHARLES W. QUIN. 12mo, 1s. 6d. cloth limp.
"A useful and handy book, containing a good deal of valuable information."—*Athenæum.*

Market Gardening.
MARKET AND KITCHEN GARDENING. By Contributors to "The Garden." Compiled by C. W. SHAW, late Editor of "Gardening Illustrated." 12mo, 3s. 6d. cloth boards. [*Just published.*
"The most valuable compendium of kitchen and market-garden work published."—*Farmer.*

Cottage Gardening.
COTTAGE GARDENING; or, Flowers, Fruits, and Vegetables or Small Gardens. By E. HOBDAY. 12mo, 1s. 6d. cloth limp.
"Contains much useful information at a small charge."—*Glasgow Herald.*

ESTATE MANAGEMENT, AUCTIONEERING, LAW, etc.

Hudson's Land Valuer's Pocket-Book.

THE LAND VALUER'S BEST ASSISTANT: Being Tables on a very much Improved Plan, for Calculating the Value of Estates. With Tables for reducing Scotch, Irish, and Provincial Customary Acres to Statute Measure. &c. By R. HUDSON, C.E. New Edition. Royal 32mo, leather, elastic band, 4s.

"This new edition includes tables for ascertaining the value of leases for any term of years; and for showing how to lay out plots of ground of certain acres in forms, square, round, &c., with valuable rules for ascertaining the probable worth of standing timber to any amount; and is of incalculable value to the country gentleman and professional man."—*Farmers' Journal.*

Ewart's Land Improver's Pocket-Book.

THE LAND IMPROVER'S POCKET-BOOK OF FORMULÆ, TABLES and MEMORANDA *required in any Computation relating to the Permanent Improvement of Landed Property.* By JOHN EWART, Land Surveyor and Agricultural Engineer. Second Edition, Revised. Royal 32mo, oblong, leather, gilt edges, with elastic band, 4s.

"A compendious and handy little volume."—*Spectator.*

Complete Agricultural Surveyor's Pocket-Book.

THE LAND VALUER'S AND LAND IMPROVER'S COMPLETE POCKET-BOOK. Consisting of the above Two Works bound together. Leather, gilt edges, with strap, 7s. 6d.

"Hudson's book is the best ready-reckoner on matters relating to the valuation of land and crops, and its combination with Mr. Ewart's work greatly enhances the value and usefulness of the latter-mentioned. . . . It is most useful as a manual for reference."—*North of England Farmer.*

Auctioneer's Assistant.

THE APPRAISER, AUCTIONEER, BROKER, HOUSE AND ESTATE AGENT AND VALUER'S POCKET ASSISTANT, for the Valuation for Purchase, Sale, or Renewal of Leases, Annuities and Reversions, and of property generally; with Prices for Inventories, &c. By JOHN WHEELER, Valuer, &c. Fifth Edition, re-written and greatly extended by C. NORRIS, Surveyor, Valuer, &c. Royal 32mo, 5s. cloth.

"A neat and concise book of reference, containing an admirable and clearly-arranged list of prices for inventories, and a very practical guide to determine the value of furniture, &c."—*Standard.*

"Contains a large quantity of varied and useful information as to the valuation for purchase, sale, or renewal of leases, annuities and reversions, and of property generally, with prices for inventories, and a guide to determine the value of interior fittings and other effects."—*Builder.*

Auctioneering.

AUCTIONEERS: *Their Duties and Liabilities.* By ROBERT SQUIBBS, Auctioneer. Demy 8vo, 10s. 6d. cloth.

"The position and duties of auctioneers treated compendiously and clearly."—*Builder.*

"Every auctioneer ought to possess a copy of this excellent work."—*Ironmonger.*

"Of great value to the profession. . . . We readily welcome this book from the fact that it treats the subject in a manner somewhat new to the profession."—*Estates Gazette.*

Legal Guide for Pawnbrokers.

THE PAWNBROKERS', FACTORS' AND MERCHANTS' GUIDE TO THE LAW OF LOANS AND PLEDGES. With the Statutes and a Digest of Cases on Rights and Liabilities, Civil and Criminal, as to Loans and Pledges of Goods, Debentures, Mercantile and other Securities. By H. C. FOLKARD, Esq., Barrister-at Law, Author of "The Law of Slander and Libel," &c. With Additions and Corrections. Fcap. 8vo, 3s. 6d. cloth.

"This work contains simply everything that requires to be known concerning the department of the law of which it treats. We can safely commend the book as unique and very nearly perfect."—*Iron.*

"The task undertaken by Mr. Folkard has been very satisfactorily performed. . . . Such explanations as are needful have been supplied with great clearness and with due regard to brevity."—*City Press.*

ESTATE MANAGEMENT, AUCTIONEERING, LAW, etc. 39

How to Invest.
HINTS FOR INVESTORS: Being an Explanation of the Mode of Transacting Business on the Stock Exchange. To which are added Comments on the Fluctuations and Table of Quarterly Average prices of Consols since 1759 Also a Copy of the London Daily Stock and Share List. By WALTER M. PLAYFORD, Sworn Broker. Crown 8vo, 2s. cloth.
"An invaluable guide to investors and speculators."—*Bullionist*

Metropolitan Rating Appeals.
REPORTS OF APPEALS HEARD BEFORE THE COURT OF GENERAL ASSESSMENT SESSIONS, from the Year 1871 to 1885. By EDWARD RYDE and ARTHUR LYON RYDE. Fourth Edition, brought down to the Present Date, with an Introduction to the Valuation (Metropolis) Act, 1869, and an Appendix by WALTER C. RYDE, of the Inner Temple, Barrister-at-Law. 8vo, 16s. cloth.
"A useful work, occupying a place mid-way between a handbook for a lawyer and a guide to the surveyor. It is compiled by a gentleman eminent in his profession as a land agent, whose speciality, it is acknowledged, lies in the direction of assessing property for rating purposes."—*Land Agents' Record*.

House Property.
HANDBOOK OF HOUSE PROPERTY. A Popular and Practical Guide to the Purchase, Mortgage, Tenancy, and Compulsory Sale of Houses and Land, including the Law of Dilapidations and Fixtures; with Examples of all kinds of Valuations, Useful Information on Buildings, and Suggestive Elucidations of Fine Art. By E. L. TARBUCK, Architect and Surveyor. Fourth Edition, Enlarged. 12mo, 5s. cloth.
"The advice is thoroughly practical."—*Law Journal*.
"For all who have dealings with house property, this is an indispensable guide."—*Decoration*.
"Carefully brought up to date, and much improved by the addition of a division on fine art. A well-written and thoughtful work."—*Land Agents Record*.

Inwood's Estate Tables.
TABLES FOR THE PURCHASING OF ESTATES, Freehold, Copyhold, or Leasehold; Annuities, Advowsons, etc., and for the Renewing of Leases held under Cathedral Churches, Colleges, or other Corporate bodies, for Terms of Years certain, and for Lives; also for Valuing Reversionary Estates, Deferred Annuities, Next Presentations, &c.; together with SMART's Five Tables of Compound Interest, and an Extension of the same to Lower and Intermediate Rates. By W. INWOOD. 23rd Edition, with considerable Additions, and new and valuable Tables of Logarithms for the more Difficult Computations of the Interest of Money, Discount, Annuities, &c., by M. FEDOR THOMAN, of the Société Crédit Mobilier of Paris. Crown 8vo, 8s. cloth.
"Those interested in the purchase and sale of estates, and in the adjustment of compensation cases, as well as in transactions in annuities, life insurances, &c., will find the present edition of eminent service."—*Engineering*.
"'Inwood's Tables' still maintain a most enviable reputation. The new issue has been enriched by large additional contributions by M. Fedor Thoman, whose carefully arranged Tables cannot fail to be of the utmost utility."—*Mining Journal*.

Agricultural and Tenant-Right Valuation.
THE AGRICULTURAL AND TENANT-RIGHT-VALUER'S ASSISTANT. A Practical Handbook on Measuring and Estimating the Contents, Weights and Values of Agricultural Produce and Timber, the Values of Estates and Agricultural Labour, Forms of Tenant-Right-Valuations, Scales of Compensation under the Agricultural Holdings Act, 1883, &c. &c. By TOM BRIGHT, Agricultural Surveyor. Crown 8vo, 3s. 6d. cloth.
"Full of tables and examples in connection with the valuation of tenant-right, estates, labour, contents and weights of timber, and farm produce of all kinds."—*Agricultural Gazette*.
"An eminently practical handbook, full of practical tables and data of undoubted interest and value to surveyors and auctioneers in preparing valuations of all kinds."—*Farmer*.

Plantations and Underwoods.
POLE PLANTATIONS AND UNDERWOODS: A Practical Handbook on Estimating the Cost of Forming, Renovating, Improving and Grubbing Plantations and Underwoods, their Valuation for Purposes of Transfer, Rental, Sale or Assessment. By TOM BRIGHT, F.S.Sc., Author of "The Agricultural and Tenant-Right-Valuer's Assistant," &c. Crown 8vo, 3s. 6d. cloth. [*Just published*.
"Very useful to those actually engaged in managing wood."—*Bell's Weekly Messenger*.
"To valuers, foresters and agents it will be a welcome aid."—*North British Agriculturist*.
"Well calculated to assist the valuer in the discharge of his duties, and of undoubted interest and use both to surveyors and auctioneers in preparing valuations of all kinds.'—*Kent Herald*.

A Complete Epitome of the Laws of this Country.

EVERY MAN'S OWN LAWYER: A Handy-Book of the Principles of Law and Equity. By A BARRISTER. Twenty-sixth Edition. Reconstructed, Thoroughly Revised, and much Enlarged. Including the Legislation of the Two Sessions of 1888, and including careful digests of *The Local Government Act,* 1888; *County Electors Act,* 1888; *County Courts Act,* 1888; *Glebe Lands Act,* 1888; *Law of Libel Amendment Act,* 1888; *Patents, Designs and Trade Marks Act,* 1888; *Solicitors Act,* 1888; *Preferential Payments in Bankruptcy Act,* 1888; *Land Charges Registration and Searches Act,* 1888; *Trustee Act,* 1888, &c. Crown 8vo, 688 pp., price 6s. 8d. (saved at every consultation!), strongly bound in cloth. *[Just published.*

*** THE BOOK WILL BE FOUND TO COMPRISE (AMONGST OTHER MATTER)—

THE RIGHTS AND WRONGS OF INDIVIDUALS—MERCANTILE AND COMMERCIAL LAW—PARTNERSHIPS, CONTRACTS AND AGREEMENTS—GUARANTEES, PRINCIPALS AND AGENTS—CRIMINAL LAW—PARISH LAW—COUNTY COURT LAW—GAME AND FISHERY LAWS—POOR MEN'S LAWSUITS—LAWS OF BANKRUPTCY—WAGERS—CHEQUES, BILLS AND NOTES—COPYRIGHT—ELECTIONS AND REGISTRATION—INSURANCE—LIBEL AND SLANDER—MARRIAGE AND DIVORCE—MERCHANT SHIPPING—MORTGAGES—SETTLEMENTS—STOCK EXCHANGE PRACTICE—TRADE MARKS AND PATENTS—TRESPASS—NUISANCES—TRANSFER OF LAND—WILLS, &c. &c. Also LAW FOR LANDLORD AND TENANT—MASTER AND SERVANT—HEIRS—DEVISEES AND LEGATEES—HUSBAND AND WIFE—EXECUTORS AND TRUSTEES—GUARDIAN AND WARD—MARRIED WOMEN AND INFANTS—LENDER, BORROWER AND SURETIES—DEBTOR AND CREDITOR—PURCHASER AND VENDOR—COMPANIES—FRIENDLY SOCIETIES—CLERGYMEN—CHURCHWARDENS—MEDICAL PRACTITIONERS—BANKERS—FARMERS—CONTRACTORS—STOCK BROKERS—SPORTSMEN—GAMEKEEPERS—FARRIERS—HORSE DEALERS—AUCTIONEERS—HOUSE AGENTS—INNKEEPERS—BAKERS—MILLERS—PAWNBROKERS—SURVEYORS—RAILWAYS AND CARRIERS—CONSTABLES—SEAMEN—SOLDIERS, &c. &c.

☞ *The following subjects may be mentioned as amongst those which have received special attention during the revision in question:*—Marriage of British Subjects Abroad; Police Constables; Pawnbrokers; Intoxicating Liquors; Licensing; Domestic Servants; Landlord and Tenant; Vendors and Purchasers; Municipal Elections; Local Elections; Corrupt Practices at Elections; Public Health and Nuisances; Highways; Churchwardens; Legal and Illegal Ritual; Vestry Meetings; Rates.

It is believed that the extensions and amplifications of the present edition, while intended to meet the requirements of the ordinary Englishman, will also have the effect of rendering the book useful to the legal practitioner in the country.

One result of the reconstruction and revision, with the extensive additions thereby necessitated, has been *the enlargement of the book by nearly a hundred and fifty pages*, while the price remains as before.

The PUBLISHERS feel every confidence, therefore, that this standard work will continue to be regarded, as hitherto, as an absolute necessity FOR EVERY MAN OF BUSINESS AS WELL AS EVERY HEAD OF A FAMILY.

*** OPINIONS OF THE PRESS.

"It is a complete code of English Law, written in plain language, which all can understand. . . . Should be in the hands of every business man, and all who wish to abolish lawyers' bills."—*Weekly Times.*

"A useful and concise epitome of the law, compiled with considerable care. —*Law Magazine.*

"A concise, cheap and complete epitome of the English law. So plainly written that he who runs may read, and he who reads may understand.'—*Figaro.*

"A dictionary of legal facts well put together. The book is a very useful one."—*Spectator.*

"A work which has long been wanted, which is thoroughly well done, and which we most cordially recommend."—*Sunday Times.*

Private Bill Legislation and Provisional Orders.

HANDBOOK FOR THE USE OF SOLICITORS AND ENGINEERS Engaged in Promoting Private Acts of Parliament and Provisional Orders, for the Authorization of Railways, Tramways, Works for the Supply of Gas and Water, and other undertakings of a like character. By L. LIVINGSTON MACASSEY, of the Middle Temple, Barrister-at-Law, and Member of the Institution of Civil Engineers; Author of "Hints on Water Supply." Demy 8vo, 950 pp., price 25s. cloth.

"The volume is a desideratum on a subject which can be only acquired by practical experience, and the order of procedure in Private Bill Legislation and Provisional Orders is followed. The author's suggestions and notes will be found of great value to engineers and others professionally engaged in this class of practice."—*Building News.*

"The author's double experience as an engineer and barrister has eminently qualified him for the task, and enabled him to approach the subject alike from an engineering and legal point of view. The volume will be found a great help both to engineers and lawyers engaged in promoting Private Acts of Parliament and Provisional Orders."—*Local Government Chronicle.*

J. OGDEN AND CO. LIMITED, PRINTERS, GREAT SAFFRON HILL, E.C.

Weale's Rudimentary Series.

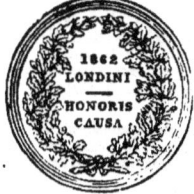

LONDON, 1862.
THE PRIZE MEDAL
Was awarded to the Publishers of
"WEALE'S SERIES."

A NEW LIST OF
WEALE'S SERIES
RUDIMENTARY SCIENTIFIC, EDUCATIONAL, AND CLASSICAL.

Comprising nearly Three Hundred and Fifty *distinct works in almost every department of Science,* Art, *and Education, recommended to the notice of* Engineers, Architects, Builders, Artisans, *and Students generally, as well as to those interested in Workmen's Libraries, Literary and Scientific Institutions, Colleges, Schools, Science Classes, &c., &c.*

☞ "WEALE'S SERIES includes Text-Books on almost every branch of Science and Industry, comprising such subjects as Agriculture, Architecture and Building, Civil Engineering, Fine Arts, Mechanics and Mechanical Engineering, Physical and Chemical Science, and many miscellaneous Treatises. The whole are constantly undergoing revision, and new editions, brought up to the latest discoveries in scientific research, are constantly issued. The prices at which they are sold are as low as their excellence is assured."—*American Literary Gazette.*

"Amongst the literature of technical education, WEALE'S SERIES has ever enjoyed a high reputation, and the additions being made by Messrs. CROSBY LOCKWOOD & SON render the series even more complete, and bring the information upon the several subjects down to the present time."—*Mining Journal.*

"It is not too much to say that no books have ever proved more popular with, or more useful to, young engineers and others than the excellent treatises comprised in WEALE'S SERIES."—*Engineer.*

"The excellence of WEALE'S SERIES is now so well appreciated, that it would be wasting our space to enlarge upon their general usefulness and value."—*Builder.*

"WEALE'S SERIES has become a standard as well as an unrivalled collection of treatises in all branches of art and science."—*Public Opinion.*

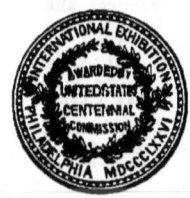

PHILADELPHIA, 1876.
THE PRIZE MEDAL
Was awarded to the Publishers for
Books: Rudimentary, Scientific,
"WEALE'S SERIES," ETC.

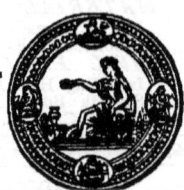

CROSBY LOCKWOOD & SON,
7, STATIONERS' HALL COURT, LUDGATE HILL, LONDON, E.C.

WEALE'S RUDIMENTARY SCIENTIFIC SERIES.

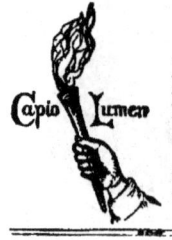

₊ The volumes of this Series are freely Illustrated with Woodcuts, or otherwise, where requisite. Throughout the following List it must be understood that the books are bound in limp cloth, unless otherwise stated; *but the volumes marked with a ‡ may also be had strongly bound in cloth boards for 6d. extra.*

N.B.—In ordering from this List it is recommended, as a means of facilitating business and obviating error, to quote the numbers affixed to the volumes, as well as the titles and prices.

CIVIL ENGINEERING, SURVEYING, ETC.

No.
31. *WELLS AND WELL-SINKING.* By JOHN GEO. SWINDELL, A.R.I.B.A., and G. R. BURNELL, C.E. Revised Edition. With a New Appendix on the Qualities of Water. Illustrated. 2s.
35. *THE BLASTING AND QUARRYING OF STONE*, for Building and other Purposes. With Remarks on the Blowing up of Bridges. By Gen. Sir JOHN BURGOYNE, Bart., K.C.B. Illustrated. 1s. 6d.
43. *TUBULAR, AND OTHER IRON GIRDER BRIDGES*, particularly describing the Britannia and Conway Tubular Bridges. By G. DRYSDALE DEMPSEY, C.E. Fourth Edition. 2s.
44. *FOUNDATIONS AND CONCRETE WORKS*, with Practical Remarks on Footings, Sand, Concrete, Béton, Pile-driving, Caissons, and Cofferdams, &c. By E. DOBSON. Fifth Edition. 1s. 6d.
60. *LAND AND ENGINEERING SURVEYING.* By T. BAKER, C.E. Fourteenth Edition, revised by Professor J. R. YOUNG. 2s.‡
80*. *EMBANKING LANDS FROM THE SEA.* With examples and Particulars of actual Embankments, &c. By J. WIGGINS, F.G.S. 2s.
81. *WATER WORKS*, for the Supply of Cities and Towns. With a Description of the Principal Geological Formations of England as influencing Supplies of Water; and Details of Engines and Pumping Machinery for raising Water. By SAMUEL HUGHES, F.G.S., C.E. New Edition. 4s.‡
118. *CIVIL ENGINEERING IN NORTH AMERICA*, a Sketch of. By DAVID STEVENSON, F.R.S.E., &c. Plates and Diagrams. 3s.
167. *IRON BRIDGES, GIRDERS, ROOFS, AND OTHER WORKS.* By FRANCIS CAMPIN, C.E. 2s. 6d.‡
197. *ROADS AND STREETS (THE CONSTRUCTION OF).* By HENRY LAW, C.E., revised and enlarged by D. K. CLARK, C.E., including pavements of Stone, Wood, Asphalte, &c. 4s. 6d.‡
203. *SANITARY WORK IN THE SMALLER TOWNS AND IN VILLAGES.* By C. SLAGG, A.M.I.C.E. Revised Edition. 3s.‡
212. *GAS-WORKS, THEIR CONSTRUCTION AND ARRANGEMENT*; and the Manufacture and Distribution of Coal Gas. Originally written by SAMUEL HUGHES, C.E. Re-written and enlarged by WILLIAM RICHARDS, C.E. Seventh Edition, with important additions. 5s. 6d.‡
213. *PIONEER ENGINEERING.* A Treatise on the Engineering Operations connected with the Settlement of Waste Lands in New Countries. By EDWARD DOBSON, Assoc. Inst. C.E. 4s. 6d.‡
216. *MATERIALS AND CONSTRUCTION;* A Theoretical and Practical Treatise on the Strains, Designing, and Erection of Works of Construction. By FRANCIS CAMPIN, C.E. Second Edition, revised. 3s.‡
219. *CIVIL ENGINEERING.* By HENRY LAW, M.Inst. C.E. Including HYDRAULIC ENGINEERING by GEO. R. BURNELL, M.Inst. C.E. Seventh Edition, revised, with large additions by D. KINNEAR CLARK, M.Inst. C.E. 6s. 6d., Cloth boards, 7s. 6d.

☞ *The ‡ indicates that these vols. may be had strongly bound at 6d. extra.*

LONDON : CROSBY LOCKWOOD AND SON,

MECHANICAL ENGINEERING, ETC.

33. *CRANES*, the Construction of, and other Machinery for Raising Heavy Bodies. By Joseph Glynn, F.R.S. Illustrated. 1s. 6d.
34. *THE STEAM ENGINE*. By Dr. Lardner. Illustrated. 1s. 6d.
59. *STEAM BOILERS:* their Construction and Management. By R. Armstrong, C.E. Illustrated. 1s. 6d.
82. *THE POWER OF WATER*, as applied to drive Flour Mills, and to give motion to Turbines, &c. By Joseph Glynn, F.R.S. 2s.‡
98. *PRACTICAL MECHANISM*, the Elements of; and Machine Tools. By T. Baker, C.E. With Additions by J. Nasmyth, C.E. 2s. 6d.‡
139. *THE STEAM ENGINE*, a Treatise on the Mathematical Theory of, with Rules and Examples for Practical Men. By T. Baker, C.E. 1s. 6d.
164. *MODERN WORKSHOP PRACTICE*, as applied to Steam Engines, Bridges, Ship-building, Cranes, &c. By J. G. Winton. Fourth Edition, much enlarged and carefully revised. 3s. 6d.‡ [*Just published*.
165. *IRON AND HEAT*, exhibiting the Principles concerned in the Construction of Iron Beams, Pillars, and Girders. By J. Armour. 2s. 6d.‡
166. *POWER IN MOTION:* Horse-Power, Toothed-Wheel Gearing, Long and Short Driving Bands, and Angular Forces. By J. Armour. 2s.‡
171. *THE WORKMAN'S MANUAL OF ENGINEERING DRAWING.* By J. Maxton. 6th Edn. With 7 Plates and 350 Cuts. 3s. 6d.‡
190. *STEAM AND THE STEAM ENGINE*, Stationary and Portable. Being an Extension of the Elementary Treatise on the Steam Engine of Mr. John Sewell. By D. K. Clark, M.I.C.E. 3s. 6d.‡
200. *FUEL*, its Combustion and Economy. By C. W. Williams. With Recent Practice in the Combustion and Economy of Fuel—Coal, Coke, Wood, Peat, Petroleum, &c.—by D. K. Clark, M.I.C.E. 3s. 6d.‡
202. *LOCOMOTIVE ENGINES.* By G. D. Dempsey, C.E.; with large additions by D. Kinnear Clark, M.I.C.E. 3s.‡
211. *THE BOILERMAKER'S ASSISTANT* in Drawing, Templating, and Calculating Boiler and Tank Work. By John Courtney. Practical Boiler Maker. Edited by D. K. Clark, C.E. 100 Illustrations. 2s.
217. *SEWING MACHINERY:* Its Construction, History, &c., with full Technical Directions for Adjusting, &c. By J. W. Urquhart, C.E. 2s.‡
223. *MECHANICAL ENGINEERING.* Comprising Metallurgy, Moulding, Casting, Forging, Tools, Workshop Machinery, Manufacture of the Steam Engine, &c. By Francis Campin, C.E. Second Edition. 2s. 6d.‡
236. *DETAILS OF MACHINERY.* Comprising Instructions for the Execution of various Works in Iron. By Francis Campin, C.E. 3s.‡
237. *THE SMITHY AND FORGE;* including the Farrier's Art and Coach Smithing. By W. J. E. Crane. Illustrated. 2s. 6d.‡
238. *THE SHEET-METAL WORKER'S GUIDE;* a Practical Handbook for Tinsmiths, Coppersmiths, Zincworkers, &c. With 94 Diagrams and Working Patterns. By W. J. E. Crane. Second Edition, revised. 1s. 6d.
251. *STEAM AND MACHINERY MANAGEMENT:* with Hints on Construction and Selection. By M. Powis Bale, M.I.M.E. 2s. 6d.‡
254. *THE BOILERMAKER'S READY-RECKONER.* By J. Courtney. Edited by D. K. Clark, C.E. 4s., limp; 5s., half-bound.
255. *LOCOMOTIVE ENGINE-DRIVING.* A Practical Manual for Engineers in charge of Locomotive Engines. By Michael Reynolds, M.S.E. Eighth Edition. 3s. 6d., limp; 4s. 6d. cloth boards.
256. *STATIONARY ENGINE-DRIVING.* A Practical Manual Engineers in charge of Stationary Engines. By Michael Reynolds, M.S.E. Third Edition. 3s. 6d. limp; 4s. 6d. cloth boards.
260. *IRON BRIDGES OF MODERATE SPAN:* their Construction and Erection. By Hamilton W. Pendred, C.E. 2s.

The ‡ *indicates that these vols. may be had strongly bound at 6d. extra.*

7, STATIONERS' HALL COURT, LUDGATE HILL, E.C.

WEALE'S RUDIMENTARY SERIES.

MINING, METALLURGY, ETC.

4. *MINERALOGY*, Rudiments of; a concise View of the General Properties of Minerals. By A. RAMSAY, F.G.S., F.R.G.S., &c. Third Edition, revised and enlarged. Illustrated. 3s. 6d.‡

117. *SUBTERRANEOUS SURVEYING*, with and without the Magnetic Needle. By T. FENWICK and T. BAKER, C.E. Illustrated. 2s. 6d. ‡

133. *METALLURGY OF COPPER*. By R. H. LAMBORN. 2s. 6d.‡

135. *ELECTRO-METALLURGY;* Practically Treated. By ALEXANDER WATT. Ninth Edition, enlarged and revised, with additional Illustrations, and including the most recent Processes. 3s. 6d.‡

172. *MINING TOOLS,* Manual of. For the Use of Mine Managers, Agents, Students, &c. By WILLIAM MORGANS. 2s. 6d.

172*. *MINING TOOLS, ATLAS* of Engravings to Illustrate the above, containing 235 Illustrations, drawn to Scale. 4to. 4s. 6d.

176. *METALLURGY OF IRON.* Containing History of Iron Manufacture, Methods of Assay, and Analyses of Iron Ores, Processes of Manufacture of Iron and Steel, &c. By H. BAUERMAN, F.G.S. Sixth Edition, revised and enlarged. 5s.‡ [*Just published.*

180. *COAL AND COAL MINING.* By WARINGTON W. SMYTH, M.A., F.R.S. Sixth Edition, revised 3s. 6d.‡

195. *THE MINERAL SURVEYOR AND VALUER'S COMPLETE GUIDE.* By W. LINTERN, Mining Engineer. Third Edition, with an Appendix on Magnetic and Angular Surveying. With Four Plates. 3s. 6d.‡ [*Just published.*

214. *SLATE AND SLATE QUARRYING*, Scientific, Practical, and Commercial. By D. C. DAVIES, F.G.S., Mining Engineer, &c. 3s.‡

264. *A FIRST BOOK OF MINING AND QUARRYING*, with the Sciences connected therewith, for Primary Schools and Self Instruction. By J. H. COLLINS, F.G.S. Second Edition, with additions. 1s. 6d.

ARCHITECTURE, BUILDING, ETC.

16. *ARCHITECTURE—ORDERS*—The Orders and their Æsthetic Principles. By W. H. LEEDS. Illustrated. 1s. 6d.

17. *ARCHITECTURE—STYLES*—The History and Description of the Styles of Architecture of Various Countries, from the Earliest to the Present Period. By T. TALBOT BURY, F.R.I.B.A., &c. Illustrated. 2s.
*** ORDERS AND STYLES OF ARCHITECTURE, *in One Vol.,* 3s. 6d.

18. *ARCHITECTURE—DESIGN*—The Principles of Design in Architecture, as deducible from Nature and exemplified in the Works of the Greek and Gothic Architects. By E. L. GARBETT, Architect. Illustrated. 2s.6d.
*** The three preceding Works, in One handsome Vol., half bound, entitled " MODERN ARCHITECTURE," *price* 6s.

22. *THE ART OF BUILDING*, Rudiments of. General Principles of Construction, Materials used in Building, Strength and Use of Materials, Working Drawings, Specifications, and Estimates. By E. DOBSON, 2s.‡

25. *MASONRY AND STONECUTTING :* Rudimentary Treatise on the Principles of Masonic Projection and their application to Construction. By EDWARD DOBSON, M.R.I.B.A., &c. 2s. 6d.‡

42. *COTTAGE BUILDING.* By C. BRUCE ALLEN, Architect. Tenth Edition, revised and enlarged. With a Chapter on Economic Cottages for Allotments, by EDWARD E. ALLEN, C.E. 2s.

45. *LIMES, CEMENTS, MORTARS, CONCRETES, MASTICS,* PLASTERING, &c. By G. R. BURNELL, C.E. Thirteenth Edition. 1s. 6d.

57. *WARMING AND VENTILATION.* An Exposition of the General Principles as applied to Domestic and Public Buildings, Mines, Lighthouses. Ships, &c. By C. TOMLINSON, F.R.S., &c. Illustrated. 3s.

☞ *The* ‡ *indicates that these vols. may be had strongly bound at* 6d. *extra.*

LONDON : CROSBY LOCKWOOD AND SON,

Architecture, Building, etc., *continued.*

111. *ARCHES, PIERS, BUTTRESSES, &c.:* Experimental Essays on the Principles of Construction. By W. BLAND. Illustrated. 1s. 6d.
116. *THE ACOUSTICS OF PUBLIC BUILDINGS;* or, The Principles of the Science of Sound applied to the purposes of the Architect and Builder. By T. ROGER SMITH, M.R.I.B.A., Architect. Illustrated. 1s. 6d.
127. *ARCHITECTURAL MODELLING IN PAPER,* the Art of. By T. A. RICHARDSON, Architect. Illustrated. 1s. 6d.
128. *VITRUVIUS — THE ARCHITECTURE OF MARCUS VITRUVIUS POLLO.* In Ten Books. Translated from the Latin by JOSEPH GWILT, F.S.A., F.R.A.S. With 23 Plates. 5s.
130. *GRECIAN ARCHITECTURE,* An Inquiry into the Principles of Beauty in; with an Historical View of the Rise and Progress of the Art in Greece. By the EARL OF ABERDEEN. 1s.
*** *The two preceding Works in One handsome Vol., half bound, entitled* "ANCIENT ARCHITECTURE." *price* 6s.
132. *THE ERECTION OF DWELLING-HOUSES.* Illustrated by a Perspective View, Plans, Elevations, and Sections of a pair of Semi-detached Villas, with the Specification, Quantities, and Estimates, &c. By S. H. BROOKS. New Edition, with Plates. 2s. 6d.‡
156. *QUANTITIES & MEASUREMENTS* in Bricklayers', Masons', Plasterers', Plumbers', Painters', Paperhangers', Gilders', Smiths', Carpenters' and Joiners' Work. By A. C. BEATON, Surveyor. New Edition. 1s. 6d.
175. *LOCKWOOD & SON'S BUILDER'S & CONTRACTOR'S* PRICE BOOK, containing the latest Prices of all kinds of Builders' Materials and Labour, and of all Trades connected with Building, &c., &c. Edited by F. T. W. MILLER, Architect. Published annually. 3s. 6d.; half bound, 4s.
182. *CARPENTRY AND JOINERY*—THE ELEMENTARY PRINCIPLES OF CARPENTRY. Chiefly composed from the Standard Work of THOMAS TREDGOLD, C.E. With a TREATISE ON JOINERY by E. WYNDHAM TARN, M.A. Fourth Edition, Revised. 3s. 6d.‡
182*. *CARPENTRY AND JOINERY. ATLAS* of 35 Plates to accompany the above. With Descriptive Letterpress. 4to. 6s.
185. *THE COMPLETE MEASURER;* the Measurement of Boards, Glass, &c.; Unequal-sided, Square-sided, Octagonal-sided, Round Timber and Stone, and Standing Timber, &c. By RICHARD HORTON. Fifth Edition. 4s.; strongly bound in leather, 5s.
187. *HINTS TO YOUNG ARCHITECTS.* By G. WIGHTWICK. New Edition. By G. H. GUILLAUME. Illustrated. 3s. 6d.‡
188. *HOUSE PAINTING, GRAINING, MARBLING, AND SIGN WRITING:* with a Course of Elementary Drawing for House-Painters, Sign-Writers, &c., and a Collection of Useful Receipts. By ELLIS A. DAVIDSON. Fifth Edition. With Coloured Plates. 5s. cloth limp; 6s. cloth boards.
189. *THE RUDIMENTS OF PRACTICAL BRICKLAYING.* In Six Sections: General Principles; Arch Drawing, Cutting, and Setting; Pointing; Paving, Tiling, Materials; Slating and Plastering; Practical Geometry, Mensuration, &c. By ADAM HAMMOND. Seventh Edition. 1s. 6d.
191. *PLUMBING.* A Text-Book to the Practice of the Art or Craft of the Plumber. With Chapters upon House Drainage and Ventilation. Fifth Edition. With 380 Illustrations. By W. P. BUCHAN. 3s. 6d.‡
192. *THE TIMBER IMPORTER'S, TIMBER MERCHANT'S,* and BUILDER'S STANDARD GUIDE. By R. E. GRANDY. 2s.
206. *A BOOK ON BUILDING, Civil and Ecclesiastical,* including CHURCH RESTORATION. With the Theory of Domes and the Great Pyramid, &c. By Sir EDMUND BECKETT, Bart., LL.D., Q.C., F.R.A.S. 4s. 6d.‡
226. *THE JOINTS MADE AND USED BY BUILDERS* in the Construction of various kinds of Engineering and Architectural Works. By WYVILL J. CHRISTY, Architect. With upwards of 160 Engravings on Wood. 3s.‡

☞ *The ‡ indicates that these vols. may be had strongly bound at 6d. extra.*

7, STATIONERS' HALL COURT, LUDGATE HILL, E.C.

Architecture, Building, etc., *continued.*

228. *THE CONSTRUCTION OF ROOFS OF WOOD AND IRON.* By E. WYNDHAM TARN, M.A., Architect. Second Edition, revised. 1s. 6d.

229. *ELEMENTARY DECORATION*: as applied to the Interior and Exterior Decoration of Dwelling-Houses, &c. By J. W. FACEY. 2s.

257. *PRACTICAL HOUSE DECORATION.* A Guide to the Art of Ornamental Painting. By JAMES W. FACEY. 2s. 6d.

⁎⁎⁎ The two preceding Works, in One handsome Vol., half-bound, entitled " HOUSE DECORATION, ELEMENTARY AND PRACTICAL," *price 5s.*

230. *HANDRAILING.* Showing New and Simple Methods for finding the Pitch of the Plank. Drawing the Moulds, Bevelling, Jointing-up, and Squaring the Wreath. By GEORGE COLLINGS. Plates and Diagrams. 1s. 6d.

247. *BUILDING ESTATES*: a Rudimentary Treatise on the Development, Sale, Purchase, and General Management of Building Land. By FOWLER MAITLAND, Surveyor. Second Edition, revised. 2s.

248. *PORTLAND CEMENT FOR USERS.* By HENRY FAIJA, Assoc. M. Inst. C.E. Second Edition, corrected. Illustrated. 2s.

252. *BRICKWORK*: a Practical Treatise, embodying the General and Higher Principles of Bricklaying, Cutting and Setting, &c. By F. WALKER. Second Edition, Revised and Enlarged. 1s. 6d.

23.
189. *THE PRACTICAL BRICK AND TILE BOOK.* Comprising: BRICK AND TILE MAKING, by E. DOBSON, A.I.C.E.; PRACTICAL BRICKLAY-
252. ING, by A. HAMMOND; BRICKWORK, by F. WALKER. 550 pp. with 270 Illustrations. 6s. Strongly half-bound.

253. *THE TIMBER MERCHANT'S, SAW-MILLER'S, AND IMPORTER'S FREIGHT-BOOK AND ASSISTANT.* By WM. RICHARDSON. With a Chapter on Speeds of Saw-Mill Machinery, &c. By M. POWIS BALE, A.M.Inst.C.E. 3s.‡

258. *CIRCULAR WORK IN CARPENTRY AND JOINERY.* A Practical Treatise on Circular Work of Single and Double Curvature. By GEORGE COLLINGS, Author of "A Treatise on Handrailing." 2s. 6d.

259. *GAS FITTING*: A Practical Handbook treating of every Description of Gas Laying and Fitting. By JOHN BLACK. With 122 Illustrations. 2s. 6d.‡

261. *SHORING AND ITS APPLICATION*: A Handbook for the Use of Students. By GEORGE H. BLAGROVE. 1s. 6d. [*Just published.*

265. *THE ART OF PRACTICAL BRICK CUTTING & SETTING.* By ADAM HAMMOND. With 90 Engravings. 1s. 6d. [*Just published.*

267. *THE SCIENCE OF BUILDING*: An Elementary Treatise on the Principles of Construction. Adapted to the Requirements of Architectural Students. By E. WYNDHAM TARN, M.A. Lond. Third Edition, Revised and Enlarged. With 59 Wood Engravings. 3s. 6d.‡ [*Just published.*

SHIPBUILDING, NAVIGATION, MARINE ENGINEERING, ETC.

51. *NAVAL ARCHITECTURE.* An Exposition of the Elementary Principles of the Science, and their Practical Application to Naval Construction. By J. PEAKE. Fifth Edition, with Plates and Diagrams. 3s. 6d.‡

53*. *SHIPS FOR OCEAN & RIVER SERVICE*, Elementary and Practical Principles of the Construction of. By H. A. SOMMERFELDT. 1s. 6d.

53.** *AN ATLAS OF ENGRAVINGS* to Illustrate the above. Twelve large folding plates. Royal 4to, cloth. 7s. 6d.

54. *MASTING, MAST-MAKING, AND RIGGING OF SHIPS*, Also Tables of Spars, Rigging, Blocks; Chain, Wire, and Hemp Ropes, &c., relative to every class of vessels. By ROBERT KIPPING, N.A. 2s.

54*. *IRON SHIP-BUILDING.* With Practical Examples and Details. By JOHN GRANTHAM, C.E. 5th Edition. 4s.

☞ *The ‡ indicates that these vols. may be had strongly bound at 6d. extra.*

LONDON : CROSBY LOCKWOOD AND SON.

Shipbuilding, Navigation, Marine Engineering, etc., *cont.*

55. *THE SAILOR'S SEA BOOK:* a Rudimentary Treatise on Navigation. By JAMES GREENWOOD, B.A. With numerous Woodcuts and Coloured Plates. New and enlarged edition. By W. H. ROSSER. 2s. 6d.‡
80. *MARINE ENGINES AND STEAM VESSELS.* By ROBERT MURRAY, C.E. Eighth Edition, thoroughly Revised, with Additions by the Author and by GEORGE CARLISLE, C.E., Senior Surveyor to the Board of Trade, Liverpool. 4s. 6d. limp; 5s. cloth boards.
83*bis.* *THE FORMS OF SHIPS AND BOATS.* By W. BLAND. Seventh Edition, Revised, with numerous Illustrations and Models. 1s. 6d.
99. *NAVIGATION AND NAUTICAL ASTRONOMY,* in Theory and Practice. By Prof. J. R. YOUNG. New Edition. 2s. 6d.
106. *SHIPS' ANCHORS,* a Treatise on. By G. COTSELL, N.A. 1s. 6d.
149. *SAILS AND SAIL-MAKING.* With Draughting, and the Centre of Effort of the Sails; Weights and Sizes of Ropes; Masting, Rigging, and Sails of Steam Vessels, &c. 12th Edition. By R. KIPPING, N.A., 2s. 6d.‡
155. *ENGINEER'S GUIDE TO THE ROYAL & MERCANTILE NAVIES.* By a PRACTICAL ENGINEER. Revised by D. F. M'CARTHY. 3s.
55 & 204. *PRACTICAL NAVIGATION.* Consisting of The Sailor's Sea-Book. By JAMES GREENWOOD and W. H. ROSSER. Together with the requisite Mathematical and Nautical Tables for the Working of the Problems. By H. LAW, C.E., and Prof. J. R. YOUNG. 7s. Half-bound.

AGRICULTURE, GARDENING, ETC.

61*. *A COMPLETE READY RECKONER FOR THE ADMEASUREMENT OF LAND,* &c. By A. ARMAN. Third Edition, revised and extended by C. NORRIS, Surveyor, Valuer, &c. 2s.
131. *MILLER'S, CORN MERCHANT'S, AND FARMER'S READY RECKONER.* Second Edition, with a Price List of Modern Flour-Mill Machinery, by W. S. HUTTON, C.E. 2s.
140. *SOILS, MANURES, AND CROPS.* (Vol. 1. OUTLINES OF MODERN FARMING.) By R. SCOTT BURN. Woodcuts. 2s.
141. *FARMING & FARMING ECONOMY,* Notes, Historical and Practical, on. (Vol. 2. OUTLINES OF MODERN FARMING.) By R. SCOTT BURN. 3s.
142. *STOCK; CATTLE, SHEEP, AND HORSES.* (Vol. 3. OUTLINES OF MODERN FARMING.) By R. SCOTT BURN. Woodcuts. 2s. 6d.
145. *DAIRY, PIGS, AND POULTRY,* Management of the. By R. SCOTT BURN. (Vol. 4. OUTLINES OF MODERN FARMING.) 2s.
146. *UTILIZATION OF SEWAGE, IRRIGATION, AND RECLAMATION OF WASTE LAND.* (Vol. 5. OUTLINES OF MODERN FARMING.) By R. SCOTT BURN. Woodcuts. 2s. 6d.

⁎ Nos. 140-1-2-5-6, *in One Vol., handsomely half-bound, entitled* " OUTLINES OF MODERN FARMING." *By* ROBERT SCOTT BURN. *Price* 12s.

177. *FRUIT TREES,* The Scientific and Profitable Culture of. From the French of DU BREUIL. Revised by GEO. GLENNY. 187 Woodcuts. 3s. 6d.‡
198. *SHEEP; THE HISTORY, STRUCTURE, ECONOMY, AND DISEASES OF.* By W. C. SPOONER, M.R.V.C., &c. Fifth Edition, enlarged, including Specimens of New and Improved Breeds. 3s. 6d.‡
201. *KITCHEN GARDENING MADE EASY.* By GEORGE M. F. GLENNY. Illustrated. 1s. 6d.‡
207. *OUTLINES OF FARM MANAGEMENT,* and the Organization of Farm Labour. By R. SCOTT BURN. 2s. 6d.‡
208. *OUTLINES OF LANDED ESTATES MANAGEMENT.* By R. SCOTT BURN. 2s. 6d.‡

⁎ Nos. 207 & 208 *in One Vol., handsomely half-bound, entitled* " OUTLINES OF LANDED ESTATES AND FARM MANAGEMENT." *By* R. SCOTT BURN. *Price* 6s.

☞ *The* ‡ *indicates that these vols. may be had strongly bound at 6d. extra.*

Agriculture, Gardening, etc., *continued.*

209. *THE TREE PLANTER AND PLANT PROPAGATOR.* A Practical Manual on the Propagation of Forest Trees, Fruit Trees, Flowering Shrubs, Flowering Plants, &c. By SAMUEL WOOD. 2s.‡

210. *THE TREE PRUNER.* A Practical Manual on the Pruning of Fruit Trees, including also their Training and Renovation; also the Pruning of Shrubs, Climbers, and Flowering Plants. By SAMUEL WOOD. 2s.‡

. Nos. 209 & 210 *in One Vol., handsomely half-bound, entitled* "THE TREE PLANTER, PROPAGATOR, AND PRUNER." By SAMUEL WOOD. *Price 5s.*

218. *THE HAY AND STRAW MEASURER :*-Being New Tables for the Use of Auctioneers, Valuers, Farmers, Hay and Straw Dealers, &c. By JOHN STEELE. Fourth Edition. 2s.

222. *SUBURBAN FARMING.* The Laying-out and Cultivation of Farms, adapted to the Produce of Milk, Butter, and Cheese, Eggs, Poultry, and Pigs. By Prof. JOHN DONALDSON and R. SCOTT BURN. 3s. 6d.‡

231. *THE ART OF GRAFTING AND BUDDING.* By CHARLES BALTET. With Illustrations. 2s. 6d.‡

232. *COTTAGE GARDENING;* or, Flowers, Fruits, and Vegetables for Small Gardens. By E. HOBDAY. 1s. 6d.

233. *GARDEN RECEIPTS.* Edited by CHARLES W. QUIN. 1s. 6d.

234. *MARKET AND KITCHEN GARDENING.* By C. W. SHAW, late Editor of "Gardening Illustrated." 3s.‡ [*Just published.*

239. *DRAINING AND EMBANKING.* A Practical Treatise, embodying the most recent experience in the Application of Improved Methods. By JOHN SCOTT, late Professor of Agriculture and Rural Economy at the Royal Agricultural College, Cirencester. With 68 Illustrations. 1s. 6d.

240. *IRRIGATION AND WATER SUPPLY.* A Treatise on Water Meadows, Sewage Irrigation, and Warping; the Construction of Wells, Ponds, and Reservoirs, &c. By Prof. JOHN SCOTT. With 34 Illus. 1s. 6d.

241. *FARM ROADS, FENCES, AND GATES.* A Practical Treatise on the Roads, Tramways, and Waterways of the Farm; the Principles of Enclosures; and the different kinds of Fences, Gates, and Stiles. By Professor JOHN SCOTT. With 75 Illustrations. 1s. 6d.

242. *FARM BUILDINGS.* A Practical Treatise on the Buildings necessary for various kinds of Farms, their Arrangement and Construction, with Plans and Estimates. By Prof. JOHN SCOTT. With 105 Illus. 2s.

243. *BARN IMPLEMENTS AND MACHINES.* A Practical Treatise on the Application of Power to the Operations of Agriculture; and on various Machines used in the Threshing-barn, in the Stock-yard, and in the Dairy, &c. By Prof. J. SCOTT. With 123 Illustrations. 2s.

244. *FIELD IMPLEMENTS AND MACHINES.* A Practical Treatise on the Varieties now in use, with Principles and Details of Construction, their Points of Excellence, and Management. By Professor JOHN SCOTT. With 138 Illustrations. 2s.

245. *AGRICULTURAL SURVEYING.* A Practical Treatise on Land Surveying, Levelling, and Setting-out; and on Measuring and Estimating Quantities, Weights, and Values of Materials, Produce, Stock, &c. By Prof. JOHN SCOTT. With 62 Illustrations. 1s. 6d.

. Nos. 239 to 245 *in One Vol., handsomely half-bound, entitled* "THE COMPLETE TEXT-BOOK OF FARM ENGINEERING." By Professor JOHN SCOTT. *Price 12s.*

250. *MEAT PRODUCTION.* A Manual for Producers, Distributors, &c. By JOHN EWART. 2s. 6d.‡

266. *BOOK-KEEPING FOR FARMERS & ESTATE OWNERS.* By J. M. WOODMAN, Chartered Accountant. 2s. 6d. cloth limp; 3s. 6d. cloth boards. [*Just published.*

☞ *The ‡ indicates that these vols. may be had strongly bound at 6d. extra.*

LONDON : CROSBY LOCKWOOD AND SON,

MATHEMATICS, ARITHMETIC, ETC.

32. *MATHEMATICAL INSTRUMENTS*, a Treatise on; Their Construction, Adjustment, Testing, and Use concisely Explained. By J. F. HEATHER, M.A. Fourteenth Edition, revised, with additions, by A. T. WALMISLEY, M.I.C.E., Fellow of the Surveyors' Institution. Original Edition, in 1 vol., Illustrated. 2s.‡ [*Just published.*

⁎⁎⁎ In ordering the above, be careful to say, "Original Edition" (No. 32), to distinguish it from the Enlarged Edition in 3 vols. (Nos. 168-9-70.)

76. *DESCRIPTIVE GEOMETRY*, an Elementary Treatise on; with a Theory of Shadows and of Perspective, extracted from the French of G. MONGE. To which is added, a description of the Principles and Practice of Isometrical Projection. By J. F. HEATHER, M.A. With 14 Plates. 2s.

178. *PRACTICAL PLANE GEOMETRY:* giving the Simplest Modes of Constructing Figures contained in one Plane and Geometrical Construction of the Ground. By J. F. HEATHER, M.A. With 215 Woodcuts. 2s.

83. *COMMERCIAL BOOK-KEEPING.* With Commercial Phrases and Forms in English, French, Italian, and German. By JAMES HADDON, M.A., Arithmetical Master of King's College School, London. 1s. 6d.

84. *ARITHMETIC*, a Rudimentary Treatise on: with full Explanations of its Theoretical Principles, and numerous Examples for Practice. By Professor J. R. YOUNG. Eleventh Edition. 1s. 6d.

84*. A KEY to the above, containing Solutions in full to the Exercises, together with Comments, Explanations, and Improved Processes, for the Use of Teachers and Unassisted Learners. By J. R. YOUNG. 1s. 6d.

85. *EQUATIONAL ARITHMETIC*, applied to Questions of Interest, Annuities, Life Assurance, and General Commerce; with various Tables by which all Calculations may be greatly facilitated. By W. HIPSLEY. 2s.

86. *ALGEBRA*, the Elements of. By JAMES HADDON, M.A. With Appendix, containing miscellaneous Investigations, and a Collection of Problems in various parts of Algebra. 2s.

86*. A KEY AND COMPANION to the above Book, forming an extensive repository of Solved Examples and Problems in Illustration of the various Expedients necessary in Algebraical Operations. By J. R. YOUNG. 1s. 6d.

88. *EUCLID*, THE ELEMENTS OF: with many additional Propositions
89. and Explanatory Notes: to which is prefixed, an Introductory Essay on Logic. By HENRY LAW, C.E. 2s. 6d.‡

⁎⁎⁎ Sold also separately, viz.:—

88. EUCLID, The First Three Books. By HENRY LAW, C.E. 1s. 6d.
89. EUCLID, Books 4, 5, 6, 11, 12. By HENRY LAW, C.E. 1s. 6d.

90. *ANALYTICAL GEOMETRY AND CONIC SECTIONS*, By JAMES HANN. A New Edition, by Professor J. R. YOUNG. 2s.‡

91. *PLANE TRIGONOMETRY*, the Elements of. By JAMES HANN, formerly Mathematical Master of King's College, London. 1s. 6d.

92. *SPHERICAL TRIGONOMETRY*, the Elements of. By JAMES HANN. Revised by CHARLES H. DOWLING, C.E. 1s.

⁎⁎⁎ Or with "The Elements of Plane Trigonometry," in One Volume, 2s. 6d.

93. *MENSURATION AND MEASURING.* With the Mensuration and Levelling of Land for the Purposes of Modern Engineering. By T. BAKER, C.E. New Edition by E. NUGENT, C.E. Illustrated. 1s. 6d.

101. *DIFFERENTIAL CALCULUS*, Elements of the. By W. S. B. WOOLHOUSE, F.R.A.S., &c. 1s. 6d.

102. *INTEGRAL CALCULUS*, Rudimentary Treatise on the. By HOMERSHAM COX, B.A. Illustrated. 1s.

136. *ARITHMETIC*, Rudimentary, for the Use of Schools and Self-Instruction. By JAMES HADDON, M.A. Revised by A. ARMAN. 1s. 6d.
137. A KEY TO HADDON'S RUDIMENTARY ARITHMETIC. By A. ARMAN. 1s. 6d.

☞ *The ‡ indicates that these vols. may be had strongly bound at 6d. extra.*

7, STATIONERS' HALL COURT, LUDGATE HILL, E.C.

WEALE'S RUDIMENTARY SERIES.

Mathematics, Arithmetic, etc., *continued.*

168. *DRAWING AND MEASURING INSTRUMENTS.* Including—I. Instruments employed in Geometrical and Mechanical Drawing, and in the Construction, Copying, and Measurement of Maps and Plans. II. Instruments used for the purposes of Accurate Measurement, and for Arithmetical Computations. By J. F. HEATHER, M.A. Illustrated. 1s. 6d
169. *OPTICAL INSTRUMENTS.* Including (more especially) Telescopes, Microscopes, and Apparatus for producing copies of Maps and Plans by Photography. By J. F. HEATHER, M.A. Illustrated. 1s. 6d.
170. *SURVEYING AND ASTRONOMICAL INSTRUMENTS.* Including—I. Instruments Used for Determining the Geometrical Features of a portion of Ground. II. Instruments Employed in Astronomical Observations. By J. F. HEATHER, M.A. Illustrated. 1s. 6d.

* *The above three volumes form an enlargement of the Author's original work "Mathematical Instruments." (See No. 32 in the Series.)*

168.⎫ *MATHEMATICAL INSTRUMENTS.* By J. F. HEATHER,
169. ⎬ M.A. Enlarged Edition, for the most part entirely re-written. The 3 Parts as
170.⎭ above, in One thick Volume. With numerous Illustrations. 4s. 6d.‡
158. *THE SLIDE RULE, AND HOW TO USE IT;* containing full, easy, and simple Instructions to perform all Business Calculations with unexampled rapidity and accuracy. By CHARLES HOARE, C.E. Fifth Edition. With a Slide Rule in tuck of cover. 2s. 6d.‡
196. *THEORY OF COMPOUND INTEREST AND ANNUITIES;* with Tables of Logarithms for the more Difficult Computations of Interest, Discount, Annuities, &c. By FÉDOR THOMAN. 4s.‡
199. *THE COMPENDIOUS CALCULATOR;* or, Easy and Concise Methods of Performing the various Arithmetical Operations required in Commercial and Business Transactions; together with Useful Tables. By D. O'GORMAN. Twenty-seventh Edition, carefully revised by C. NORRIS. 2s. 6d., cloth limp; 3s. 6d., strongly half-bound in leather.
204. *MATHEMATICAL TABLES,* for Trigonometrical, Astronomical, and Nautical Calculations; to which is prefixed a Treatise on Logarithms. By HENRY LAW, C.E. Together with a Series of Tables for Navigation and Nautical Astronomy. By Prof. J. R. YOUNG. New Edition. 4s.
204*. *LOGARITHMS.* With Mathematical Tables for Trigonometrical, Astronomical, and Nautical Calculations. By HENRY LAW, M.Inst.C.E. New and Revised Edition. (Forming part of the above Work). 3s.
221. *MEASURES, WEIGHTS, AND MONEYS OF ALL NATIONS,* and an Analysis of the Christian, Hebrew, and Mahometan Calendars. By W. S. B. WOOLHOUSE, F.R.A.S., F.S.S. Sixth Edition. 2s.‡
227. *MATHEMATICS AS APPLIED TO THE CONSTRUCTIVE ARTS.* Illustrating the various processes of Mathematical Investigation, by means of Arithmetical and Simple Algebraical Equations and Practical Examples. By FRANCIS CAMPIN, C.E. Second Edition. 3s.‡

PHYSICAL SCIENCE, NATURAL PHILOSOPHY, ETC.

1. *CHEMISTRY.* By Professor GEORGE FOWNES, F.R.S. With an Appendix on the Application of Chemistry to Agriculture. 1s.
2. *NATURAL PHILOSOPHY,* Introduction to the Study of. By C. TOMLINSON. Woodcuts. 1s. 6d.
6. *MECHANICS,* Rudimentary Treatise on. By CHARLES TOMLINSON. Illustrated. 1s. 6d.
7. *ELECTRICITY;* showing the General Principles of Electrical Science, and the purposes to which it has been applied. By Sir W. SNOW HARRIS, F.R.S., &c. With Additions by R. SABINE, C.E., F.S.A. 1s. 6d.
7*. *GALVANISM.* By Sir W. SNOW HARRIS. New Edition by ROBERT SABINE, C.E., F.S.A. 1s. 6d.
8. *MAGNETISM;* being a concise Exposition of the General Principles of Magnetical Science. By Sir W. SNOW HARRIS. New Edition, revised by H. M. NOAD, Ph.D. With 165 Woodcuts. 3s. 6d.‡

☞ *The ‡ indicates that these vols. may be had strongly bound at 6d. extra*

LONDON : CROSBY LOCKWOOD AND SON,

Physical Science, Natural Philosophy, etc., *continued.*

11. *THE ELECTRIC TELEGRAPH;* its History and Progress; with Descriptions of some of the Apparatus. By R. SABINE, C.E., F.S.A. 3s.
12. *PNEUMATICS,* including Acoustics and the Phenomena of Wind Currents. for the Use of Beginners By CHARLES TOMLINSON, F.R.S. Fourth Edition, enlarged. Illustrated. 1s. 6d. [*Just published.*
72. *MANUAL OF THE MOLLUSCA;* a Treatise on Recent and Fossil Shells. By Dr. S. P. WOODWARD, A.L.S. Fourth Edition. With Appendix by RALPH TATE, A.L.S., F.G.S. With numerous Plates and 300 Woodcuts. 6s. 6d. Cloth boards, 7s. 6d.
96. *ASTRONOMY.* By the late Rev. ROBERT MAIN, M.A. Third Edition, by WILLIAM THYNNE LYNN, B.A., F.R.A.S. 2s.
97. *STATICS AND DYNAMICS,* the Principles and Practice of; embracing also a clear development of Hydrostatics, Hydrodynamics, and Central Forces. By T. BAKER, C.E. Fourth Edition. 1s. 6d.
138. *TELEGRAPH,* Handbook of the; a Guide to Candidates for Employment in the Telegraph Service. By R. BOND. 3s.‡
173. *PHYSICAL GEOLOGY,* partly based on Major-General PORTLOCK's "Rudiments of Geology." By RALPH TATE, A.L.S., &c. Woodcuts. 2s.
174. *HISTORICAL GEOLOGY,* partly based on Major-General PORTLOCK's "Rudiments." By RALPH TATE, A.L.S., &c. Woodcuts. 2s. 6d.
173 *RUDIMENTARY TREATISE ON GEOLOGY,* Physical and
& Historical. Partly based on Major-General PORTLOCK's "Rudiments of
174. Geology." By RALPH TATE, A.L.S., F.G.S., &c. In One Volume. 4s. 6d.‡
183 *ANIMAL PHYSICS,* Handbook of. By Dr. LARDNER, D.C.L.,
& formerly Professor of Natural Philosophy and Astronomy in University
184. College, Lond. With 520 Illustrations. In One Vol. 7s. 6d., cloth boards.
*** *Sold also in Two Parts, as follows :—*
183. ANIMAL PHYSICS. By Dr. LARDNER. Part I., Chapters I.—VII. 4s.
184. ANIMAL PHYSICS. By Dr. LARDNER. Part II., Chapters VIII.—XVIII. 3s.

FINE ARTS.

20. *PERSPECTIVE FOR BEGINNERS.* Adapted to Young Students and Amateurs in Architecture, Painting, &c. By GEORGE PYNE. 2s.
40. *GLASS STAINING, AND THE ART OF PAINTING ON GLASS.* From the German of Dr. GESSERT and EMANUEL OTTO FROMBERG. With an Appendix on THE ART OF ENAMELLING. 2s. 6d.
69. *MUSIC,* A Rudimentary and Practical Treatise on. With numerous Examples. By CHARLES CHILD SPENCER. 2s. 6d.
71. *PIANOFORTE,* The Art of Playing the. With numerous Exercises & Lessons from the Best Masters. By CHARLES CHILD SPENCER. 1s. 6d.
69-71. *MUSIC & THE PIANOFORTE.* In one vol. Half bound, 5s.
181. *PAINTING POPULARLY EXPLAINED,* including Fresco, Oil, Mosaic, Water Colour, Water-Glass, Tempera, Encaustic, Miniature, Painting on Ivory, Vellum, Pottery, Enamel, Glass, &c. With Historical Sketches of the Progress of the Art by THOMAS JOHN GULLICK, assisted by JOHN TIMBS, F.S.A. Fifth Edition, revised and enlarged. 5s.‡
186. *A GRAMMAR OF COLOURING,* applied to Decorative Painting and the Arts. By GEORGE FIELD. New Edition, enlarged and adapted to the Use of the Ornamental Painter and Designer. By ELLIS A. DAVIDSON. With two new Coloured Diagrams, &c. 3s.‡
246. *A DICTIONARY OF PAINTERS, AND HANDBOOK FOR PICTURE AMATEURS;* including Methods of Painting, Cleaning, Relining and Restoring, Schools of Painting, &c. With Notes on the Copyists and Imitators of each Master. By PHILIPPE DARYL. 2s. 6d.‡

☞ *The ‡ indicates that these vols. may be had strongly bound at 6d. extra.*

7, STATIONERS' HALL COURT, LUDGATE HILL, E.C.

INDUSTRIAL AND USEFUL ARTS.

23. *BRICKS AND TILES*, Rudimentary Treatise on the Manufacture of. By E. Dobson, M.R.I.B.A. Illustrated, 3s.‡
67. *CLOCKS, WATCHES, AND BELLS*, a Rudimentary Treatise on. By Sir Edmund Beckett, LL.D., Q.C. Seventh Edition, revised and enlarged. 4s. 6d. limp; 5s. 6d. cloth boards.
83**. *CONSTRUCTION OF DOOR LOCKS*. Compiled from the Papers of A. C. Hobbs, and Edited by Charles Tomlinson, F.R.S. 2s. 6d.
162. *THE BRASS FOUNDER'S MANUAL;* Instructions for Modelling, Pattern-Making, Moulding, Turning, Filing, Burnishing, Bronzing, &c. With copious Receipts, &c. By Walter Graham. 2s.‡
205. *THE ART OF LETTER PAINTING MADE EASY*. By J. G. Badenoch. Illustrated with 12 full-page Engravings of Examples. 1s. 6d.
215. *THE GOLDSMITH'S HANDBOOK*, containing full Instructions for the Alloying and Working of Gold. By George E. Gee, 3s.‡
225. *THE SILVERSMITH'S HANDBOOK*, containing full Instructions for the Alloying and Working of Silver. By George E. Gee. 3s.‡
*** *The two preceding Works, in One handsome Vol., half-bound, entitled "* The Goldsmith's & Silversmith's Complete Handbook." *7s.*
249. *THE HALL-MARKING OF JEWELLERY PRACTICALLY CONSIDERED*. By George E. Gee. 3s.‡
224. *COACH BUILDING*, A Practical Treatise, Historical and Descriptive. By J. W. Burgess. 2s. 6d.‡
235. *PRACTICAL ORGAN BUILDING*. By W. E. Dickson, M.A., Precentor of Ely Cathedral. Illustrated. 2s. 6d.‡
262. *THE ART OF BOOT AND SHOEMAKING*, including Measurement, 'Last-fitting, Cutting-out, Closing and Making. By John Bedford Leno. Numerous Illustrations. Third Edition. 2s.
263. *MECHANICAL DENTISTRY:* A Practical Treatise on the Construction of the Various Kinds of Artificial Dentures, with Formulæ, Tables, Receipts, &c. By Charles Hunter. Third Edition. 3s.‡

MISCELLANEOUS VOLUMES.

36. *A DICTIONARY OF TERMS used in ARCHITECTURE, BUILDING, ENGINEERING, MINING, METALLURGY, ARCHÆOLOGY, the FINE ARTS, &c.* By John Weale. Fifth Edition. Revised by Robert Hunt, F.R.S. Illustrated. 5s. limp; 6s. cloth boards.
50. *THE LAW OF CONTRACTS FOR WORKS AND SERVICES.* By David Gibbons. Third Edition, enlarged. 3s.‡
112. *MANUAL OF DOMESTIC MEDICINE*. By R. Gooding, B.A., M.D. A Family Guide in all Cases of Accident and Emergency. 2s.‡
112*. *MANAGEMENT OF HEALTH*. A Manual of Home and Personal Hygiene. By the Rev. James Baird, B.A. 1s.
150. *LOGIC*, Pure and Applied. By S. H. Emmens. 1s. 6d.
153. *SELECTIONS FROM LOCKE'S ESSAYS ON THE HUMAN UNDERSTANDING*. With Notes by S. H. Emmens. 2s.
154. *GENERAL HINTS TO EMIGRANTS*. 2s.
157. *THE EMIGRANT'S GUIDE TO NATAL*. By Robert James Mann, F.R.A.S., F.M.S. Second Edition. Map. 2s.
193. *HANDBOOK OF FIELD FORTIFICATION*. By Major W. W. Knollys, F.R.G.S. With 163 Woodcuts. 3s.‡
194. *THE HOUSE MANAGER:* Being a Guide to Housekeeping. Practical Cookery, Pickling and Preserving, Household Work, Dairy Management, &c. By An Old Housekeeper. 3s. 6d.‡
194, *HOUSE BOOK (The).* Comprising :—I. The House Manager. 112 & By an Old Housekeeper. II. Domestic Medicine. By R. Gooding, M.D. 112*. III. Management of Health. By J. Baird. In One Vol., half-bound, 6s.

☞ *The ‡ indicates that these vols. may be had strongly bound at 6d. extra.*

LONDON: CROSBY LOCKWOOD AND SON.

EDUCATIONAL AND CLASSICAL SERIES.

HISTORY.

1. **England, Outlines of the History of;** more especially with reference to the Origin and Progress of the English Constitution. By WILLIAM DOUGLAS HAMILTON, F.S.A., of Her Majesty's Public Record Office. 4th Edition, revised. 5s.; cloth boards, 6s.
5. **Greece, Outlines of the History of;** in connection with the Rise of the Arts and Civilization in Europe. By W. DOUGLAS HAMILTON, of University College, London, and EDWARD LEVIEN, M.A., of Balliol College, Oxford. 2s. 6d.; cloth boards, 3s. 6d.
7. **Rome, Outlines of the History of:** from the Earliest Period to the Christian Era and the Commencement of the Decline of the Empire. By EDWARD LEVIEN, of Balliol College, Oxford. Map, 2s. 6d.; cl. bds. 3s. 6d.
9. **Chronology of History, Art, Literature, and Progress,** from the Creation of the World to the Present Time. The Continuation by W. D. HAMILTON, F.S.A. 3s.; cloth boards, 3s. 6d.
50. **Dates and Events in English History,** for the use of Candidates in Public and Private Examinations. By the Rev. E. RAND. 1s.

ENGLISH LANGUAGE AND MISCELLANEOUS.

11. **Grammar of the English Tongue, Spoken and Written.** With an Introduction to the Study of Comparative Philology. By HYDE CLARKE, D.C.L. Fourth Edition. 1s. 6d.
12. **Dictionary of the English Language,** as Spoken and Written. Containing above 100,000 Words. By HYDE CLARKE, D.C.L. 3s. 6d.; cloth boards, 4s. 6d.; complete with the GRAMMAR, cloth bds., 5s. 6d.
48. **Composition and Punctuation,** familiarly Explained for those who have neglected the Study of Grammar. By JUSTIN BRENAN. 18th Edition. 1s. 6d.
49. **Derivative Spelling-Book:** Giving the Origin of Every Word from the Greek, Latin, Saxon, German, Teutonic, Dutch, French, Spanish, and other Languages; with their present Acceptation and Pronunciation. By J. ROWBOTHAM, F.R.A.S. Improved Edition. 1s. 6d.
51. **The Art of Extempore Speaking:** Hints for the Pulpit, the Senate, and the Bar. By M. BAUTAIN, Vicar-General and Professor at the Sorbonne. Translated from the French. 8th Edition, carefully corrected. 2s. 6d.
53. **Places and Facts in Political and Physical Geography,** for Candidates in Examinations. By the Rev. EDGAR RAND, B.A. 1s.
54. **Analytical Chemistry,** Qualitative and Quantitative, a Course of. To which is prefixed, a Brief Treatise upon Modern Chemical Nomenclature and Notation. By WM. W. PINK and GEORGE E. WEBSTER. 2s.

THE SCHOOL MANAGERS' SERIES OF READING BOOKS,

Edited by the Rev. A. R. GRANT, Rector of Hitcham, and Honorary Canon of Ely; formerly H.M. Inspector of Schools.
INTRODUCTORY PRIMER, 3d.

	s. d.		s. d.
FIRST STANDARD	0 6	FOURTH STANDARD	1 2
SECOND „	0 10	FIFTH „	1 6
THIRD „	1 0	SIXTH „	1 6

LESSONS FROM THE BIBLE. Part I. Old Testament. 1s.
LESSONS FROM THE BIBLE. Part II. New Testament, to which is added THE GEOGRAPHY OF THE BIBLE, for very young Children. By Rev. C. THORNTON FORSTER. 1s. 2d. *⁎* Or the Two Parts in One Volume. 2s.

7, STATIONERS' HALL COURT, LUDGATE HILL, E.C.

14   WEALE'S EDUCATIONAL AND CLASSICAL SERIES.

FRENCH.

24. **French Grammar.** With Complete and Concise Rules on the Genders of French Nouns. By G. L. STRAUSS, Ph.D. 1s. 6d.
25. **French-English Dictionary.** Comprising a large number of New Terms used in Engineering, Mining, &c. By ALFRED ELWES. 1s. 6d.
26. **English-French Dictionary.** By ALFRED ELWES. 2s.
25,26. **French Dictionary** (as above). Complete, in One Vol., 3s.; cloth boards, 3s. 6d. *⁎* Or with the GRAMMAR, cloth boards, 4s. 6d.
47. **French and English Phrase Book:** containing Introductory Lessons, with Translations, several Vocabularies of Words, a Collection of suitable Phrases, and Easy Familiar Dialogues. 1s. 6d.

GERMAN.

39. **German Grammar.** Adapted for English Students, from Heyse's Theoretical and Practical Grammar, by Dr. G. L. STRAUSS. 1s. 6d.
40. **German Reader:** A Series of Extracts, carefully culled from the most approved Authors of Germany; with Notes, Philological and Explanatory. By G. L. STRAUSS, Ph.D. 1s.
41-43. **German Triglot Dictionary.** By N. E. S. A. HAMILTON. In Three Parts. Part I. German-French-English. Part II. English-German-French. Part III. French-German-English. 3s., or cloth boards, 4s.
41-43 & 39. **German Triglot Dictionary** (as above), together with German Grammar (No. 39), in One Volume, cloth boards, 5s.

ITALIAN.

27. **Italian Grammar,** arranged in Twenty Lessons, with a Course of Exercises. By ALFRED ELWES. 1s. 6d.
28. **Italian Triglot Dictionary,** wherein the Genders of all the Italian and French Nouns are carefully noted down. By ALFRED ELWES. Vol. 1. Italian-English-French. 2s. 6d.
30. **Italian Triglot Dictionary.** By A. ELWES. Vol. 2. English-French-Italian. 2s. 6d.
32. **Italian Triglot Dictionary.** By ALFRED ELWES. Vol. 3. French-Italian-English. 2s. 6d.
28,30,32. **Italian Triglot Dictionary** (as above). In One Vol., 7s. 6d Cloth boards.

SPANISH AND PORTUGUESE.

34. **Spanish Grammar,** in a Simple and Practical Form. With a Course of Exercises. By ALFRED ELWES. 1s. 6d.
35. **Spanish-English and English-Spanish Dictionary.** Including a large number of Technical Terms used in Mining, Engineering, &c. with the proper Accents and the Gender of every Noun. By ALFRED ELWES 4s.; cloth boards, 5s. *⁎* Or with the GRAMMAR, cloth boards, 6s.
55. **Portuguese Grammar,** in a Simple and Practical Form. With a Course of Exercises. By ALFRED ELWES. 1s. 6d.
56. **Portuguese-English and English-Portuguese Dictionary.** Including a large number of Technical Terms used in Mining, Engineering, &c., with the proper Accents and the Gender of every Noun. By ALFRED ELWES. Second Edition, Revised, 5s.; cloth boards, 6s. *⁎* Or with the GRAMMAR, cloth boards, 7s.

HEBREW.

46*. **Hebrew Grammar.** By Dr. BRESSLAU. 1s. 6d.
44. **Hebrew and English Dictionary,** Biblical and Rabbinical; containing the Hebrew and Chaldee Roots of the Old Testament Post-Rabbinical Writings. By Dr. BRESSLAU. 6s.
46. **English and Hebrew Dictionary.** By Dr. BRESSLAU. 3s.
44,46,46*. **Hebrew Dictionary** (as above), in Two Vols., complete, with the GRAMMAR. cloth boards, 12s.

LONDON: CROSBY LOCKWOOD AND SON,

LATIN.

19. **Latin Grammar.** Containing the Inflections and Elementary Principles of Translation and Construction. By the Rev. THOMAS GOODWIN, M.A., Head Master of the Greenwich Proprietary School. 1s. 6d.
20. **Latin-English Dictionary.** By the Rev. THOMAS GOODWIN, M.A. 2s.
22. **English-Latin Dictionary;** together with an Appendix of French and Italian Words which have their origin from the Latin. By the Rev. THOMAS GOODWIN, M.A. 1s. 6d.
20,22. **Latin Dictionary** (as above). Complete in One Vol., 3s. 6d. cloth boards, 4s. 6d. *⁎* Or with the GRAMMAR, cloth boards, 5s. 6d.

LATIN CLASSICS. With Explanatory Notes in English.

1. **Latin Delectus.** Containing Extracts from Classical Authors, with Genealogical Vocabularies and Explanatory Notes, by H. YOUNG. 1s. 6d.
2. **Cæsaris Commentarii de Bello Gallico.** Notes, and a Geographical Register for the Use of Schools, by H. YOUNG. 2s.
3. **Cornelius Nepos.** With Notes. By H. YOUNG. 1s.
4. **Virgilii Maronis Bucolica et Georgica.** With Notes on the Bucolics by W. RUSHTON, M.A., and on the Georgics by H. YOUNG. 1s. 6d.
5. **Virgilii Maronis Æneis.** With Notes, Critical and Explanatory, by H. YOUNG. New Edition, revised and improved With copious Additional Notes by Rev. T. H. L. LEARY, D.C.L., formerly Scholar of Brasenose College, Oxford. 3s.
5*. —— Part 1. Books i.—vi., 1s. 6d.
5** —— Part 2. Books vii.—xii., 2s.
6. **Horace;** Odes, Epode, and Carmen Sæculare. Notes by H. YOUNG. 1s. 6d.
7. **Horace;** Satires, Epistles, and Ars Poetica. Notes by W. BROWNRIGG SMITH, M.A., F.R.G.S. 1s. 6d.
8. **Sallustii Crispi Catalina et Bellum Jugurthinum.** Notes, Critical and Explanatory, by W. M. DONNE, B.A., Trin. Coll., Cam. 1s. 6d.
9. **Terentii Andria et Heautontimorumenos.** With Notes, Critical and Explanatory, by the Rev. JAMES DAVIES, M.A. 1s. 6d.
10. **Terentii Adelphi, Hecyra, Phormio.** Edited, with Notes, Critical and Explanatory, by the Rev. JAMES DAVIES, M.A. 2s.
11. **Terentii Eunuchus, Comœdia.** Notes, by Rev. J. DAVIES, M.A. 1s. 6d.
12. **Ciceronis Oratio pro Sexto Roscio Amerino.** Edited, with an Introduction, Analysis, and Notes, Explanatory and Critical, by the Rev. JAMES DAVIES, M.A. 1s. 6d.
13. **Ciceronis Orationes in Catilinam, Verrem, et pro Archia.** With Introduction, Analysis, and Notes, Explanatory and Critical, by Rev. T. H. L. LEARY, D.C.L. formerly Scholar of Brasenose College, Oxford. 1s. 6d.
14. **Ciceronis Cato Major, Lælius, Brutus, sive de Senectute, de Amicitia, de Claris Oratoribus Dialogi.** With Notes by W. BROWNRIGG SMITH M.A., F.R.G.S. 2s.
16. **Livy:** History of Rome. Notes by H. YOUNG and W. B. SMITH, M.A. Part 1. Books i., ii., 1s. 6d.
16*. —— Part 2. Books iii., iv., v., 1s. 6d.
17. —— Part 3. Books xxi., xxii., 1s. 6d.
19. **Latin Verse Selections,** from Catullus, Tibullus, Propertius, and Ovid. Notes by W. B. DONNE, M.A., Trinity College, Cambridge. 2s.
20. **Latin Prose Selections,** from Varro, Columella, Vitruvius, Seneca, Quintilian, Florus, Velleius Paterculus, Valerius Maximus Suetonius, Apuleius, &c. Notes by W. B. DONNE, M.A. 2s.
21. **Juvenalis Satiræ.** With Prolegomena and Notes by T. H. S. ESCOTT, B.A., Lecturer on Logic at King's College, London. 2s.

GREEK.

14. **Greek Grammar,** in accordance with the Principles and Philological Researches of the most eminent Scholars of our own day. By HANS CLAUDE HAMILTON. 1s. 6d.

15,17. **Greek Lexicon.** Containing all the Words in General Use, with their Significations, Inflections, and Doubtful Quantities. By HENRY R. HAMILTON. Vol. 1. Greek-English, 2s. 6d.; Vol. 2. English-Greek, 2s. Or the Two Vols. in One, 4s. 6d.: cloth boards, 5s.

14,15. **Greek Lexicon** (as above). Complete, with the GRAMMAR, in 17. One Vol., cloth boards, 6s.

GREEK CLASSICS. With Explanatory Notes in English.

1. **Greek Delectus.** Containing Extracts from Classical Authors, with Genealogical Vocabularies and Explanatory Notes, by H. YOUNG. New Edition, with an improved and enlarged Supplementary Vocabulary, by JOHN HUTCHISON, M.A., of the High School, Glasgow. 1s. 6d.

2, 3. **Xenophon's Anabasis;** or, The Retreat of the Ten Thousand. Notes and a Geographical Register, by H. YOUNG. Part 1. Books i. to iii., 1s. Part 2. Books iv. to vii., 1s.

4. **Lucian's Select Dialogues.** The Text carefully revised, with Grammatical and Explanatory Notes, by H. YOUNG. 1s. 6d.

5-12. **Homer, The Works of.** According to the Text of BAEUMLEIN. With Notes, Critical and Explanatory, drawn from the best and latest Authorities, with Preliminary Observations and Appendices, by T. H. L. LEARY, M.A., D.C.L.

THE ILIAD: Part 1. Books i. to vi., 1s. 6d.   Part 3. Books xiii. to xviii., 1s. 6d.
Part 2. Books vii. to xii., 1s. 6d.   Part 4. Books xix. to xxiv., 1s. 6d.
THE ODYSSEY: Part 1. Books i. to vi., 1s. 6d   Part 3. Books xiii. to xviii., 1s. 6d.
Part 2. Books vii. to xii., 1s. 6d.   Part 4. Books xix. to xxiv., and Hymns, 2s.

13. **Plato's Dialogues:** The Apology of Socrates, the Crito, and the Phædo. From the Text of C. F. HERMANN. Edited with Notes, Critical and Explanatory, by the Rev. JAMES DAVIES, M.A. 2s.

14-17. **Herodotus, The History of,** chiefly after the Text of GAISFORD. With Preliminary Observations and Appendices, and Notes, Critical and Explanatory, by T. H. L. LEARY, M.A., D.C.L.
Part 1. Books i., ii. (The Clio and Euterpe), 2s.
Part 2. Books iii., iv. (The Thalia and Melpomene), 2s.
Part 3. Books v.-vii. (The Terpsichore, Erato, and Polymnia), 2s.
Part 4. Books viii., ix. (The Urania and Calliope) and Index, 1s. 6d.

18. **Sophocles:** Œdipus Tyrannus. Notes by H. YOUNG. 1s.

20. **Sophocles:** Antigone. From the Text of DINDORF. Notes, Critical and Explanatory, by the Rev. JOHN MILNER, B.A. 2s.

23. **Euripides:** Hecuba and Medea. Chiefly from the Text of DINDORF. With Notes, Critical and Explanatory, by W. BROWNRIGG SMITH, M.A., F.R.G.S. 1s. 6d.

26. **Euripides:** Alcestis. Chiefly from the Text of DINDORF. With Notes, Critical and Explanatory, by JOHN MILNER, B.A. 1s. 6d.

30. **Æschylus:** Prometheus Vinctus: The Prometheus Bound. From the Text of DINDORF. Edited, with English Notes, Critical and Explanatory, by the Rev. JAMES DAVIES, M.A. 1s.

32. **Æschylus:** Septem Contra Thebes: The Seven against Thebes. From the Text of DINDORF. Edited, with English Notes, Critical and Explanatory, by the Rev. JAMES DAVIES, M.A. 1s.

40. **Aristophanes:** Acharnians. Chiefly from the Text of C. H. WEISE. With Notes, by C. S. T. TOWNSHEND, M.A. 1s. 6d.

41. **Thucydides:** History of the Peloponnesian War. Notes by H. YOUNG. Book 1. 1s. 6d.

42. **Xenophon's Panegyric on Agesilaus.** Notes and Introduction by LL. F. W. JEWITT. 1s. 6d.

43. **Demosthenes.** The Oration on the Crown and the Philippics. With English Notes. By Rev. T. H. L. LEARY, D.C.L., formerly Scholar of Brasenose College, Oxford. 1s. 6d.

CROSBY LOCKWOOD AND SON, 7, STATIONERS' HALL COURT, E.C.

Lightning Source UK Ltd.
Milton Keynes UK
UKOW05n0015070617
302820UK00001B/59/P